Marine Bioactive Peptides II: Structure, Function, and Therapeutic Potential

Marine Bioactive Peptides II: Structure, Function, and Therapeutic Potential

Editor

Tatiana V. Ovchinnikova

MDPI • Basel • Beijing • Wuhan • Barcelona • Belgrade • Manchester • Tokyo • Cluj • Tianjin

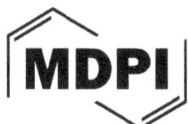

Editor
Tatiana V. Ovchinnikova
Institute of Bioorganic
Chemistry, Russian Academy of
Sciences
Russia

Editorial Office
MDPI
St. Alban-Anlage 66
4052 Basel, Switzerland

This is a reprint of articles from the Special Issue published online in the open access journal *Marine Drugs* (ISSN 1660-3397) (available at: http://www.mdpi.com).

For citation purposes, cite each article independently as indicated on the article page online and as indicated below:

LastName, A.A.; LastName, B.B.; LastName, C.C. Article Title. *Journal Name* **Year**, *Volume Number*, Page Range.

ISBN 978-3-0365-2524-2 (Hbk)
ISBN 978-3-0365-2525-9 (PDF)

© 2021 by the authors. Articles in this book are Open Access and distributed under the Creative Commons Attribution (CC BY) license, which allows users to download, copy and build upon published articles, as long as the author and publisher are properly credited, which ensures maximum dissemination and a wider impact of our publications.

The book as a whole is distributed by MDPI under the terms and conditions of the Creative Commons license CC BY-NC-ND.

Contents

About the Editor vii

Tatiana V. Ovchinnikova
Marine Peptides: Structure, Bioactivities, and a New Hope for Therapeutic Application
Reprinted from: *Mar. Drugs* **2021**, *19*, 407, doi:10.3390/md19080407 1

Rebeca Alvariño, Eva Alonso, Louis Bornancin, Isabelle Bonnard, Nicolas Inguimbert, Bernard Banaigs and Luis M. Botana
Biological Activities of Cyclic and Acyclic B-Type Laxaphycins in SH-SY5Y Human Neuroblastoma Cells
Reprinted from: *Mar. Drugs* **2020**, *18*, 364, doi:10.3390/md18070364 7

Fadia S. Youssef, Mohamed L. Ashour, Abdel Nasser B. Singab and Michael Wink
A Comprehensive Review of Bioactive Peptides from Marine Fungi and Their Biological Significance
Reprinted from: *Mar. Drugs* **2019**, *17*, 559, doi:10.3390/md17100559 29

Thomas C. N. Leung, Zhe Qu, Wenyan Nong, Jerome H. L. Hui and Sai Ming Ngai
Proteomic Analysis of the Venom of Jellyfishes *Rhopilema esculentum* and *Sanderia malayensis*
Reprinted from: *Mar. Drugs* **2020**, *18*, 655, doi:10.3390/md18120655 53

Gang Gao, Yanbing Wang, Huiming Hua, Dahong Li and Chunlan Tang
Marine Antitumor Peptide Dolastatin 10: Biological Activity, Structural Modification and Synthetic Chemistry
Reprinted from: *Mar. Drugs* **2021**, *19*, 363, doi:10.3390/md19070363 71

Qi-Ting Zhang, Ze-Dong Liu, Ze Wang, Tao Wang, Nan Wang, Ning Wang, Bin Zhang and Yu-Fen Zhao
Recent Advances in Small Peptides of Marine Origin in Cancer Therapy
Reprinted from: *Mar. Drugs* **2021**, *19*, 115, doi:10.3390/md19020115 101

Pavel V. Panteleev, Andrey V. Tsarev, Victoria N. Safronova, Olesia V. Reznikova, Ilia A. Bolosov, Sergei V. Sychev, Zakhar O. Shenkarev and Tatiana V. Ovchinnikova
Structure Elucidation and Functional Studies of a Novel β-hairpin Antimicrobial Peptide from the Marine Polychaeta *Capitella teleta*
Reprinted from: *Mar. Drugs* **2020**, *18*, 620, doi:10.3390/md18120620 131

Ilia A. Krenev, Ekaterina S. Umnyakova, Igor E. Eliseev, Yaroslav A. Dubrovskii, Nikolay P. Gorbunov, Vladislav A. Pozolotin, Alexei S. Komlev, Pavel V. Panteleev, Sergey V. Balandin, Tatiana V. Ovchinnikova, Olga V. Shamova and Mikhail N. Berlov
Antimicrobial Peptide Arenicin-1 Derivative Ar-1-(C/A) as Complement System Modulator
Reprinted from: *Mar. Drugs* **2020**, *18*, 631, doi:10.3390/md18120631 151

Guo-Xu Zhao, Xiu-Rong Yang, Yu-Mei Wang, Yu-Qin Zhao, Chang-Feng Chi and Bin Wang
Antioxidant Peptides from the Protein Hydrolysate of Spanish Mackerel (*Scomberomorous niphonius*) Muscle by in Vitro Gastrointestinal Digestion and Their In Vitro Activities
Reprinted from: *Mar. Drugs* **2019**, *17*, 531, doi:10.3390/md17090531 165

Linda Kornstad Nygård, Ingunn Mundal, Lisbeth Dahl, Jūratė Šaltytė Benth and Anne Marie Mork Rokstad
Limited Benefit of Marine Protein Hydrolysate on Physical Function and Strength in Older Adults: A Randomized Controlled Trial
Reprinted from: *Mar. Drugs* **2021**, *19*, 62, doi:10.3390/md19020062 . . . . **183**

Milica Pavlicevic, Elena Maestri and Marta Marmiroli
Marine Bioactive Peptides—An Overview of Generation, Structure and Application with a Focus on Food Sources
Reprinted from: *Mar. Drugs* **2020**, *18*, 424, doi:10.3390/md18080424 . . . . **197**

About the Editor

Tatiana V. Ovchinnikova, Head of the Science-Educational Centre, M.M. Shemyakin & Yu.A. Ovchinnikov Institute of Bioorganic Chemistry, Russian Academy of Sciences; Full Professor, Department of Bioorganic Chemistry, M.V. Lomonosov Moscow State University. She received her degree in Chemistry with Honors at the University of Kyiv (Ukraine) and then completed her Ph.D. in Bioorganic Chemistry at M.M. Shemyakin & Yu.A. Ovchinnikov Institute of Bioorganic Chemistry (Moscow, Russia). She obtained a Second Doctorate (Habilitation) degree in Bioorganic Chemistry and Biotechnology in 2011. Her research interests focus on discovery, isolation, structural elucidation, functional characterization, structure–function relationship analysis, and the evaluation of the therapeutic potential of novel antimicrobial and host defense peptides of animal and plant origin, investigation of their antimicrobial and anticancer activity, as well as mechanisms of their participation in innate immunity, screening of marine organisms for the discovery of novel peptides with high activities against microorganisms and transformed human cells, bioengineering of peptide molecules with improved therapeutic potency and efficacy for using in medicine and veterinary, design of innovative antibiotics and anticancer drugs. She has published over 450 scientific papers, reviews, book chapters, patents, and communications at national and international conferences, including over 150 peer-reviewed publications in international journals.

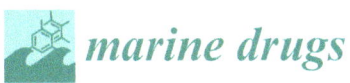

Editorial

Marine Peptides: Structure, Bioactivities, and a New Hope for Therapeutic Application

Tatiana V. Ovchinnikova [1,2,3]

[1] M.M. Shemyakin & Yu.A. Ovchinnikov Institute of Bioorganic Chemistry, The Russian Academy of Sciences, Miklukho-Maklaya Str. 16/10, 117997 Moscow, Russia; ovch@ibch.ru; Tel.: +7-495-336-44-44
[2] Department of Bioorganic Chemistry, Faculty of Biology, Lomonosov Moscow State University, 119234 Moscow, Russia
[3] Department of Biotechnology, Sechenov First Moscow State Medical University, 119991 Moscow, Russia

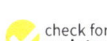

Citation: Ovchinnikova, T.V. Marine Peptides: Structure, Bioactivities, and a New Hope for Therapeutic Application. *Mar. Drugs* **2021**, *19*, 407. https://doi.org/10.3390/md19080 407

Received: 14 July 2021
Accepted: 20 July 2021
Published: 23 July 2021

Publisher's Note: MDPI stays neutral with regard to jurisdictional claims in published maps and institutional affiliations.

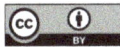

Copyright: © 2021 by the author. Licensee MDPI, Basel, Switzerland. This article is an open access article distributed under the terms and conditions of the Creative Commons Attribution (CC BY) license (https:// creativecommons.org/licenses/by/ 4.0/).

Over the last years, plethora of bioactive peptides have been isolated from organisms which live in sea water. Taking in account that more than two-thirds of the global surface area is covered with the oceans, marine species constitute above a half of the total biodiversity. Long-term evolution of marine organisms was advanced in the midst of pathogens, and efficient defense mechanisms were the necessary condition of their survival. Many marine peptides play a key role in host defense as evolutionary ancient components of innate immunity system [1]. They are involved in basic mechanisms of living organisms survival, including growth, defense, reproduction, and homeostasis. Protective peptides were isolated from many marine invertebrates and vertebrates. Their antibacterial, antifungal, antiviral, antitumor, antioxidative, antihypertensive, antiatherosclerotic, anticoagulant, antidiabetic, analgesic, immune-modulating, and neuroprotective properties attract increasing attention of pharmaceutical, cosmeceutical, and nutraceutical industries which focus on the design of innovative antibiotics, anticancer drugs, analgesics, medicines for neurological disorders, etc.

Marine peptides are multifarious in structure and biological properties. The Special Issue «Marine Bioactive Peptides II: Structure, Function, and Therapeutic Potential» was aimed to collect papers on present-day information regarding structural elucidation, functional characterization, and therapeutic potential evaluation of peptides from marine organisms. Getting started with this book, we hope to assemble an interesting edition that would highlight new developments and current trends in marine peptide research.

Cyanobacteria are Gram-negative organisms, also called blue-green algae. They appeared over 3.5 billion years ago and live all over the world including fresh and ocean water, deserts and ice shelves. This evolutionary success is related to their ability to produce a wide variety of secondary metabolites [2]. Lipopeptides laxaphycins have been isolated from several species of cyanobacteria including *Hormothamnion enteromorphoides*, *Anabaena torulosa*, *Lyngbya confervoides* and *Anabaena laxa* [3]. In particular, laxaphycins B and B3, and acyclolaxaphycins B and B3 were isolated from the marine cyanobacteria Anabaena torulosa. In this Special Issue, two new acyclic compounds, [des-(Ala4-Hle5)] acyclolaxaphycins B and B3, were purified from the herviborous gastropod (sea hare) Stylocheilus striatus, and structures of both compounds were elucidated [4]. Activities of all the six peptides were determined towards SH-SY5Y human neuroblastoma cells. In this Special Issue, pro-apoptotic properties of cyclic laxaphycins B were indicated. Acyclic laxaphycins affected on autophagy-related protein expression by increasing AMPK phosphorylation and inhibiting mTOR. Gastropod-derived acyclic compounds were shown to undergo a biotransformation (ring opening and amino acid residues deletion) that had not been previously described [4].

Marine fungi represent a valuable source of bioactive peptides. In this Special Issue, the review [5] summarized data on structures and biological activities of 131 peptides isolated from 17 fungal genera including *Acremonium, Ascotricha, Aspergillus, Asteromyces, Ceratodictyon, Clonostachs, Emericella, Exserohilum, Microsporum, Metarrhizium, Penicillium, Scytalidium, Simplicillium, Stachylidium, Talaromyces, Trichoderma,* and *Zygosporium*. 35 marine peptides revealed cytotoxic activities against different cancer cells, 23 ones displayed pronounced antimicrobial and antiviral activities. For example, asperterrestide A exerted the antiviral activity against influenza H1N1 and H3N2 virus strains. Some of the *Aspergillus* peptides revealed anti-inflammatory properties via inhibiting IL-10 expression of the LPS-induced THP-1 cells. Antidiabetic and lipid-lowering activities were also demonstrated some fungal peptides, such as terrelumamides A and B, which improved insulin sensitivity as determined by the utilization of mesenchymal cells of a bone marrow origin obtained from human adopting an adipogenesis model. Psychrophilin G exhibited a pronounced lipid-reducing activity. Simplicilliumtide D displayed an antifouling effect against the larvae of *Bugula neritina*. However, 47% of the isolated peptides did not show the examined biological activities and thus required further in-depth study [5].

Jellyfish are venomous marine invertebrates of the phylum Cnidaria. All members of this ancient phylum are generally toxic (jellyfish, sea anemones, hydra, and corals) [6]. The toxins of these mostly marine animals are of ever-increasing biomedical interest. In this Special Issue, the putative toxins of two species of jellyfish (*Rhopilema esculentum* Kishinouye, 1891, also known as a flame jellyfish, and Amuska jellyfish *Sanderia malayensis* Goette, 1886) were identified in nematocysts [7]. Using nano-flow liquid chromatography tandem mass spectrometry (nLC–MS/MS), in total 3000 proteins were found in the nematocysts in each of the above two jellyfish species. 40 and 41 putative toxins were identified in *R. esculentum* and *S. malayensis*, respectively. All the toxins were further classified into 8 families in accordance with their predicted functions. The most dominant toxins (>60%) were identified as hemostasis-impairing ones and proteases. For the first time ever, the authors studied the proteomes of nematocysts from two jellyfish species [7]. Earlier, this group reported high-quality de novo reference genomes for the above jellyfish, as well as their transcriptomes [8]. Herein, the authors identifed the putative toxins in these two jellyfish species at the protein level.

Many bioactive peptides were identified in the immune, neuroendocrine, and gut systems of mollusks [9]. The marine peptide Dolastatin 10 (Dol-10) was isolated from the Indian Ocean mollusk *Dolabella auricularia* [10]. The peptide induces apoptosis of lung cancer cells and other tumor cells at nanomolar concentrations. Dol-10 and its derivatives are highly effective in vitro towards L1210 leukemia cells, small cell lung cancer NCI-H69 cells, human prostate cancer DU-145 cells, etc. [11]. Dol-10 has been developed into commercial drugs for treating some specific lymphomas. With the implementation of Dol-10 derivatives and antibody-drug conjugates (ADCs), anticancer activity and tumor targeting were essentially improved, and the systemic toxicity was reduced. Adcetris® has been approved for the treatment of anaplastic large T-cell systemic malignant lymphoma and Hodgkin lymphoma [11]. Thus, Dol-10 is one of the most medically valuable marine peptides discovered up to now. By modifying the chemical structure of Dol-10 and combining the peptide with the application of ADCs technology, new antitumor drug candidates can be developed. In this Special Issue, the authors summarized data on biological activities and chemical structures of Dol-10 derivatives [11]. In their comprehensive review, the authors analyzed synthetic work with Dol-10 in the last 35 years, which provides the input for the development of novel antitumor drugs on the basis of marine peptides.

Molecular mechanisms of anticancer action of marine peptides are still obscure. Nevertheless, several marine peptides have been applied in preclinical treatment. This Special Issue presents the comprehensive review [12] that highlights mechanisms of anticancer action of linear and cyclic peptides from marine organisms. More than 10,000 bioactive molecules have been isolated from marine organisms [13]. Over recent years, many natural and synthetic peptides were characterized, and special databases were established, including database of anticancer peptides and proteins The CancerPPD [14]. 49 marine-derived bioactive compounds or their derivatives have been applied for clinical trials or approved for the market [15]. 11 marine drugs were approved for the market by European and American drug authorities. Four of them are anticancer drugs: Cytosar-U, Yondelis, Halaven, and Adcetris [12]. The review focus on small anticancer peptides of marine origin and molecular mechanisms of their action with a view to the future development of novel marine antitumor agents.

The large majority of polychaeta species are marine animals that inhabit all oceans and seas from the Arctic to the Antarctic. Marine polychaeta is an underinvestigated class of invertebrates in the context of discovery of new host defense peptides. Papers included in this Special Issue deal with marine polychaeta, providing good examples of their biological potential. The peptides arenicins and capitellacin, were isolated from *Arenicola marina* [16] and *Capitella teleta* [17], respectively. Earlier, structure-function relationships of arenicins have been extensively investigated [18–25]. Arenicin was shown to modulate the human complement system [26]. Here, the authors reported the property change in arenicin-1 derivative Ar-1-(C/A) structure and its antimicrobial, hemolytic and complement-modulating activities in comparison with those of the natural peptide. Despite the absence of a disulfide bond, the peptide possessed all important functional features, but its hemolytic activity reduced [26]. The use of marine peptides as new complement modulators has several advantages. These molecules are relatively small, and the immune response to them is limited. They do not resemble human peptides, which allows to avoid cross-reactivity and side effects. Besides, this approach promotes antimicrobial effects, taking into account the inhibited complement system [26]. In this Special Issue, a novel BRICHOS-domain related AMP from the marine polychaeta *Capitella teleta*, named capitellacin, was reported [17]. The peptide exhibits high homology with β-hairpin marine peptides tachyplesins and polyphemusins from the horseshoe crabs. The β-hairpin structure of capitellacin was proved by CD and NMR spectroscopy. In aqueous solution the peptide adopts a monomeric right-handed twisted β-hairpin without significant amphipathicity. Moreover, the peptide retains this conformation in membrane environment. Capitellacin displays a pronounced antimicrobial activity in vitro against a wide panel of bacteria including drug-resistant strains. In contrast to other known β-hairpin antimicrobial peptides, capitellacin acts via non-lytic mechanism at concentrations inhibiting bacterial growth. Molecular mechanism of the peptide antimicrobial action does not seem to be related to the inhibition of bacterial translation. A low cytotoxicity towards human cells and high antibacterial cell selectivity as compared to tachyplesin-1 make capitellacin a promising candidate compound for design of a novel anti-infective drug [17].

The Spanish mackerel *Scomberomorous niphonius* belongs to the Scombridae family and is distributed in the Western North Pacific, including the East China Sea, the Yellow Sea, and the Bohai Sea of China. Recently, some bioactive ingredients have been prepared from the skins and bones of the Spanish mackerel [27]. Among them, antioxidant peptides (APs) are of particular interest. Eight APs including GPY, GPTGE, PFGPD, GPTGAKG, PYGAKG, GATGPQG, GPFGPM, and YGPM have been earlier isolated from the skin of the Spanish mackerel [28]. In this Special Issue, the authors reported isolation and characterization of APs from the protein hydrolysate of the Spanish mackerel muscle obtained by in vitro gastrointestinal (GI) digestion and evaluated biological properties of the isolated peptides [29]. The proteins of the Spanish mackerel muscle were hydrolyzed with different enzymes and by in vitro GI digestion. Four novel APs, designated as SMP-3, SMP-7, SMP-10, and SMP-11, were isolated and identified as PELDW, WPDHW, FGYDWW, and YLHFW, respectively. All these peptides displayed high radical scavenging activity, lipid peroxidation inhibition ability, and protective effects on plasmid DNA (pBR322DNA) against oxidative damage induced by H_2O_2 [29].

Marine peptides are approved as a food ingredient in Norway. The peptide compounds are manufactured by hydrolysis of the Atlantic cod Gadus morhua fillet [30]. The tablets are produced by Flexipharma AS and based on the marine peptide compound 565952 P from Firmenich Bjørge Biomarin AS. The double-blinded, randomized, controlled trial of the marine protein hydrolysate (MPH) was used to evaluate its effect o on measures of physical function and strength in the elderly. This is one of the first long-term studies of MPH and age-related changes in muscle health. Despite a limited benefit of marine protein hydrolysate on physical function and strength in older adults was delivered, the authors came to the conclusion that a daily intake of 3 g MPH for 6 to 12 months would prevent loss of physical performance, compared with a placebo [30].

In this Special Issue, the review [31] analyzes structural features and biological activities of 253 peptides, mainly from marine food sources. The authors aimed to present the current state-of-art in marine peptides structures, biological activities, and applications, and also to compare them with those isolated from other animal food sources. In summary, the authors concluded that marine organisms have proven to be invaluable sources of peptides with unique structures and diverse bioactivities [31].

The papers included in this Special Issue deal with various marine-derived peptides, providing an informative view of their biomedical potential. The initial call resulted in 32 submissions, and 19 of them were accepted and included in the Special Issue I [32]. Following the success of the first Special Issue, we invited researchers in the field to contribute to the second edition entitled "Marine bioactive peptides II: structure, function, and therapeutic potential". A range of new marine peptides were isolated and characterized. Most of them displayed broad-spectrum biological activities and therapeutic potential for clinical trials in humans. All the papers presented in this Special Issue II underlined the central role of bioactive peptides in innate immunity of marine organisms as well as their potential for human health care.

In conclusion, the Guest Editor thanks all the Authors who contributed to this Special Issue, all the Reviewers for evaluating the submitted manuscripts, and the Editorial board of *Marine Drugs*, especially Prof. Dr. Orazio Taglialatela-Scafati, Editor-in-Chief of this journal for his continuous help in turning this Special Issue into reality.

Funding: This research received no external funding.

Conflicts of Interest: The author declares no conflict of interest.

References

1. Hancock, R.E.W.; Brown, K.L.; Mookherjee, N. Host defence peptides from invertebrates –Emerging antimicrobial strate-gies. *Immunobiology* 2006, *211*, 315–322. [CrossRef]
2. Rastogi, P.; Sinha, R.P. Biotechnological and industrial significance of cyanobacterial secondary metabolites. *Biotechnol. Adv.* 2009, *27*, 521–539. [CrossRef]
3. Bornancin, L.; Boyaud, F.; Mahiout, Z.; Bonnard, I.; Mills, S.C.; Banaigs, B.; Inguimbert, N. Isolation and Synthesis of Lax-aphycin B-Type Peptides: A Case Study and Clues to Their Biosynthesis. *Mar. Drugs* 2015, *13*, 7285–7300. [CrossRef]
4. Alvariño, R.; Alonso, E.; Bornancin, L.; Bonnard, I.; Inguimbert, N.; Banaigs, B.; Botana, L.M. Biological Activities of Cyclic and Acyclic B-Type Laxaphycins in SH-SY5Y Human Neuroblastoma Cells. *Mar. Drugs* 2020, *18*, 364. [CrossRef] [PubMed]
5. Youssef, F.S.; Ashour, M.I..; Singab, A.N.B.; Wink, M. A Comprehensive Review of Bioactive Peptides from Marine Fungi and Their Biological Significance. *Mar. Drugs* 2019, *17*, 559. [CrossRef]
6. Turk, T.; Kem, W.R. The phylum Cnidaria and investigations of its toxins and venoms until 1990. *Toxicon* 2009, *54*, 1031–1037. [CrossRef] [PubMed]
7. Leung, T.C.N.; Qu, Z.; Nong, W.; Hui, J.H.L.; Ngai, S.M. Proteomic Analysis of the Venom of Jellyfishes *Rhopilema esculentum* and *Sanderia malayensis*. *Mar. Drugs* 2020, *18*, 655. [CrossRef] [PubMed]
8. Nong, W.; Cao, J.; Li, Y.; Qu, Z.; Sun, J.; Swale, T.; Yip, H.Y.; Qian, P.Y.; Qiu, J.-W.; Kwan, H.S.; et al. Jellyfish genomes reveal distinct homeobox gene clusters and conservation of small RNA processing. *Nat. Commun.* 2020, *11*, 1–11. [CrossRef] [PubMed]
9. Tascedda, F.; Ottaviani, E. Biologically active peptides in mollusks. *Invertebr. Surviv. J.* 2016, *13*, 186–190.
10. Pettit, G.R.; Kamano, Y.; Herald, C.L.; Tuinman, A.A.; Boettner, F.E.; Kizu, H.; Schmidt, J.M.; Baczynskyj, L.; Tomer, K.B.; Bontems, R.J. The isolation and structure of a remarkable marine animal antineoplastic constituent: Dolastatin. *J. Am. Chem. Soc.* 1987, *109*, 6883–6885. [CrossRef]
11. Gao, G.; Wang, Y.; Hua, H.; Li, D.; Tang, C. Marine Antitumor Peptide Dolastatin 10: Biological Activity, Structural Modification and Synthetic Chemistry. *Mar. Drugs* 2021, *19*, 363. [CrossRef]
12. Zhang, Q.; Liu, Z.; Wang, Z.; Wang, T.; Wang, N.; Wang, N.; Zhang, B.; Zhao, Y. Recent Advances in Small Peptides of Ma-rine Origin in Cancer Therapy. *Mar. Drugs* 2021, *19*, 115. [CrossRef]
13. Dyshlovoy, S.A.; Honecker, F. Marine Compounds and Cancer: 2017 Updates. *Mar. Drugs* 2018, *16*, 41. [CrossRef] [PubMed]

14. Atul, T.; Abhishek, T.; Priya, A.; Sudheer, G.; Minakshi, S.; Deepika, M.; Anshika, J.; Sandeep, S.; Ankur, G.; Raghava, G.P.S. CancerPPD: A database of anticancer peptides and proteins. *Nucleic Acids Res.* **2015**, *43*, 837–843.
15. Wang, C.; Zhang, G.J.; Liu, W.D.; Yang, X.Y.; Zhu, N.; Shen, J.M.; Wang, Z.C.; Liu, Y.; Cheng, S.; Yu, G.L.; et al. Recent pro-gress in research and development of marine drugs. *Chin. J. Mar. Drugs* **2019**, *38*, 35–69.
16. Ovchinnikova, T.V.; Aleshina, G.M.; Balandin, S.V.; Krasnosdembskaya, A.D.; Markelov, M.L.; Frolova, E.I.; Leonova, Y.F.; Tagaev, A.A.; Krasnodembsky, E.G.; Kokryakov, V.N. Purification and primary structure of two isoforms of arenicin, a novel antimicrobial peptide from marine polychaeta Arenicola marina. *FEBS Lett.* **2004**, *577*, 209–214. [CrossRef]
17. Panteleev, P.V.; Tsarev, A.V.; Safronova, V.N.; Reznikova, O.V.; Bolosov, I.A.; Sychev, S.V.; Shenkarev, Z.O.; Ovchinnikova, T.V. Structure Elucidation and Functional Studies of a Novel β-hairpin Antimicrobial Peptide from the Marine Polychaeta *Capitella teleta*. *Mar. Drugs* **2020**, *18*, 620. [CrossRef] [PubMed]
18. Ovchinnikova, T.V.; Shenkarev, Z.O.; Nadezhdin, K.D.; Balandin, S.; Zhmak, M.N.; Kudelina, I.A.; Finkina, E.I.; Kokryakov, V.N.; Arseniev, A.S. Recombinant expression, synthesis, purification, and solution structure of arenicin. *Biochem. Biophys. Res. Commun.* **2007**, *360*, 156–162. [CrossRef] [PubMed]
19. Ovchinnikova, T.V.; Shenkarev, Z.O.; Balandin, S.V.; Nadezhdin, K.D.; Paramonov, A.S.; Kokryakov, V.N.; Arseniev, A.S. Molecular insight into mechanism of antimicrobial action of the β-hairpin peptide arenicin: Specific oligomerization in de-tergent micelles. *Biopolymers* **2008**, *89*, 455–464. [CrossRef]
20. Andrä, J.; Jakovkin, I.; Grötzinger, J.; Hecht, O.; Krasnodembskaya, A.; Goldmann, T.; Gutsmann, T.; Leippe, M. Structure and mode of action of the antimicrobial peptide arenicin. *Biochem. J.* **2008**, *410*, 113–122. [CrossRef] [PubMed]
21. Shenkarev, Z.O.; Balandin, S.V.; Trunov, K.I.; Paramonov, A.S.; Sukhanov, S.V.; Barsukov, L.I.; Arseniev, A.S.; Ovchinnikova, T.V. Molecular mechanism of action of β-hairpin antimicrobial peptide arenicin: Oligomeric structure in DPC micelles and pore formation in planar lipid bilayers. *Biochemistry* **2011**, *50*, 6255–6265. [CrossRef] [PubMed]
22. Panteleev, P.V.; Bolosov, I.A.; Balandin, S.V.; Ovchinnikova, T.V. Design of antimicrobial peptide arenicin analogs with improved therapeutic indices. *J. Pept. Sci.* **2014**, *21*, 105–113. [CrossRef] [PubMed]
23. Panteleev, P.V.; Bolosov, I.A.; Ovchinnikova, T.V. Bioengineering and functional characterization of arenicin shortened an-alogs with enhanced antibacterial activity and cell selectivity. *J. Pept. Science* **2016**, *22*, 82–91. [CrossRef] [PubMed]
24. Panteleev, P.V.; Myshkin, M.Y.; Shenkarev, Z.O.; Ovchinnikova, T.V. Dimerization of the antimicrobial peptide arenicin plays a key role in the cytotoxicity but not in the antibacterial activity. *Biochem. Biophys. Res. Commun.* **2017**, *482*, 1320–1326. [CrossRef] [PubMed]
25. Orlov, D.S.; Shamova, O.V.; Eliseev, I.E.; Zharkova, M.S.; Chakchir, O.B.; Antcheva, N.; Zachariev, S.; Panteleev, P.V.; Kokryakov, V.N.; Ovchinnikova, T.V.; et al. Redesigning Arenicin-1, an Antimicrobial Peptide from the Marine Poly-chaeta Arenicola marina, by Strand Rearrangement or Branching, Substitution of Specific Residues, and Backbone Lineari-zation or Cyclization. *Marine Drugs* **2019**, *17*, 376. [CrossRef] [PubMed]
26. Krenev, I.A.; Umnyakova, E.S.; Eliseev, I.E.; Dubrovskii, Y.A.; Gorbunov, N.P.; Pozolotin, V.A.; Komlev, A.S.; Panteleev, P.V.; Balandin, S.V.; Ovchinnikova, T.V.; et al. Antimicrobial Peptide Arenicin-1 Derivative Ar-1-(C/A) as Complement System Modulator. *Mar. Drugs* **2020**, *18*, 631. [CrossRef] [PubMed]
27. Sable, R.; Parajuli, P.; Jois, S. Peptides, Peptidomimetics, and Polypeptides from Marine Sources: A Wealth of Natural Sources for Pharmaceutical Applications. *Mar. Drugs* **2017**, *15*, 124. [CrossRef]
28. Zhang, J.B.; Wang, Y.M.; Chi, C.F.; Sun, K.L.; Wang, B. Eight peptides from collagen hydrolysate fraction of Spanish macke-rel (Scomberomorus niphonius) skin: Isolation, identification, and antioxidant activity in vitro. *Mar. Drugs* **2019**, *17*, 224. [CrossRef]
29. Zhao, G.-X.; Yang, X.-R.; Wang, Y.-M.; Zhao, Y.-Q.; Chi, C.-F.; Wang, B. Antioxidant Peptides from the Protein Hydrolysate of Spanish Mackerel (*Scomberomorus niphonius*) Muscle by in Vitro Gastrointestinal Digestion and Their in Vitro Activities. *Mar. Drugs* **2019**, *17*, 531. [CrossRef]
30. Nygård, L.; Mundal, I.; Dahl, L.; Šaltytė Benth, J.; Rokstad, A. Limited Benefit of Marine Protein Hydrolysate on Physical Function and Strength in Older Adults: A Randomized Controlled Trial. *Mar. Drugs* **2021**, *19*, 62. [CrossRef]
31. Pavlicevic, M.; Maestri, E.; Marmiroli, M. Marine Bioactive Peptides—An Overview of Generation, Structure and Application with a Focus on Food Sources. *Mar. Drugs* **2020**, *18*, 424. [CrossRef] [PubMed]
32. Ovchinnikova, T.V. Structure, Function, and Therapeutic Potential of Marine Bioactive Peptides. *Mar. Drugs* **2019**, *17*, 505. [CrossRef] [PubMed]

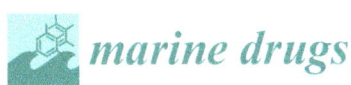

Article

Biological Activities of Cyclic and Acyclic B-Type Laxaphycins in SH-SY5Y Human Neuroblastoma Cells

Rebeca Alvariño [1], Eva Alonso [1,2,*], Louis Bornancin [3], Isabelle Bonnard [3,4], Nicolas Inguimbert [3,4], Bernard Banaigs [3,4] and Luis M. Botana [1]

1. Departamento de Farmacología, Facultad de Veterinaria, Universidad de Santiago de Compostela, 27003 Lugo, Spain; rebeca.alvarino@usc.es (R.A.); luis.botana@usc.es (L.M.B.)
2. Fundación Instituto de Investigación Sanitario Santiago de Compostela (FIDIS), Hospital Universitario Lucus Augusti, 27003 Lugo, Spain
3. PSL Research University: EPHE-UPVD-CNRS, USR 3278 CRIOBE, Université de Perpignan, 52 Avenue Paul Alduy, 66860 Perpignan, France; lbornan@dtu.dk (L.B.); isabelle.bonnard@univ-perp.fr (I.B.); nicolas.inguimbert@univ-perp.fr (N.I.); banaigs@univ-perp.fr (B.B.)
4. Laboratoire d'Excellence "CORAIL", Université de Perpignan Via Domitia, 58 Avenue Paul Alduy, 66860 Perpignan, France
* Correspondence: eva.alonso.lopez@sergas.es; Tel.: +34982822233

Received: 8 June 2020; Accepted: 13 July 2020; Published: 15 July 2020

Abstract: Laxaphycins are a family of non-ribosomal lipopeptides that have been isolated from several cyanobacteria. Some of these compounds have presented cytotoxic activities, but their mechanism of action is poorly understood. In this work, the already described laxaphycins B and B3, and acyclolaxaphycins B and B3 were isolated from the marine cyanobacteria *Anabaena torulosa*. Moreover, two new acyclic compounds, [des-(Ala[4]-Hle[5])] acyclolaxaphycins B and B3, were purified from the herviborous gastropod *Stylocheilus striatus*, with this being the first description of biotransformed laxaphycins. The structure of these new compounds was elucidated, together with the absolute configuration of acyclolaxaphycins B and B3. The bioactivities of the six peptides were determined in SH-SY5Y human neuroblastoma cells. Laxaphycins B and B3 were cytotoxic (IC$_{50}$: 1.8 and 0.8 µM, respectively) through the induction of apoptosis. In comparison, acyclic laxaphycins did not show cytotoxicity but affected mitochondrial functioning, so their effect on autophagy-related protein expression was analyzed, finding that acyclic peptides affected this process by increasing AMPK phosphorylation and inhibiting mTOR. This work confirms the pro-apoptotic properties of cyclic laxaphycins B and is the first report indicating the effects on autophagy of their acyclic analogs. Moreover, gastropod-derived compounds presented ring opening and amino-acids deletion, a biotransformation that had not been previously described.

Keywords: biotransformation; laxaphycin; autophagy; apoptosis; cyanobacteria

1. Introduction

The phylum Cyanobacteria includes photosynthetic prokaryotes from terrestrial, freshwater and marine ecosystems. These Gram-negative organisms, also called blue-green algae, appeared on Earth over 3.5 billion years ago and can live as colonial or unicellular forms in almost all habitats (deserts, ice shelves, as endosymbionts, etc.). This high degree of adaptation is related to their ability to produce a wide range of secondary metabolites [1,2]. A significant part of these compounds are complex cyclic peptides, depsipeptides or lipopeptides that contain unusual amino acids and multiple N-methylations [3]. Many of these molecules are produced through non-ribosomal peptide synthase (NRPS) and/or polyketide synthase (PKS) enzymatic systems. The enzymes are organized in modules, each one carrying out the addition of a subpart of the final molecule and generating a great diversity of compounds [4,5]. As a result, non-ribosomal peptides exhibit a broad spectrum of biological activities, including, anticancer, antifungal and antimicrobial properties [6]. Furthermore, cyclic peptides are less flexible than their linear counterparts, and contain non-proteinogenic amino acids, two characteristics that give them greater selectivity and better resistance to hydrolysis by exo- and endopeptidases.

Laxaphycins are a large family of lipopeptides synthetized through a hybrid PKS/NRPS pathway by different species of cyanobacteria [7]. These compounds have been obtained from specimens of *Hormothamnion enteromorphoides*, *Anabaena torulosa*, *Lyngbya confervoides* and *Anabaena laxa* collected worldwide. The fact that different species could produce similar metabolites suggests horizontal gene transfer or an ancient common parent between them. Therefore, these peptides have been selected by evolution in both freshwater and oceanic cyanobacteria and may confer to them an ecological advantage. Laxaphycins are divided in two sub-families: laxaphycin A-type, undecapeptides with a segregation of hydrophobic and hydrophilic residues; and laxaphycin B-type, dodecapeptides in which hydrophobic and hydrophilic residues are alternated [8]. Laxaphycin B-type members such as laxaphycins B, B2 and B3 have presented antifungal, antimicrobial and cytotoxic activities [9–12]. Laxaphycin A-type compounds have shown weak cytotoxicity, with the exception of the compound hormothamnin A [13]. Moreover, we have recently reported evidence that points to an activation of the autophagic flux by laxaphycin A peptides [14].

Autophagy is a regulated process that leads to the clearance of misfolded or damaged proteins and dysfunctional organelles. This cellular machinery is activated by a variety of signals such as nutrient starvation, oxidative stress and energy depletion. Cells can degrade damaged components and restore substrates for energy metabolism through this pathway [15]. At basal levels, autophagy maintains cellular homeostasis and is an important mechanism in cell growth and development. This process plays an important role in many pathologies such as cancer, diabetes and neurodegenerative diseases [16]. Therefore, much effort has been made in the search for new compounds capable of targeting the autophagic flux [17,18].

When the autophagic flux is initiated, the mammalian target of rapamycin (mTOR), considered the master cell growth regulator, is inhibited. This inhibition leads to the activation of the Unc-51-like kinase 1 (ULK1) complex, which in turn stimulates the Beclin1-VPS34 complex. The components of this complex are phosphorylated and trigger the elongation of the phagophore. Two systems control this process: the ATG5-ATG12 and the microtubule-associated light chain 3 (LC3). During this step, LC3I is converted to LC3II, the lipidated form, considered the signature of the autophagic membranes [19]. Finally, the autophagosome undergoes maturation and fuses with the lysosome, leading to the formation of the autolysosome, with an internal acidic and hydrolytic environment that degrades the damaged cellular components [20,21].

Adenosine monophosphate-activated protein kinase (AMPK) is an important energy sensor in cells and plays a key role in the activation of autophagy due to the significance of this process in the generation of metabolic intermediates to maintain ATP levels. AMPK is activated when energy levels decrease and can trigger autophagic flux either by phosphorylating the ULK1 complex or through the regulation of mTOR activity [22].

The human neuroblastoma cell line SH-SY5Y is a useful model for assessing neurotoxic and neuroprotective compounds, since these cells express intact genes implied in reactive oxygen species (ROS) metabolism, or calcium and mitochondrial signaling [23].

In this study, the biological activities of six B-type laxaphycins were analyzed in SH-SY5Y cells (Figure 1). The already known laxaphycins B (**1**) and B3 (**2**), and acyclolaxaphycins B (**3**) and B3 (**4**) were obtained from a marine specimen of *A. torulosa*, whereas two new acyclic compounds, [des-(Ala^4-Hle^5)] acyclolaxaphycin B (**5**) and [des-(Ala^4-Hle^5)] acyclolaxaphycin B3 (**6**), were isolated from the herbivorous gastropod *Stylocheilus striatus*. The absolute configurations of **3** and **4**, as well as the complete structural elucidation of the new diet-derived peptides **5** and **6** are also provided.

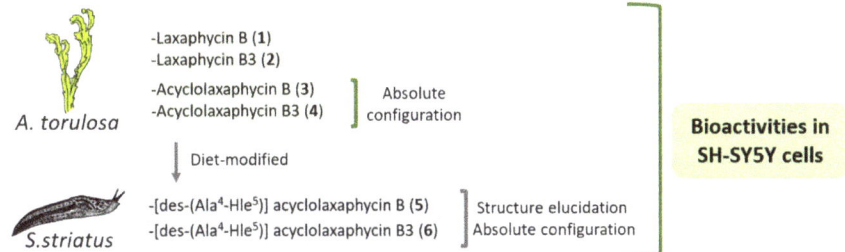

Figure 1. Scheme of laxaphycin B sources and compound analysis

2. Results

2.1. Structure Elucidation of Peptides **3**, **4**, **5** and **6**

S. striatus was collected on A. cf torulosa in the lagoon of Moorea, French Polynesia, sealed underwater in a bag, freeze-dried and extracted. The crude extract was fractionated using flash chromatography and the resulting fraction containing new peptides was subjected to HPLC purification to yield compounds **5** (2.5 mg) and **6** (5 mg) as a white, amorphous powder. Compounds **5** and **6** responded positively to a ninhydrin test, suggesting a non-blocked N-terminus. The already described laxaphycins B (**1**) and B3 (**2**) [9], and acyclolaxaphycins B (**3**) and B3 (**4**) were repurified from A. torulosa as described in [7] (Figure 2).

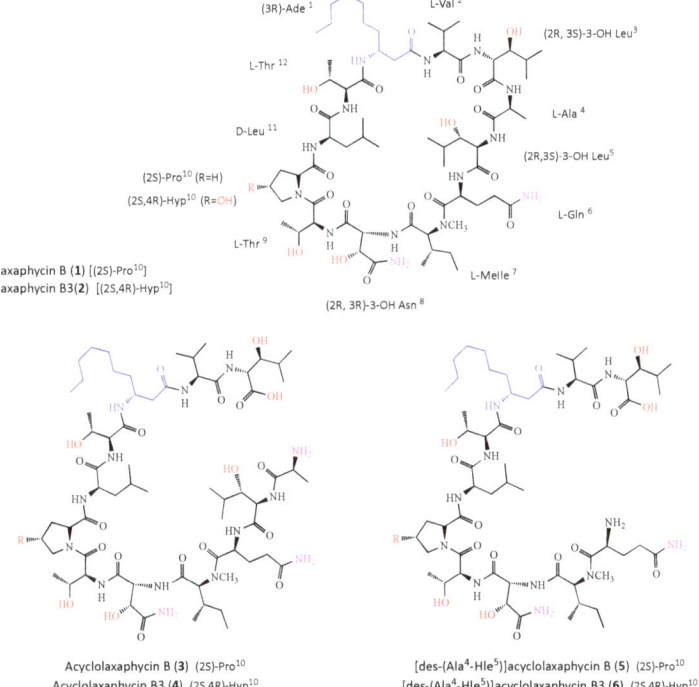

Figure 2. Chemical structures of laxaphycin B-type compounds. As for (**1**) and (**2**), R=H for (**3**) and (**5**), and R=OH for (**4**) and (**6**).

Using the positive high-resolution electrospray ionization mass spectrometry (HRESIMS) spectra, the molecular formula was determined to be $C_{56}H_{100}N_{12}O_{17}$ (*m/z* 1213.7509) [M + H]$^+$ for compound **5** and $C_{56}H_{100}N_{12}O_{18}$ (*m/z* 1229.7972) [M + H]$^+$ for compound **6**.

All the NMR experiments were conducted in DMSO-*d6*. The signal distribution pattern observed in the ^{1}H-NMR spectrum of **5** and **6** was characteristic of lipopeptides, displaying amide NH signals (δ_H 7.40–7.90), CαH signals (δ_H 3.5–4.7), aliphatic CH2 (δ_H 1.1–1.3) and CH$_3$ signals (δ_H 0.7–0.9).

- [des-(Ala^4-Hle^5)] acyclolaxaphycin B (**5**)

In the NH proton region, seven doublets and two singlets were observed. The values of chemical shifts (Table 1) were reported using 2D-NMR spectra including correlation spectroscopy (COSY), total correlation spectroscopy (TOCSY), rotating frame nuclear magnetic resonance spectroscopy (ROESY), heteronuclear single quantum correlation (HSQC), HSQC-TOCSY, and heteronuclear multiple bond correlation (HMBC) (Figures S1–S8). Analysis of TOCSY correlations (Figure S4) revealed the presence of 10 amino acid residues: N-methylisoleucine (N-MeIle), 3-hydroxyasparagine (Has), two threonines (Thr), proline (Pro), leucine (Leu), β-aminodecanoic acid (β-Ade), valine (Val) and 3-hydroxyleucine (Hle). In comparison with laxaphycin B, analyses of TOCSY and HSQC (Figure S6) spectra revealed the absence of typical correlations within alanine and within one of the two hydroxyleucines, suggesting the lack of these two residues in **5**.

Table 1. NMR spectroscopic data for [des-(Ala^4-Hle^5)] acyclolaxaphycin B (**5**) and [des-(Ala^4-Hle^5)] acyclolaxaphycin B3 (**6**) (303 K) in DMSO-d6.

		[des-(Ala^4-Hle^5)] Acyclolaxaphycin B (5)		[des-(Ala^4-Hle$_5$)] Acyclolaxaphycin B3 (6)	
		^{13}C	^{1}H	^{13}C	^{1}H
		δ (ppm)	δ (ppm)	δ (ppm)	δ (ppm)
Gln^1	NH$_2$			NH	
	CαH	53.01	4.50	CαH 53.15	4.51
	CβH$_2$	29.95	1.88	CβH$_2$ 29.91	1.90
	CγH$_2$	28.76	2.20	CγH$_2$ 29.12	2.20
	CON	174.24		CONH 174.27	
	NH$_2$		6.74/7.30		
	CO	172.85		CO 172.90	
N-MeILe^2	NCH$_3$	29.53	2.88	NCH$_3$ 29.60	2.88
	CαH	59.75	4.73	CαH 59.68	4.73
	CβH	31.00	1.94	CβH 31.12	1.92
	CγH$_2$	23.59	0.92/1.31	CγH$_2$ 24.02	0.89/1.29
	Cγ'H$_3$	15.16	0.78	Cγ'H$_3$ 15.20	0.78
	CδH$_3$	10.32	0.81	CδH$_3$ 10.41	0.80
	CO	169.71		CO 169.76	
Has^3	NH		7.49	NH	7.52
	CαH	55.12	4.62	CαH 55.36	4.63
	CβH	70.84	4.37	CβH 70.91	4.37
	OH			OH	
	CONH$_2$	173.26		CONH$_2$ 173.29	
	NH$_2$		7.27/7.35	NH$_2$	7.28/7.35
	CO	168.73		CO 168.79	
Thr^4	NH		7.50	NH	7.46
	CαH	54.99	4.57	CαH 55.25	4.56
	CβH	66.37	3.99	CβH 66.40	3.98
	OH			OH	
	CγH$_3$	18.34	1.01	CγH$_3$ 18.42	1.01
	CO	168.95		CO 169.02	

Table 1. *Cont.*

		[des-(Ala⁴-Hle⁵)] Acyclolaxaphycin B (5)		[des-(Ala⁴-Hle₅)] Acyclolaxaphycin B3 (6)	
		^{13}C	^{1}H	^{13}C	^{1}H
		δ (ppm)	δ (ppm)	δ (ppm)	δ (ppm)
Pro⁵/Hyp⁵	CαH	59.89	4.39	CαH 59.23	4.40
	CβH₂	28.91	1.84/2.03	CβH₂ 37.69	1.87/2.04
	CγH₍₂₎	24.07	1.81/1.89	CγH 68.41	4.29
	OH			OH	
	CδH₂	47.36	3.64/3.76	CδH₂ 55.78	3.59/3.78
	CO	170.38		CO 171.45	
Leu⁶	NH		7.89	NH	7.88
	CαH	51.63	4.28	CαH 51.61	4.27
	CβH₂	40.15	1.46/1.54	CβH₂ 40.38	1.48/1.55
	CγH	23.89	1.59	CγH 24.03	1.60
	CδH₃	22.91	0.85	CδH₃ 22.96	0.86
	Cδ'H₃	21.26	0.83	Cδ'H₃ 21.34	0.83
	CO	172.12		CO 172.27	
Thr⁷	NH		7.80	NH	7.75
	CαH	58.50	4.07	CαH 58.47	4.09
	CβH	66.37	3.99	CβH 66.43	3.98
	OH			OH	
	CγH₃	19.62	0.99	CγH₃ 19.66	0.99
	CO	169.17		CO 169.74	
β-Ade⁸	NH		7.56	NH	7.57
	CαH₂	39.92	2.36	CαH₂ 40.29	2.36
	CβH	46.30	4.00	CβH 46.35	4.02
	CγH₂	33.19	1.35/1.41	CγH₂ 33.31	1.34/1.40
	CδH₂	28.72	1.20	CδH₂ 28.86	1.20
	CεH₂	28.60	1.20	CεH₂ 28.75	1.20
	CζH₂	25.37	1.20	CζH₂ 25.41	1.20
	Cη H₂	31.20	1.20	Cη H₂ 31.26	1.20
	Cθ H₂	22.01	1.24	Cθ H₂ 22.15	1.25
	CιH₃	13.84	0.85	CιH₃ 13.97	0.84
	CO	170.23		CO 170.45	
Val⁹	NH		7.89	NH	7.90
	CαH	57.73	4.23	CαH 57.73	4.26
	CβH₂	29.88	2.03	CβH₂ 30.35	2.03
	CγH₃	19.28	0.82	CγH₃ 19.25	0.82
	Cγ'H₃	17.67	0.81	Cγ'H₃ 17.77	0.81
	CO	170.57		CO 170.85	
Hle¹⁰	NH		7.55	NH	7.59
	CαH	54.87	4.27	Cα 54.85	4.30
	CβH	75.89	3.52	CβH 76.02	3.51
	OH			OH	
	CγH	30.52	1.53	CγH 30.73	1.51
	CδH₃	19.22	0.82	CδH₃ 19.119	0.88
	Cδ'H₃	19.16	0.77	Cδ'H₃ 19.12	0.76
	CO	172.02		CO 172.09	

The remaining non-identified spin system was identified as a glutamine residue with the presence of two carbonyl signals at 172.85 and 174.24 ppm, and by HMBC (Figure S8) correlation from Hα (δ_H4.50) to Cβ (δ_C29.95), from Hβ (δ_H1.88) to Cα (δ_C53.01) and Cγ (δ_C28.76) and from Hγ (δ_H2.20) to Cβ (δ_C29.95) and Cδ (δ_C174.24). However, the poor resolutions of glutamine correlation signals in 2D-NMR (HMBC, HSQC and ROESY) did not allow us to assign the two NH₂ signals. This might be explained by the presence of multiple conformations in solution due to an increase in the flexibility of the N-terminal residue. The HMBC spectrum provided information on sequence-specific assignments. Indeed, the cross-peaks between carbonyl carbons (residue i) and NH, NCH$_3$ protons or Hα (residue i + 1) suggested the presence of two partial sequences including Gln-N-MeIle-Has-Thr (fragment 1) and Pro-Leu-Thr-β-Ade-Val-Hle (fragment 2). Analysis of the ROESY spectra (Figure S5) revealed a correlation between Hα ($δ_H$4.57) of Thr^4 and Hδ ($δ_H$3.64/3.76) of Pro^5, assembling fragments 1 and 2 and establishing the complete sequence as Gln-N-MeIle-Has-Thr-Pro-Leu-Thr-β-Ade-Val-Hle. Even if it does not constitute evidence, the lack of HMBC or ROESY correlations between Gln and Hle, observable in the case of laxaphycins B (**1**) and B3 (**2**), suggested that the peptide is linear. Positive arguments are provided by the molecular formula determined to be $C_{56}H_{100}N_{12}O_{17}$ by HRMS and by a positive response to a ninhydrin test suggesting a non-blocked N-terminus.

- [des-(Ala^4-Hle^5)] acyclolaxaphycin B3 (**6**)

ESIMS-MS fragmentation of compound **6** led us to a y6-y8 ion series shifted to a higher mass by 16 amu in comparison to that of **5**, suggesting that the variable residue could be Pro. Compound **6** showed remarkable NMR spectral similarities (Figures S9–S16) to **5**, being the most significant differences being the presence of an additional hydroxyl group on proline (Hγ at 4.29 ppm vs. two Hγ at 1.81 and 1.89 ppm for [des-(Ala^4-Hle^5)] acyclolaxaphycin B (**5**); Cγ at 68.41 ppm vs. 24.07 ppm for **5**; Cβ and Cδ were also deblinded by the presence of the hydroxyl function (Δδ 8.8 and 8.4 ppm, respectively)). The NMR spectral analysis (Table 1) established the complete sequence as Gln-N-MeIle-Has-Thr-Hyp-Leu-Thr-β-Ade-Val-Hle.

ESIMS-MS fragmentations for **5** and **6** were consistent with the proposed amino acid sequences and the presence of y ions at m/z 416.3143 (y3), 517.3628 (y4), 727.5011 (y6), 828.5375 (y7) and 958.5770 (y8), and b ions at m/z 487.2525 (b4) and 256.1671 (b2) for compound **5**, as well as y ions at m/z 416.3174 (y3), 517.3633 (y4), 743.4884 (y6), 844.5478 (y7) and 974.5867 (y8), and b ions at m/z 814.4389 (b7), 487.2570 (b4) and 256.1678 (b2) for compound **6** (Figure 3).

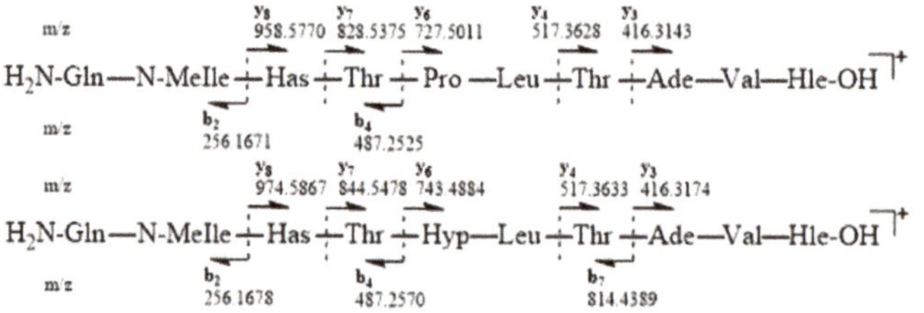

Figure 3. Electrospray ionization mass spectrometry (ESIMS/MS) fragmentation of [des-(Ala4-I Ile5)] acyclolaxaphycins B (**5**) and B3 (**6**)

2.2. Absolute Configuration of Peptides 3, 4, 5 and 6

The absolute configuration of each amino acid residue in compounds **3–6** was established using the advanced Marfey's method after hydrolysis [24,25]. The LC-MS comparison between the Marfey's derivatives of the acid hydrolysate of laxaphycin B and those of acyclolaxaphycin B (**3**) established the 2S configuration of Val, Ala, Gln, Pro, N-MeIle, the 2R configuration of Leu, as well as the 3R configuration of Ade. The Marfey's analysis of the four stereoisomers of standard threonine revealed the (2S,3R) configuration of both threonines present in acyclolaxaphycin B (**3**). The Marfey's method also revealed the 2R configuration of the two 3-hydroxyleucines. The absolute configuration of Cβ of both 3-hydroxyleucines (2R,3S) was established through NOESY correlations between the Hγ and the NH observed.

As previously described [9], the elution order of the 3-hydroxyasparagine (HAsp), which results from the acid hydrolysis of Has, is another exception of Marfey's rule. Indeed, the D-FDLA-(2R)-HAsp derivative elutes after the L-FDLA-(2R)-HAsp derivative. Thus, we established that the Cα configuration of the Has residue was 2R. The configuration of the Cβ of Has was established to be 3R by a comparison with laxaphycin B Marfey's derivatives. Therefore, the complete structure of acyclolaxaphycin B (3) was established as (2S)- Ala-(2R,3S)- Hle-(2S)- Gln-(2S)-N-MeIle-(2R,3R)-Has-(2S,3R)-Thr-(2S)-Pro-(2R)-Leu-(2S,3R)-Thr-(3R)-Ade-(2S)-Val-(2R,3S)-Hle.

Regarding acyclolaxaphycin B3 (4), the configuration of Val, Ala, Gln, N-MeIle, Leu, Ade, Has, Thr (x2) and Hle (x2) were found to be the same as for acyclophycin B (3). The absolute configuration of the Cα of the Hyp residue appeared to be (2S) and a comparison with laxaphycin B3 derivative enabled the Cγ configuration to be assigned to 4R, establishing the complete structure as (2S)-Ala-(2R,3S)-Hle-(2S)-Gln-(2S)-N-MeIle-(2R,3R)-Has-(2S,3R)-Thr-(2S,4R)-Hyp-(2R)-Leu-(2S,3R)-Thr-(3R)-Ade-(2S)-Val-(2R,3S)-Hle.

The chromatographic comparison between the Marfey's derivatives of the acid hydrolysate of [des-(Ala^4-Hle^5)] acyclolaxaphycin B (5) and those of acyclophycin B (3) established the 2S configuration of Val, Gln, Pro, N-MeIle, the 2R configuration of Leu, as well as the 3R configuration of Ade, and the (2R,3R) configuration of Has, (2S,3R) of Thr (x2), and (2R,3S) of Hle. The complete structure of 5 was defined as (2S)-Gln-(2S)-N-MeIle-(2R,3R)-Has-(2S,3R)-Thr-(2S)-Pro-(2R)-Leu-(2S,3R)-Thr-(3R)-Ade-(2S)-Val-(2R,3S)-Hle.

With regard to [des-(Ala^4-Hle^5)] acyclolaxaphycin B3 (6), the configuration of Val, Gln, N-MeIle, Leu, Ade, Has, Thr (x2) and Hle (x2) were found to be the same as for 5. The absolute configuration of the Cα of the Hyp residue appeared to be (2S) and a comparison with laxaphycin B3 derivative enabled the Cγ configuration to be assigned to 4R, establishing the complete structure as (2S)-Gln-(2S)-N-MeIle-(2R,3R)-Has-(2S,3R)-Thr-(2S,4R)-Hyp-(2R)-Leu-(2S,3R)-Thr-(3R)-Ade-(2S)-Val-(2R,3S)-Hle.

2.3. Effects of B-Type Laxaphycins on Cell Viability and Mitochondrial Function

In order to make an initial evaluation of compounds activity, their effect on cell viability, metabolic activity and mitochondrial function were tested. Cell viability was assessed by monitoring lactate dehydrogenase (LDH) levels in cells supernatant [26], cell metabolic activity was analyzed with MTT (3-(4, 5-dimethyl thiazol-2-yl)-2, 5-diphenyl tetrazolium bromide) [27], and tetramethylrhodamine methyl ester (TMRM) dye was used to determine the mitochondrial membrane potential ($\Delta\Psi_m$). The effect of laxaphycins over reactive oxygen species (ROS) and ATP levels was also monitored.

Cyclic compounds (1 and 2) turned out to be cytotoxic to neuroblastoma cells (Figure 4). Their half maximal inhibitory concentrations (IC$_{50}$) were calculated for LDH and MTT assays. In LDH test, compound 2 presented an IC$_{50}$ value of 0.8 μM, 95% confidence interval (CI): 0.24–3.0 μM, R^2: 0.90, being was slightly more cytotoxic than compound 1 (IC$_{50}$=1.8 μM, 95% CI: 0.65–5.1, R^2: 0.93) (Figure 4a,f). The same was observed in MTT assay, compound 2 was the most toxic (IC$_{50}$ =0.15 μM, 95 % CI: 0.06–0.37 μM, R^2: 0.91), whereas compound 1 presented an IC$_{50}$ of 0.3 μM (CI: 0.14–0.66, R^2: 0.94) (Figure 4b,g). As expected, cyclic laxaphycins depolarized the mitochondria and reduced ROS and ATP levels at toxic concentrations (Figure 4c–e,h–j).

Acyclic laxaphycins obtained from A. torulosa (compounds 3 and 4) did not display cytotoxicity at any of the concentrations tested (Figure 5a,f). Laxaphycin 3 significantly augmented cell metabolic activity at 0.1 and 1 μM and produced a decrease in $\Delta\Psi_m$ (Figure 5b,c). This compound also reduced ROS and ATP levels at the highest concentrations (Figure 5d,e). Interestingly, the reduction in ATP was observed at 6 h, but it was recovered at 24 h, reaching levels of control cells. Compound 4 presented similar results, depolarizing the mitochondrial membrane at 10 μM, and diminishing ROS release and ATP levels at 6 h (Figure 5h–j).

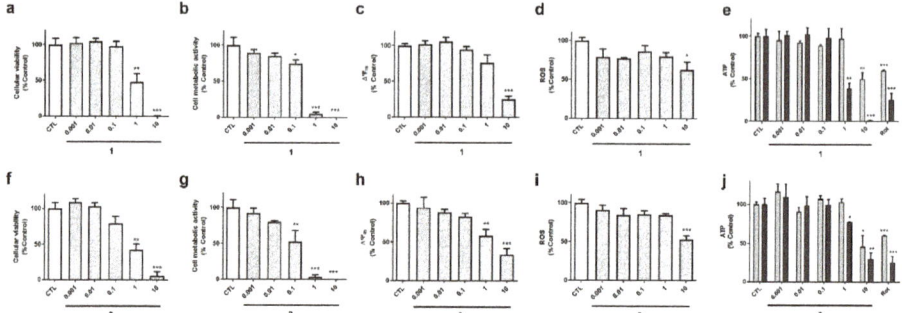

Figure 4. Effect of cyclic laxaphycins B on cell viability and mitochondrial function. SH-SY5Y cells were treated with compounds **1** (a–e) and **2** (f–j) for 24 h. Then, cell viability was determined with LDH test, cell metabolic activity with MTT assay, $\Delta\Psi_m$ with tetramethylrhodamine methyl ester (TMRM) dye, reactive oxygen species (ROS) levels with carboxy-H_2DCFDA and ATP levels with a commercial kit. ATP levels were assessed both at 6 h (light bars) and 24 h (dark bars). Concentration expressed in µM. Mean ± SEM of three experiments performed by triplicate. Values are presented as percentage of control cells. * $p < 0.05$, ** $p < 0.01$, *** $p < 0.001$

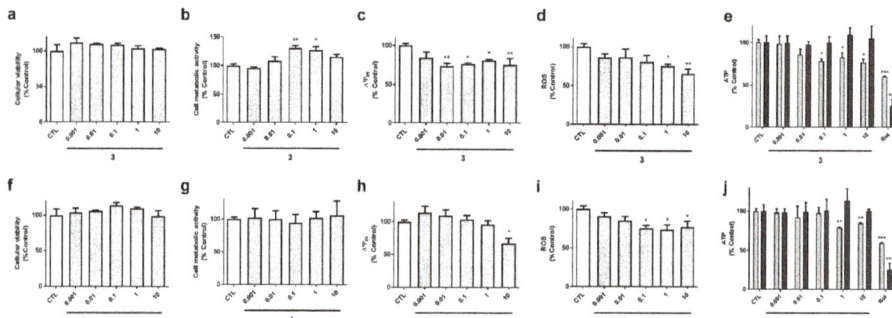

Figure 5. Effect of acyclic compounds isolated from *A. torulosa* on SH-SY5Y cells. Compounds **3** (a–e) and **4** (f–j) were added to neuroblastoma cells for 24 h and cellular viability, metabolic activity, $\Delta\Psi_m$, ROS release and ATP levels were determined. The levels of ATP were assessed at 6 and 24 h (light and dark bars, respectively). Concentration expressed in µM. Mean ± SEM of three experiments performed by triplicate. Values are presented as percentage of control cells. * $p < 0.05$, ** $p < 0.01$, *** $p < 0.001$

The biological activities of compounds **5** and **6**, isolated from the gastropod *S. striatus*, were also determined (Figure 6). These laxaphycins did not show effects on cell survival (Figure 6a,f). Compound **5** increased cell metabolic activity, depolarized the mitochondria and reduced ROS levels at the highest concentrations (Figure 6b–d). With respect to ATP, its levels were reduced by **5** after a 6 h incubation, and recovered at 24 h (Figure 6 e). Laxaphycin **6** only affected to ROS and ATP levels (Figure 6i–j), it decreased ROS release and reduced ATP content at 6 h, recovering it after 24 h, as happened with the other acyclic laxaphycins.

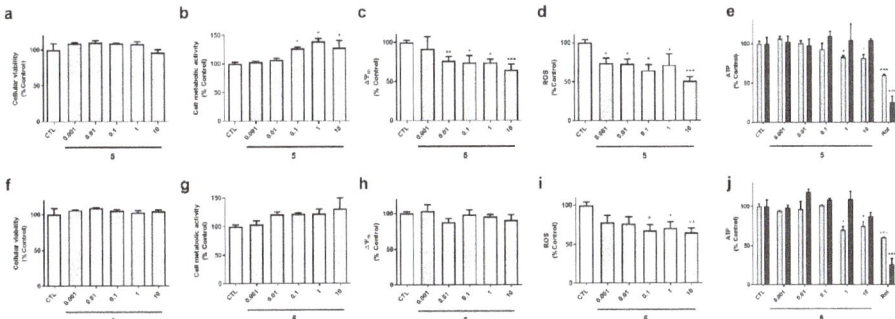

Figure 6. Effect of acyclic compounds obtained from *S. striatus* on cell viability and mitochondrial function in human neuroblastoma cells. SH-SY5Y cells were treated with compounds **5** (a–e) and **6** (f–j) for 24 h and their effects on cell viability, metabolic activity, $\Delta\Psi_m$, ROS and ATP levels were assessed with LDH assay, MTT test, TMRM dye, carboxy-H_2DCFDA and a commercial kit, respectively. ATP assay was performed at 6 h (light bars) and 24 h (dark bars). Concentration expressed in µM. Mean ± SEM of three experiments performed by triplicate. Values are presented as percentage of control cells. * $p < 0.05$, ** $p < 0.01$, *** $p < 0.01$

2.4. Cyclic Laxaphycin-B Peptides Induce Apoptosis in SH-SY5Y Cells

In view of the cytotoxicity displayed by cyclic laxaphycins **1** and **2** in LDH and MTT assays, the type of cell death produced by compounds was determined. SH-SY5Y cells were treated with compounds for 24 h. Laxaphycins **1** and **2** were used at IC_{50} values obtained from MTT assay (0.3 and 0.15 µM, respectively). Otherwise, acyclic laxaphycins **3**, **4**, **5** and **6** were tested at 10 µM. Cells were co-stained with Annexin V-Fluorescein (FITC) and propidium iodide (PI) and the fluorescence was analyzed by flow cytometry (Figure 7a). The percentages of apoptotic cells, including early apoptotic cells (Annexin V positive and PI negative) and late apoptotic cells (Annexin V positive and PI positive), and necrotic cells (Annexin V negative and PI positive) were calculated. Cells treated with compounds **1** and **2** produced a significant decrease in cell survival (around 60% of control cells). The values of Annexin-V-positive cells in these treatments confirmed that cyclic B-type laxaphycins triggered an apoptotic process. The addition of **1** and **2** produced a 50.4% ± 4.8% ($p < 0.001$) and 46.4% ± 4.8% ($p < 0.001$) of apoptotic cells, respectively. As expected, treatment with staurosporine (STS) also generated apoptosis in neuroblastoma cells (63.3% ± 3.2%, $p < 0.001$). On the other hand, acyclic laxaphycins did not show any significant effect on cell viability, agreeing with our previous results.

To confirm the results obtained with flow cytometry, the activity of caspase 3 was analyzed. This enzyme is an executioner caspase, involved both in intrinsic and extrinsic apoptosis, which targets several apoptotic substrates and initiates a cascade of events that results in cell death [28]. SH-SY5Y cells were treated with laxaphycins for 24 h at the same concentrations used in flow cytometry assays and caspase 3 activity was evaluated in cell lysates. As Figure 7b shows, compounds **1** (0.3 µM) and **2** (0.15 µM) produced a significant increase in the activity of the executioner caspase (about 20% of control cells). Once again, acyclic laxaphycins did not affect to caspase 3 activity, which is in agreement with the results of flow cytometry. STS addition also augmented the enzymatic activity of the caspase (157.8% ± 6%, $p < 0.001$).

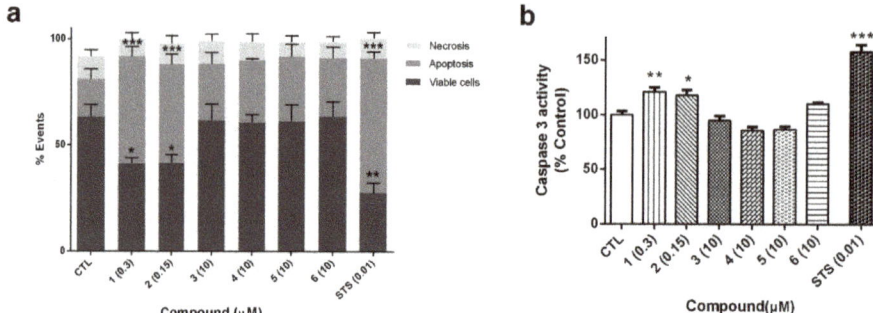

Figure 7. Cyclic laxaphycin B peptides induce apoptotic cell death in neuroblastoma cells. (**a**) Cells were treated for 24 h with compounds and stained with Annexin V-FITC and propidium iodide, and the fluorescence was analyzed by flow cytometry. Staurosporine (STS) was used as positive control. Apoptosis include early and late apoptotic cells. Data are expressed as percentage of total cells. (**b**) The activity of caspase 3 after treatment with laxaphycins during 24 h was assessed with a commercial kit. Results are expressed as percentage of control cells. Mean ± SEM of three independent experiments. * $p < 0.05$, ** $p < 0.01$, *** $p < 0.001$

2.5. Acyclic B-Type Laxaphycins Affect to Autophagy in Human Neuroblastoma Cells

Considering the results obtained with acyclic B-type laxaphycins in the mitochondrial function and our previous work with A-type laxaphycins [14], we decided to evaluate the effect of these compounds on the autophagic flux. With this purpose, SH-SY5Y cells were treated with laxaphycins B for 24 h, and the expression of proteins involved in autophagy was determined by Western blot. Bafilomycin A1 (Baf A1), an inhibitor of the fusion of autophagosomes and lysosomes, rapamycin (Rap), a mTOR inhibitor, and compound C (Comp C), an AMPK inhibitor, were used as positive controls in these assays [29]. Firstly, the effect of compounds on AMPK activation was determined, since this kinase is known to activate autophagy under circumstances of energy depletion [30]. Acyclic peptides produced a significant increase in the activation of AMPK, with compound **6** being the most active (Figure 8a). As expected, Comp C at 1 µM inhibited kinase activity. Then, we analyzed the expression of mTOR, considered the master regulator of the autophagic process. Cyclic laxaphycins **1** and **2** did not affect to the protein expression, whereas the acyclic peptides produced a significant reduction in its activation (Figure 8b). Treatment with 0.1 µM Rap also reduced mTOR activation.

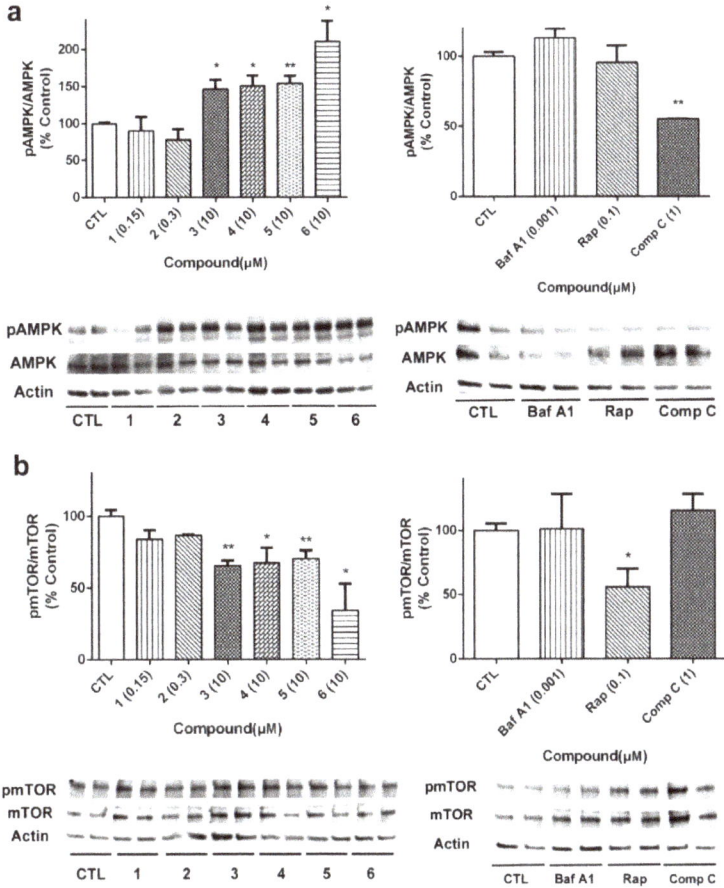

Figure 8. Analysis of autophagy initiation-related proteins in SH-SY5Y cells treated with B-type laxaphycins. Compounds were added for 24 h and the protein expression of (**a**) AMPK and (**b**) mTOR was determined by Western blot. Left panels show the results of compounds and right panels present the results of the positive controls bafilomycin A1 (Baf A1), rapamycin (Rap) and compound C (Comp C). The activation of AMPK and mTOR was analyzed as the ratio between phosphorylated/total protein levels. Protein expression levels are normalized by β-actin. Values are mean ± SEM of three replicates performed in duplicate, expressed as percentage of control cells. * $p < 0.05$, ** $p < 0.01$

The activation of p70 S6 kinase, an mTOR downstream target, was also determined (Figure 9a). The cyclic peptide **2** and the acyclic laxaphycins **4** and **6** diminished p70 S6 phosphorylation, reaching percentages among 53.5%–78.6% of untreated cells. Next, we analyzed the expression of beclin 1, a component of the complex that starts autophagosome formation [31]. As can be seen in Figure 9b, acyclic compounds **3**, **4**, **5** and **6** generated an increase in beclin1 expression. Treatment with the autophagy activator Rap also augmented its expression.

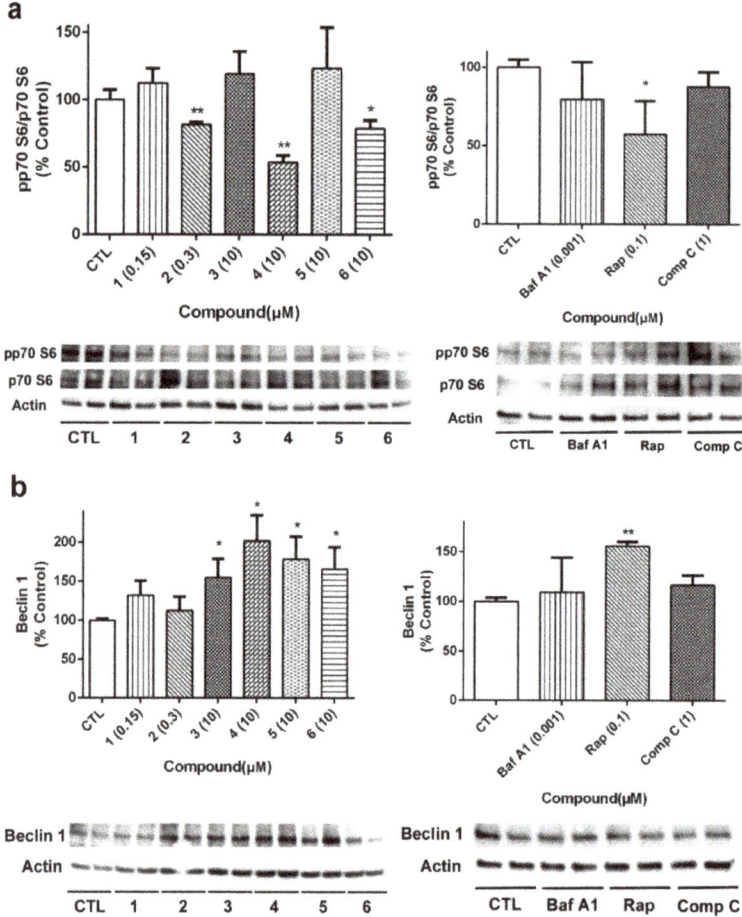

Figure 9. Analysis of p70 S6 kinase and Beclin 1 expression in neuroblastoma cells after treatment with B-type laxaphycins. The protein expression of (**a**) p70 S6 and (**b**) beclin 1 was determined by Western blot. Left panels show the results of compounds and right panels present the results of the positive controls bafilomycin A1 (Baf A1), rapamycin (Rap) and compound C (Comp C). The activation of the kinase was analyzed as the ratio between phosphorylated/total protein levels. Protein expression levels are normalized by β-actin. Values are mean ± SEM of three replicates performed in duplicate, expressed as percentage of control cells. * $p < 0.05$, ** $p < 0.01$

Beclin 1 is implicated in other cellular mechanisms, such as apoptosis, so its quantification must be complemented with other proteins involved in autophagy [29]. In our case, the expression of LC3 and p62 was analyzed to further confirm the effects of laxaphycins over autophagy (Figure 10). As Figure 10a shows, LC3II/I ratio was increased when acyclic laxaphycins were added to neuroblastoma cells, confirming our previous results. Treatment with Baf A1 and Rap also increased LC3II/I ratio. With regard to p62, whose degradation is related to autophagy, treatment with acyclic laxaphycins produced a significant decrease in its expression, with levels between 37.7–48.6% of untreated cells, a greater degradation than that produced by Rap (Figure 10b). In summary, these results suggest that acyclic laxaphycins B affect to the autophagic flux in human neuroblastoma cells, which is probably mediated by their effects on mitochondria.

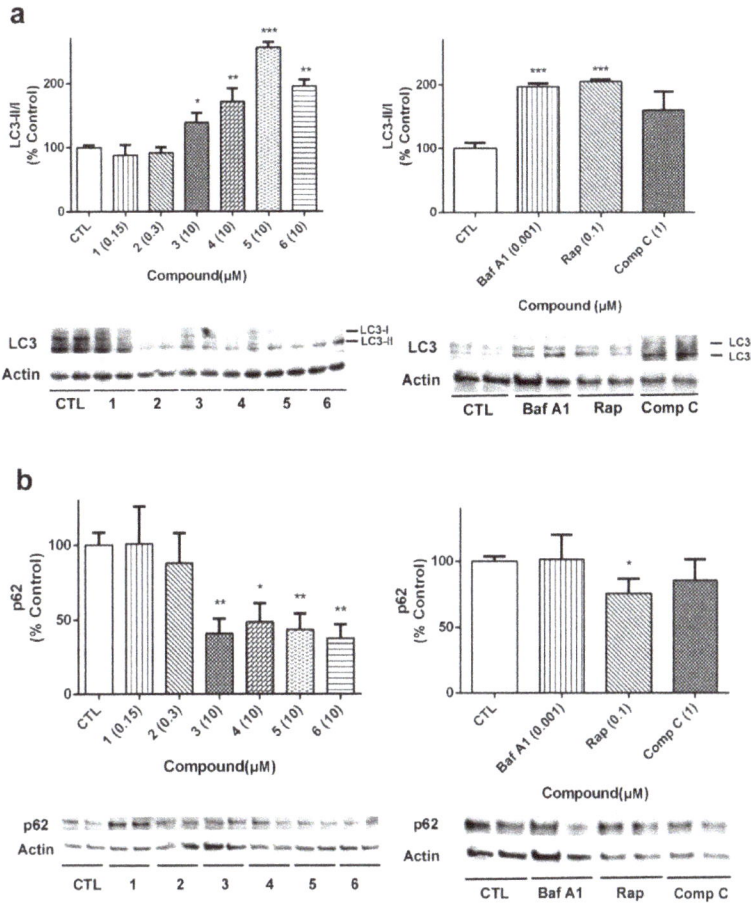

Figure 10. Determination of the effect of laxaphycins B on LC3 and p62 expression. SH-SY5Y cells were treated with compounds for 24 h and protein expression was analysed by Western blot. (**a**) LC3 expression, calculated as the ratio between LC3II (the lipidated form) and LC3I (the soluble form). (**b**) p62 expression. Left panels show the results of compounds and right panels present the results of the positive controls bafilomycin A1 (Baf A1), rapamycin (Rap) and compound C (Comp C). Protein expression levels are normalized by β-actin. Values are mean ± SEM of three replicates performed in duplicate, expressed as percentage of control cells. * $p < 0.05$, ** $p < 0.01$, *** $p < 0.001$

3. Discussion

Laxaphycins are a large family of lipopeptides synthetized through a hybrid PKS/NRPS pathway by different cyanobacteria species. These peptides, selected by evolution in both freshwater and oceanic cyanobacteria, may confer to these primary producers an ecological advantage.

Laxaphycins are divided into two sub-families, laxaphycin A-type and laxaphycin B-type peptides. Laxaphycin B-type members such as laxaphycins B, B2, and B3 have presented antifungal, antimicrobial and cytotoxic activities [9–12], while laxaphycin A-type compounds have shown only weak cytotoxicity [10,12,14].

Here we describe the complete structural elucidation of four acyclic B-type laxaphycins, two of them (**3** and **4** with ring opening) corresponding to the acyclic analogues of laxaphycins B and B3, isolated from the cyanobacteria *A. torulosa*, and the other two (**5** and **6** with ring opening and deletion of two amino-acids) are diet-derived compounds isolated from the herbivorous gastropod *S. striatus* that feeds on the cyanobacteria. It is not unlikely that these acyclolaxaphycins B ensued from an adaptive biotransformation mechanism from a specific herbivorous species [32]. Cyclic lipopeptides are relatively widespread in cyanobacteria, but such biotransformation, ring opening and amino-acids deletion, had never been described.

Moreover, this study is the first description of the effects on mitochondria and autophagy produced by acyclic B-type laxaphycins, and also confirms that the toxic effects of cyclic laxaphycins B are mediated by an apoptotic process. The cytotoxicity of cyclic laxaphycins had been tested in previous works in which laxaphycin B showed cytotoxic effects against a panel of cancer cell lines ($IC_{50} < 2$ µM), and both compounds (laxaphycins B and B3) had displayed toxicity towards drug-sensitive and multidrug-resistant tumor cell lines ($IC_{50} \approx 1$ µM) [9]. Our results in neuroblastoma cells are in agreement with these previous assays, with IC_{50} values of 1.8 and 0.8 µM for laxaphycins B and B3, respectively. A previous work had hypothesized that laxaphycin B toxicity could be mediated by the inhibition of topoisomerase II [10]. The inhibition of this enzyme causes DNA disorders that enhance apoptotic cell death [33]. In the current work, we provide new data that support the triggering of an apoptotic process by laxaphycins B and B3, as indicated by Annexin V staining and caspase 3 activation. The results obtained in p70 S6 kinase, whose inhibition is involved both in autophagy and apoptosis activation [34,35], suggest a different mechanism of action of these cyclic peptides, since only laxaphycin B3 reduced the phosphorylation of this enzyme. On the other hand, the biological activities of acyclic B-type laxaphycins had not been tested so far. Our results suggest that these compounds affect the mitochondrial function, producing a decrease in ATP levels, which may lead to the activation of AMPK. Moreover, acyclic laxaphycins have an impact on the autophagic flux, as evidenced by their effect on the expression of proteins related to this cellular event. Further experiments will help us to clarify if the effect on autophagy is being produced by the activation of AMPK.

AMPK is activated when ATP levels decrease, and maintains energy homeostasis through the inhibition of energy-consuming processes, such as protein and lipid biosynthesis, and the activation of ATP-producing pathways, such as glucose metabolism and mitochondrial biogenesis. Moreover, when an energy depletion occurs, AMPK triggers the autophagic flux, since this catabolic process provides energy and substrates for the synthesis of new biomolecules [22]. Thus, increasing AMPK activity will be a good strategy to increase cellular energy and avoid energetic failure in vulnerable cells. There are several examples of indirect AMPK activators that act through the decrease of ATP levels. Natural compounds such as quercetin, resveratrol, genistein and curcumin activate the kinase by targeting components of the oxidative phosphorylation and increasing the AMP/ATP ratio [36]. However, the most studied AMPK activator is the biguanide metformin, in clinical use for the treatment of Type 2 diabetes mellitus. Metformin inhibits the complex I of mitochondrial respiratory chain, reducing the proton gradient, the production of ROS and ATP levels. This leads to the activation of AMPK and the subsequent increase in glucose uptake [37]. Along with their use as antidiabetic agents, the therapeutic application of AMPK activators has been expanded to the treatment of cancer, inflammation and neurodegeneration [38].

The phosphorylation of mTOR, considered the main regulator of autophagy, was also inhibited by treatment with acyclic laxaphycins B. mTOR plays a central role in integrating growth signals and controlling their physiological effects at a cellular level. Its activation upregulates anabolic processes such as synthesis of proteins, lipids and nucleotides, and downregulates catabolic mechanisms such as autophagy. However, mTOR hyperactivation is linked to several diseases such as cancer, since the kinase promotes tumor growth and proliferation, as well as diabetes, in which it contributes to insulin resistance [39]. Currently, mTOR inhibitors are in clinical use as immunosuppressants and anti-cancer drugs, and due to crucial role of the kinase in many illnesses, it is expected that mTOR inhibitors may have a broader application for other diseases [40,41].

Along with these illnesses, there is substantial evidence of autophagy dysregulation in neurodegenerative diseases, such as alterations in mTOR and beclin 1 expression, and accumulation of defective autophagosomes [42]. In this context, the activation of the autophagic flux has emerged as a therapeutic approach for these pathologies, because it represents a major pathway for clearance of aggregated proteins and damaged organelles. Several compounds such as metformin or Rap have shown promising effects in vivo [42], and the activation of mitophagy has been recently related to a reduction in cognitive deficits in Alzheimer's disease models [43]. Therefore, the stimulation of autophagy maybe a good strategy to face neurodegeneration. However, the use of activators must be handled carefully, as an excessive autophagy can lead to the destruction of essential cellular machinery [44]. In addition, intervention in early phases of the diseases would be more favorable than in an advanced state [21]. The results obtained with acyclic B-type laxaphycins in the human neuroblastoma cell line SH-SY5Y, which maintains certain characteristics of neuronal cells [23], could be used as a starting point to analyse their neuroprotective effects. In this sense it would be interesting to study the ability of laxaphycins to cross the blood brain barrier (BBB). There are several examples of non-ribosomal peptides capable of penetrating the BBB, such as polymyxins [45] and some cyanotoxins [46], which can reach the brain through specific peptide transporters. Moreover, the lipidic nature of laxaphycins could allow the compounds to cross the BBB, as lipid solubility is a crucial factor that facilitates transport across the barrier [47].

On the other hand, the data obtained in this work show a clear correlation among the chemical structure and the biological activities of laxaphycins B. Cyclic laxaphycins produce apoptotic cell death and exhibit a greater cytotoxicity than their acyclic analogues. Also, the results obtained in p70 S6 kinase with the cyclic laxaphycin B3 and their acyclic analogs suggest that the presence of an OH group in R is a key structural feature to the inhibition of this enzyme. Due to the supply problem associated with marine compounds, the chemical synthesis of B-type laxaphycins would be a good strategy for their pharmacological use. Laxaphycin B total synthesis has been previously published [48], as well as the synthesis of two simplified analogues of the parent compound [7], which opens a door for future synthesis of acyclic laxaphycins, which will help to better understand the structure-activity relationship of B-type laxaphycins.

In summary, this work provides new data that confirm the pro-apoptotic effects produced by cyclic laxaphycins B, and describes for first time the complete structural elucidation of four B-type acyclic laxaphycins and their biological activities. The acyclic peptides affect mitochondrial function and have an effect on the expression of key proteins involved in autophagic flux, suggesting an involvement of the compounds in the activation of this mechanism. Further experiments will help to clarify the mechanism of action of the B-type laxaphycins and the structural requirements for these activities.

4. Materials and Methods

4.1. Chemicals and Solutions

EnzCheck® Caspase-3 Assay Kit, TMRM, 5-(and-6)-carboxy-2′,7′-dichlorodihydrofluorescein diacetate (carboxy-H_2DCFDA), Pierce™ Protease Inhibitor Mini Tablets and Pierce™ Phosphatase Inhibitor Mini Tablets were purchased from Thermo Fisher Scientific (Waltham, MA, USA). Annexin V-FITC Apoptosis Detection Kit was obtained from Immunostep (Salamanca, Spain). Rap, Comp C and Baf A1 were obtained from Abcam (Cambridge, UK). Other chemicals were reagent grade and were purchased from Sigma-Aldrich (Madrid, Spain).

4.2. Organism Collection

The cyanobacterium *Anabaena torulosa*, as well as the herbivorous gastropod *Stylocheilus striatus*, were collected by SCUBA diving at a depth of 1–5 m in Moorea Atoll, French Polynesia (S 17°29′22″, W 149°54′17″) in Pacific Ocean. The cyanobacterium and the gastropod samples were sealed independently underwater in a bag with seawater and then frozen and freeze-dried.

4.3. HPLC and LC-MS Analyses

HPLC-PDA-ELSD analyses were performed with a Waters Alliance HPLC system (W 2695) coupled to a photodiodes array detector (PDA Waters 2998) and an evaporative light scattering detector (Waters ELSD 2424). The analyses were performed on a reversed-phase column (Thermo Hypersil Gold C-18, 150 × 2.1 mm, 3 µm) employing a gradient of 10% to 100% CH_3CN over 40 min followed by 25 min at 100% CH_3CN (all solvents buffered with 0.1% formic acid) with a flow rate of 0.3 mL/min. Semi-preparative HPLC purifications were performed on a binary HPLC pump system Waters 1525 with a dual λ absorbance detector Waters 2487, equipped with a reverse phase column (Interchim UP5ODB.25M, 250 × 10 mm, 5 µm) using isocratic elution (H_2O-CH_3CN) at a flow rate of 3 mL/min.

4.4. Compound Isolation and Purification

Six hundred grams of freeze-dried *A*. cf *torulosa* and 4.24 g of *S. striatus* (6 specimens) were extracted, separately but in the same manner, with a mixture of CH_3OH-CH_2Cl_2 (1:1) and sonicated during 10 minutes to yield two organic extracts after evaporation under reduced pressure. Then the two crude extracts (38 g and 4 g, respectively) were subjected to flash RP18 silica gel column eluted with H_2O (A), H_2O-CH_3CN (20:80) (B) and CH_3OH-CH_2Cl_2 (80:20) (C) to afford 3 fractions (A, B and C). Fractions B, from *A. torulosa* and *S. Striatus*, were fractioned, in turn, with flash chromatography and RP18 silica gel column with a gradient of H_2O-CH_3CN to give 7 sub-fractions. Fraction B4 from the organic extract of *S. striatus* subjected to HPLC purification (Phenomenex Gemini C6-phenyl, 110Å, 250 × 10 mm, 5 µm) and eluted with 28% CH_3CN in H2O with 0.1% formic acid at a flow rate of 4 mL/min, gave compounds **5** (2.5 mg) and **6** (5 mg). Laxaphycin A was found in sub-fraction B5, but none of the already described laxaphycins B or B3 could be detected. Fraction B4 from the organic extract of *A. torulosa* was eluted with 38% CH_3CN and gave compounds **3** (3 mg) and **4** (4 mg). Laxaphycins A, B (**1**) and B3 (**2**) were found respectively in sub-fraction B6 and B5.

4.5. Mass Spectrometry and NMR Spectroscopy

LC-MS analyses were carried out using a Thermo Fisher Scientific LC-MS device, Accela HPLC coupled to an LCQ Fleet equipped with an electrospray ionization source and a 3D ion-trap analyzer. High-resolution ESI mass spectra were obtained on a Bruker Thermo Scientific Q-Tof Maxis mass spectrometer using electrospray ionization in positive mode. Compounds were solubilized in MeOH at 1 µg/mL and infused in mass spectrometer (collision energy: 50 eV).

1D-NMR and 2D-NMR experiments were acquired on a Brucker Avance 800 spectrometer equipped with a cryogenic probe (5 mm), all compounds solubilized in DMSO-*d6* (500 µL) at 303 K. All chemical shifts were calibrated on the residual solvent peak (DMSO-*d6*, 2.50 ppm (^1H) and 39.5 ppm (^{13}C). The chemical shifts (δ), reported in parts per million (ppm) are referenced relatively to TMS.

4.6. Advanced Marfey's Analyses

The Marfey's analyses were carried out on compounds **3, 4, 5** and **6**. Approximately 0.3 mg of each compound were hydrolyzed with 1 mL of 6 N HCl for 20 h at 110 °C in sealed glass vials. The cooled hydrolysate mixtures were evaporated to dryness and traces of HCl were removed from the reaction mixtures by repeated evaporation. Each hydrolysate mixture was dissolved in H_2O (100 µL). 110 µL of acetone, 20 µL of 1 N $NaHCO_3$ and 20 µL of 1% L or D/L FDLA (1-fluoro-2,4-dinitrophenyl-5-L-leucinamide) in acetone were added to each 50 µL aliquot. The mixtures were then heated to 40 °C for 1 h. The cooled solutions were neutralized with 1 N HCl (20 µL), and then dried in vacuo. The residues were dissolved in 1:1 CH_3CN-H_2O and then analyzed by LC-MS. LC-MS analyses were performed on a reversed-phase column (Thermo Hypersil Gold C-18, 150 × 2.1 mm, 3 µm) with two linear gradients: (1) from 20% CH_3CN-80% 0.01 M formic acid to 60% CH_3CN-40% 0.01 M formic acid at 0.3 mL/min over 70 min and (2) from 10% CH_3CN-90% 0.01 M formic acid to 50% CH_3CN-50% 0.01 M formic acid at 0.3 mL/min over 70 min, then to 80% CH_3CN-20% over 10 min.

The configuration of the α carbon for each residue can be assigned in accordance with the elution order of the D- and L-FDLA derivatives [24,25]: amino acids for which the D-FDLA analogue elutes first have a D configuration, whereas those for which the L-FDLA analogue elutes first have an L configuration. Furthermore, the hydrolysates were compared to that of laxaphycin B.

4.7. Cell Culture

SH-SY5Y human neuroblastoma cell line was obtained from American Type Culture Collection (ATCC), number CRL2266. Cells were cultured in Dulbecco´s modified Eagle´s medium: Nutrient Mix F-12 (DMEM/F-12) with 10% fetal bovine serum (FBS), 1% glutamax, 100 U/mL penicillin and 100 µg/mL streptomycin. Cells were maintained at 37 °C in a humidified atmosphere of 5% CO_2 and 95% air and dissociated weekly using 0.05% trypsin/EDTA. All the reagents were obtained from Thermo Fischer Scientific.

4.8. Cytotoxicity Assay

Cell viability was assessed with the LDH test [14]. Cells were seeded in 96-well plates and exposed to different compound concentrations (0.001–10 µM). Cells were incubated with compounds at 37 °C in humidified 5% CO_2/95% air atmosphere for 24 h. Quillaja bark saponin was used as cellular death control. Then, cell medium was collected and LDH release was evaluated. Pierce™ LDH-Cytotoxicity Assay Kit (Thermo Fisher Scientific) was used for LDH determination. Absorbance was measured at 490 nm to determine LDH release to the medium. Experiments were carried out in triplicate at least three independent times.

4.9. Metabolic Activity Evaluation

The effect of laxaphycins on cell metabolic activity was evaluated by MTT (3-(4, 5-dimethyl thiazol-2-yl)-2, 5-diphenyl tetrazolium bromide) assay [27,49]. SH-SY5Y cells were cultured in 96-well plates and treated with compounds at concentrations ranging from 0.001 to 10 µM for 24 h. Next, cells were rinsed three times and incubated for 1 h with MTT (500 µg/mL) dissolved in saline buffer. MTT excess was washed and cells were disaggregated with 5% sodium dodecyl sulfate. Absorbance of the colored formazan salt was measured at 595 nm in a spectrophotometer plate reader. Cell death control signal was subtracted from the other data.

4.10. Mitochondrial Membrane Potential Measurement

$\Delta\Psi_m$ was evaluated with TMRM assay as previously described [49]. SH-SY5Y cells were seeded in 96-well plates at 5×10^4 cells per well. After 24 h, cells were treated with compounds (0.001–10 µM) for 24 h. Next, cells were washed twice with saline solution and incubated with 1 µM TMRM for 30 min. Then human neuroblastoma cells were solubilized with 50% DMSO–50% water. Fluorescence values were measured at 535 nm excitation, 590 nm emission with a plate reader. At least three independent replicates were performed in triplicate.

4.11. Evaluation of Reactive Oxygen Species and ATP Levels

ROS production was assessed with the fluorescence dye carboxy-H_2DCFDA (5-(and-6)-carboxy-2′,7′-dichlorodihydrofluorescein diacetate) [49]. SH-SY5Y cells were seeded in 96-well plates and allowed to grow for 24 h. Then, cells were treated with laxaphycins (0.001–10 µM) for 24 h and ROS levels were measured. SH-SY5Y cells were washed twice with serum-free medium and loaded with 20 µM carboxy-H_2DCFDA. Next, the plate was incubated for 1 h at 37 °C. After this time, phosphate buffered saline (PBS) was added to each well during 30 min. The fluorescence was read at 495 nm excitation and 527 nm emission. Experiments were carried out at least three times.

ATP levels were determined with the Luminescent ATP Detection Kit (Abcam), following manufacturer´s instructions. Briefly, human neuroblastoma cells were cultured in 96-well plates at

5×10^4 cells per well. Cells were treated with compounds as described above during 6 and 24 h, Then, cells were lysed and 50 µL of substrate solution were added to each well. The plate was incubated for 5 min, and the luminescence was measured in a plate reader. Rot at 1 µM was used as positive control.

4.12. Flow Cytometry Analysis

The Annexin V-FITC Apoptosis Detection Kit was used to determine the cell death produced by compounds as previously described [50]. SH-SY5Y cells were seeded in 12-well plates at 1×10^6 per well and incubated for 24 h with laxaphycins. Then, cells were washed with PBS and resuspended in Annexin binding buffer containing Annexin V-FITC and PI. Cells were incubated for 15 min at room temperature, resuspended in PBS and filtered. The fluorescence was determined by flow cytometry using the ImageStreamMKII (Amnis Corporation, Luminex Corp, Austin, TX, USA). 10,000 events were analyzed with IDEAS Application 6.0 software (Amnis Corporation, Luminex Corp, Austin, TX, USA). STS (Sigma Aldrich) at 0.01 µM was used as control in this assay.

4.13. Evaluation of Caspase 3 Activity

The detection of caspase 3 activity was carried out with the EnzCheck® Caspase-3 Assay Kit. Neuroblastoma cells were cultured in 12-well plates at 1×10^6 cells per well and treated with compounds. After 24 h, cells were lysed and an aliquot was collected to quantify protein concentration by the Bradford method. Then, the assay was performed following manufacturer's instructions. Briefly, 50 µL of each sample were mixed with equal volume of Z-DEVD-AMC substrate and incubated for 30 min at room temperature. Then, fluorescence at 342 nm excitation and 441 nm emission was measured. Caspase 3 activity data were corrected by protein concentration values. STS (0.01 µM) was used as positive control.

4.14. Western Blotting

SH-SY5Y cells were seeded in 12-well plates and treated with laxaphycins for 24 h. Next, cells were washed with PBS and lysis buffer (50mM Tris HCl, 150 mM NaCl, 1mM EDTA and 1% Triton x-100, supplemented with a complete phosphatase/protease inhibitor cocktail) was added to each well. Cells were scrapped, sonicated and centrifuged at 13,000 rpm at 4 °C for 20 min.

For p62 quantification, cells were lysed as previously described, with modifications [14]. A hypotonic buffer (20 mM Tris-HCl, pH 7.4, 10 mM NaCl, 3 mM $MgCl_2$, containing a complete phosphatase/protease inhibitor cocktail) was added to each well. Then, cells were incubated for 15 min on ice, sonicated and centrifuged at 3000 rpm at 4 °C for 15 min.

In both cases, the supernatant was collected as the cytosolic fraction and quantified with the Bradford method. Samples containing 15 µg were used for electrophoresis, resolved in 4–20% sodium dodecyl sulphate polyacrylamide gel (Biorad, Madrid, Spain). Proteins were transferred to PVDF membranes (Merck Millipore) with a Trans-Blot® semi-dry transfer cell (Biorad). Membrane blocking and antibody incubation was performed in Snap i.d. system (Merck Millipore). Protein bands were detected with Supersignal West Pico Luminiscent Substrate and Supersignal West Femto Maximum Sensitivity Substrate (Thermo Fisher Scientific). Chemiluminiscence was determined with Diversity GeneSnap system and software (Syngene) [51]. LC3 II/I was detected with the primary antibody anti-LC3 II/I (1:1000, Abcam), the primary antibody anti-pmTOR (Ser2448) (1:1000, Merck Millipore) was used to recognize phospho-mTOR and the total levels of the kinase were determined with anti-mTOR antibody (1:10000, Abcam), beclin-1 was detected with anti-beclin-1 primary antibody (1:1000, Merck Millipore), p62 was quantified with anti-p62 antibody (1:1000, Merck Millipore), anti-phospho-p70 S6 kinase (Thr389) (1:1000, Merck Millipore) was used to detect phospho- p70 and the total levels were quantified using anti-p70 S6 kinase antibody (1:1000, Merck Millipore), anti-phospho-AMPK (Thr172) (1:500, Merck Millipore) was used to recognize the phosphorylated state of the kinase, and the total expression of the enzyme was detected with anti-AMPK antibody (1:500, Merck Millipore). Protein levels were normalized using β-Actin (1:20,000, Millipore). Baf A1

(0.001 µM) [29], Rap (0.1 µM) [52] and Comp C (1 µM) [53] were used as controls for autophagic flux measurements. All the experiments were performed at least three times in duplicate.

4.15. Statistical Analysis

Data are presented as mean ± SEM. Statistical differences were evaluated by one-way ANOVA or Student´s *t*-tests with Graph Pad Prism 6 software. Statistical significance was considered at $p < 0.05$.

Supplementary Materials: The following are available online at http://www.mdpi.com/1660-3397/18/7/364/s1, Figure S1: 1H-NMR spectrum of [des-(Ala4-Hle5)] acyclolaxaphycin B (5) in DMSO (303K), Figure S2: 13C-NMR spectrum of [des-(Ala4-Hle5)] acyclolaxaphycin B (5) in DMSO (303K), Figure S3: DEPT135-NMR spectrum of [des-(Ala4-Hle5)] acyclolaxaphycin B (5) in DMSO (303K), Figure S4: TOCSY spectrum of [des-(Ala4-Hle5)] acyclolaxaphycin B (5) in DMSO (303K), Figure S5: ROESY spectrum of [des-(Ala4-Hle5)] acyclolaxaphycin B (5) in DMSO (303K), Figure S6: HSQC spectrum of [des-(Ala4-Hle5)] acyclolaxaphycin B (5) in DMSO (303K), Figure S7: HSQC-TOCSY spectrum of [des-(Ala4-Hle5)] acyclolaxaphycin B (5) in DMSO (303K), Figure S8: HMBC spectrum of [des-(Ala4-Hle5)] acyclolaxaphycin B (5) in DMSO (303K), Figure S9: 1H-NMR spectrum of [des-(Ala4-Hle5)] acyclolaxaphycin B3 (6) in DMSO (303K), FigureS10: 13C-NMR spectrum of [des-(Ala4-Hle5)] acyclolaxaphycin B3 (6) in DMSO (303K), Figure S11: DEPT135-NMR spectrum of [des-(Ala4-Hle5)] acyclolaxaphycin B3 (6) in DMSO (303K), Figure S12: TOCSY spectrum of [des-(Ala4-Hle5)] acyclolaxaphycin B3 (6) in DMSO (303K), Figure S13: ROESYspectrum of [des-(Ala4-Hle5)] acyclolaxaphycin B3 (6) in DMSO (303K), Figure S14: HSQCspectrum of [des-(Ala4-Hle5)] acyclolaxaphycin B3 (6) in DMSO (303K), FigureS15: HSQC-TOCSYspectrum of [des-(Ala4-Hle5)] acyclolaxaphycin B3 (6) in DMSO (303K), Figure S16: HMBCspectrum of [des-(Ala4-Hle5)] acyclolaxaphycin B3 (6) in DMSO (303K).

Author Contributions: Funding acquisition, L.M.B.; investigation, R.A., E.A., L.B., I.B., N.I. and B.B.; supervision, E.A. and L.M.B.; writing—original draft, R.A.; writing—review and editing, E.A., B.B and L.M.B. All authors have read and agreed to the published version of the manuscript.

Funding: Financial support was provided to LB, IB, NI and BB by the Laboratoire d'Excellence (LabEx) "CORAIL" (Keymicals and Cyanodiv) and the GDR CNRS 3658 MediatEC (https://www.gdr-mediatec.cnrs.fr/english-version/). Chromatographic, spectroscopic, and structural analyses were performed using the facilities of the Biodiversité et Biotechnologies Marines platform at the University of Perpignan (Bio2Mar, http://bio2mar.obs-banyuls.fr/fr/index.html).

Acknowledgments: The research leading to these results has received funding from the following FEDER cofunded-grants. From Consellería de Cultura, Educación e Ordenación Universitaria, Xunta de Galicia, 2017 GRC GI-1682 (ED431C 2017/01). From CDTI and Technological Funds, supported by Ministerio de Economía, Industria y Competitividad, AGL2016-78728-R (AEI/FEDER, UE), ISCIII/PI16/01830 and RTC-2016-5507-2, ITC-20161072. From European Union POCTEP 0161-Nanoeaters -1-E-1, Interreg AlertoxNet EAPA-317-2016, Interreg Agritox EAPA-998-2018, and H2020 778069-EMERTOX. We thank Olivier Thomas and Stephane Greff for HRMS facilities and Christian Roumestand for NMR measurements.

Conflicts of Interest: The authors declare no conflict of interest.

References

1. Liu, L.; Rein, K.S. New peptides isolated from Lyngbya species: A review. *Mar. Drugs* **2010**, *8*, 1817–1837. [CrossRef] [PubMed]
2. Rastogi, P.; Sinha, R.P. Biotechnological and industrial significance of cyanobacterial secondary metabolites. *Biotechnol. Adv.* **2009**, *27*, 521–539. [CrossRef] [PubMed]
3. Vinothkumar, S.; Parameswaran, P.S. Recent advances in marine drug research. *Biotechnol. Adv.* **2013**, *31*, 1826–1845. [CrossRef] [PubMed]
4. Jones, A.C.; Monroe, E.A.; Eisman, E.B.; Gerwick, L.; Sherman, D.H.; Gerwick, W.H. The unique mechanistic transformations involved in the biosynthesis of modular natural products from marine cyanobacteria. *Nat. Prod. Rep.* **2010**, *27*, 1048–1065. [CrossRef] [PubMed]
5. Condurso, H.L.; Bruner, S.D. Structure and noncanonical chemistry of nonribosomal peptide biosynthetic machinery. *Nat. Prod. Rep.* **2012**, *29*, 1099–1110. [CrossRef]
6. Agrawal, S.; Acharya, D.; Adholeya, A.; Barrow, C.J.; Deshmukh, S.K. Nonribosomal Peptides from Marine Microbes and Their Antimicrobial and Anticancer Potential. *Front. Pharmacol.* **2017**, *8*, 828. [CrossRef]
7. Bornancin, L.; Boyaud, F.; Mahiout, Z.; Bonnard, I.; Mills, S.C.; Banaigs, B.; Inguimbert, N. Isolation and Synthesis of Laxaphycin B-Type Peptides: A Case Study and Clues to Their Biosynthesis. *Mar. Drugs* **2015**, *13*, 7285–7300. [CrossRef]

8. Banaigs, B.; Bonnard, I.; Witczak, A.; Inguimbert, N. Marine Peptide Secondary Metabolites. In *Outstanding Marine Molecules*; La Barre, S., Kornprobst, J., Eds.; Wiley-VCH Verlag GmbH & Co: Baden-Württemberg, Germany, 2014; pp. 285–318.
9. Bonnard, I.; Rolland, M.; Salmon, J.M.; Debiton, E.; Barthomeuf, C.; Banaigs, B. Total structure and inhibition of tumor cell proliferation of laxaphycins. *J. Med. Chem.* **2007**, *50*, 1266–1279. [CrossRef]
10. Gbankoto, A.; Vigo, J.; Dramane, K.; Banaigs, B.; Aina, E.; Salmon, J.M. Cytotoxic effect of Laxaphycins A and B on human lymphoblastic cells (CCRF-CEM) using digitised videomicrofluorometry. *In Vivo* **2005**, *19*, 577–582.
11. Frankmolle, W.P.; Larsen, L.K.; Caplan, F.R.; Patterson, G.M.; Knubel, G.; Levine, I.A.; Moore, R.E. Antifungal cyclic peptides from the terrestrial blue-green alga Anabaena laxa. I. Isolation and biological properties. *J. Antibiot.* **1992**, *45*, 1451–1457. [CrossRef]
12. Frankmolle, W.P.; Knubel, G.; Moore, R.E.; Patterson, G.M. Antifungal cyclic peptides from the terrestrial blue-green alga Anabaena laxa. II. Structures of laxaphycins A, B, D and E. *J. Antibiot.* **1992**, *45*, 1458–1466. [CrossRef] [PubMed]
13. Cai, W.; Matthew, S.; Chen, Q.Y.; Paul, V.J.; Luesch, H. Discovery of new A- and B-type laxaphycins with synergistic anticancer activity. *Bioorg. Med. Chem.* **2018**, *26*, 2310–2319. [CrossRef] [PubMed]
14. Bornancin, L.; Alonso, E.; Alvarino, R.; Inguimbert, N.; Bonnard, I.; Botana, L.M.; Banaigs, B. Structure and biological evaluation of new cyclic and acyclic laxaphycin-A type peptides. *Bioorg. Med. Chem.* **2019**, *27*, 1966–1980. [CrossRef] [PubMed]
15. Zare-Shahabadi, A.; Masliah, E.; Johnson, G.V.; Rezaei, N. Autophagy in Alzheimer's disease. *Rev. Neurosci.* **2015**, *26*, 385–395. [CrossRef]
16. Saha, S.; Panigrahi, D.P.; Patil, S.; Bhutia, S.K. Autophagy in health and disease: A comprehensive review. *Biomed Pharm.* **2018**, *104*, 485–495. [CrossRef]
17. Russo, M.; Russo, G.L. Autophagy inducers in cancer. *Biochem. Pharm.* **2018**, *153*, 51–61. [CrossRef]
18. Thellung, S.; Corsaro, A.; Nizzari, M.; Barbieri, F.; Florio, T. Autophagy Activator Drugs: A New Opportunity in Neuroprotection from Misfolded Protein Toxicity. *Int. J. Mol. Sci.* **2019**, *20*, 901. [CrossRef]
19. Liu, H.; Dai, C.; Fan, Y.; Guo, B.; Ren, K.; Sun, T.; Wang, W. From autophagy to mitophagy: The roles of P62 in neurodegenerative diseases. *J. Bioenerg. Biomembr.* **2017**, *49*, 413–422. [CrossRef]
20. Dikic, I.; Elazar, Z. Mechanism and medical implications of mammalian autophagy. *Nat. Rev. Mol. Cell Biol.* **2018**, *19*, 349–364. [CrossRef]
21. Li, Q.; Liu, Y.; Sun, M. Autophagy and Alzheimer's Disease. *Cell Mol. Neurobiol.* **2017**, *37*, 377–388. [CrossRef]
22. Tamargo-Gomez, I.; Marino, G. AMPK: Regulation of Metabolic Dynamics in the Context of Autophagy. *Int. J. Mol. Sci.* **2018**, *19*, 3812. [CrossRef] [PubMed]
23. Krishna, A.; Biryukov, M.; Trefois, C.; Antony, P.M.; Hussong, R.; Lin, J.; Heinaniemi, M.; Glusman, G.; Koglsberger, S.; Boyd, O.; et al. Systems genomics evaluation of the SH-SY5Y neuroblastoma cell line as a model for Parkinson's disease. *BMC Genom.* **2014**, *15*, 1154. [CrossRef]
24. Fujii, K.; Ikai, Y.; Oka, H.; Suzuki, M.; Harada, K. A nonempirical method using LC/MS for determination of the absolute configuration of constituent amino acids in a peptide: Combination of Marfey's method with mass spectrometry and its practical application. *Anal. Chem.* **1997**, *69*, 5146–5151. [CrossRef]
25. Fujii, K.; Ikai, Y.; Mayumi, T.; Oka, H.; Suzuki, M.; Harada, K. A nonempirical method using LC/MS for determination of the absolute configuration of constituent amino acids in a peptide: Elucidation of limitations of Marfey's method and of its separation mechanism. *Anal. Chem.* **1997**, *69*, 3346–3352. [CrossRef]
26. Weyermann, J.; Lochmann, D.; Zimmer, A. A practical note on the use of cytotoxicity assays. *Int. J. Pharm.* **2005**, *288*, 369–376. [CrossRef]
27. Bernas, T.; Dobrucki, J. Mitochondrial and Nonmitochondrial Reduction of MTT: Interaction of MTT With TMRE, JC-1, and NAO Mitochondrial Fluorescent Probes. *Cytometry* **2002**, *47*. [CrossRef] [PubMed]
28. D'Arcy, M.S. Cell death: a review of the major forms of apoptosis, necrosis and autophagy. *Cell Biol. Int.* **2019**, *43*, 582–592. [CrossRef] [PubMed]
29. Klionsky, D.J.; Abdelmohsen, K.; Abe, A.; Abedin, M.J.; Abeliovich, H.; Acevedo Arozena, A.; Adachi, H.; Adams, C.M.; Adams, P.D.; Adeli, K.; et al. Guidelines for the use and interpretation of assays for monitoring autophagy (3rd edition). *Autophagy* **2016**, *12*, 1–222. [CrossRef]
30. Morgunova, G.V.; Klebanov, A.A. Age-related AMP-activated protein kinase alterations: From cellular energetics to longevity. *Cell Biochem. Funct.* **2019**, *37*, 169–176. [CrossRef]

31. Menon, M.B.; Dhamija, S. Beclin 1 Phosphorylation - at the Center of Autophagy Regulation. *Front. Cell Dev. Biol.* **2018**, *6*, 137. [CrossRef]
32. Bornancin, L.; Bonnard, I.; Mills, S.C.; Banaigs, B. Chemical mediation as a structuring element in marine gastropod predator-prey interactions. *Nat. Prod. Rep.* **2017**, *34*, 644–676. [CrossRef] [PubMed]
33. Lin, R.K.; Ho, C.W.; Liu, L.F.; Lyu, Y.L. Topoisomerase IIbeta deficiency enhances camptothecin-induced apoptosis. *J. Biol. Chem.* **2013**, *288*, 7182–7192. [CrossRef] [PubMed]
34. Fenton, T.R.; Gout, I.T. Functions and regulation of the 70kDa ribosomal S6 kinases. *Cell Biol.* **2011**, *43*, 47–59. [CrossRef] [PubMed]
35. Tavares, M.R.; Pavan, I.C.; Amaral, C.L.; L, M.; AD, L.; FM, S. The S6K Protein Family in Health and Disease. *Life Sci.* **2015**, *131*, 1–10. [CrossRef] [PubMed]
36. Kim, J.; Yang, G.; Kim, Y.; Ha, J. AMPK activators: Mechanisms of action and physiological activities. *Exp Mol. Med.* **2016**, *48*, e224. [CrossRef]
37. Vial, G.; Detaille, D.; Guigas, B. Role of Mitochondria in the Mechanism(s) of Action of Metformin. *Front. Endocrinol.* **2019**, *10*, 294. [CrossRef]
38. Zaks, I.; Getter, T.; Gruzman, A. Activators of AMPK: Not just for type II diabetes. *Future Med. Chem.* **2014**, *6*, 1325–1353. [CrossRef]
39. Boutouja, F.; Stiehm, C.M.; Platta, H.W. mTOR: A Cellular Regulator Interface in Health and Disease. *Cells* **2019**, *8*, 18. [CrossRef]
40. Evangelisti, C.; Cenni, V.; Lattanzi, G. Potential therapeutic effects of the MTOR inhibitors for preventing ageing and progeria-related disorders. *Br. J. Clin. Pharm.* **2016**, *82*, 1229–1244. [CrossRef]
41. Verges, B.; Cariou, B. mTOR inhibitors and diabetes. *Diabetes Res. Clin. Pract.* **2015**, *110*, 101–108. [CrossRef]
42. Uddin, M.S.; Mamun, A.A.; Labu, Z.K.; Hidalgo-Lanussa, O.; Barreto, G.E.; Ashraf, G.M. Autophagic dysfunction in Alzheimer's disease: Cellular and molecular mechanistic approaches to halt Alzheimer's pathogenesis. *J. Cell Physiol.* **2019**, *234*, 8094–8112. [CrossRef] [PubMed]
43. Fang, E.F.; Hou, Y.; Palikaras, K.; Adriaanse, B.A.; Kerr, J.S.; Yang, B.; Lautrup, S.; Hasan-Olive, M.M.; Caponio, D.; Dan, X.; et al. Mitophagy inhibits amyloid-beta and tau pathology and reverses cognitive deficits in models of Alzheimer's disease. *Nat. Neurosci.* **2019**, *22*, 401–412. [CrossRef] [PubMed]
44. Doherty, J.; Baehrecke, E.H. Life, death and autophagy. *Nat. Cell Biol.* **2018**, *20*, 1110–1117. [CrossRef]
45. Dai, C.; Xiao, X.; Li, J.; Ciccotosto, G.D.; Cappai, R.; Tang, S.; Schneider-Futschik, E.K.; Hoyer, D.; Velkov, T.; Shen, J. Molecular Mechanisms of Neurotoxicity Induced by Polymyxins and Chemoprevention. *ACS Chem. Neurosci.* **2019**, *10*, 120–131. [CrossRef] [PubMed]
46. Hinojosa, M.G.; Gutierrez-Praena, D.; Prieto, A.I.; Guzman-Guillen, R.; Jos, A.; Camean, A.M. Neurotoxicity induced by microcystins and cylindrospermopsin: A review. *Sci. Total Environ.* **2019**, *668*, 547–565. [CrossRef]
47. Smith, D.E.; Johanson, C.E.; Keep, R.F. Peptide and peptide analog transport systems at the blood-CSF barrier. *Adv. Drug Deliv. Rev.* **2004**, *56*, 1765–1791. [CrossRef]
48. Boyaud, F.; Mahiout, Z.; Lenoir, C.; Tang, S.; Wdzieczak-Bakala, J.; Witczak, A.; Bonnard, I.; Banaigs, B.; Ye, T.; Inguimbert, N. First total synthesis and stereochemical revision of laxaphycin B and its extension to lyngbyacyclamide A. *Org. Lett.* **2013**, *15*, 3898–3901. [CrossRef]
49. Alvariño, R.; Alonso, E.; Tribalat, M.A.; Gegunde, S.; Thomas, O.P.; Botana, L.M. Evaluation of the Protective Effects of Sarains on H2O2-Induced Mitochondrial Dysfunction and Oxidative Stress in SH-SY5Y Neuroblastoma Cells. *Neurotox Res.* **2017**, *32*, 368–380. [CrossRef]
50. Levert, A.; Alvarino, R.; Bornancin, L.; Abou Mansour, E.; Burja, A.M.; Geneviere, A.M.; Bonnard, I.; Alonso, E.; Botana, L.; Banaigs, B. Structures and Activities of Tiahuramides A-C, Cyclic Depsipeptides from a Tahitian Collection of the Marine Cyanobacterium Lyngbya majuscula. *J. Nat. Prod.* **2018**, *81*, 1301–1310. [CrossRef]
51. Alvariño, R.; Alonso, E.; Lacret, R.; Oves-Costales, D.; Genilloud, O.; Reyes, F.; Alfonso, A.; Botana, L.M. Streptocyclinones A and B ameliorate Alzheimer's disease pathological processes in vitro. *Neuropharmacology* **2018**, *141*, 283–295. [CrossRef]

52. Tan, X.; Azad, S.; Ji, X. Hypoxic Preconditioning Protects SH-SY5Y Cell against Oxidative Stress through Activation of Autophagy. *Cell Transpl.* **2018**, *27*, 1753–1762. [CrossRef] [PubMed]
53. Greco, S.J.; Sarkar, S.; Johnston, J.M.; Tezapsidis, N. Leptin regulates tau phosphorylation and amyloid through AMPK in neuronal cells. *Biochem. Biophys. Res. Commun.* **2009**, *380*, 98–104. [CrossRef] [PubMed]

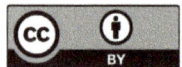

© 2020 by the authors. Licensee MDPI, Basel, Switzerland. This article is an open access article distributed under the terms and conditions of the Creative Commons Attribution (CC BY) license (http://creativecommons.org/licenses/by/4.0/).

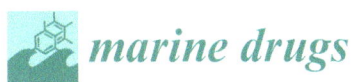

Review

A Comprehensive Review of Bioactive Peptides from Marine Fungi and Their Biological Significance

Fadia S. Youssef [1], Mohamed L. Ashour [1,2], Abdel Nasser B. Singab [1,*] and Michael Wink [3,*]

1. Department of Pharmacognosy, Faculty of Pharmacy, Ain-Shams University, Cairo 11566, Egypt; fadiayoussef@pharma.asu.edu.eg (F.S.Y.); ashour@pharma.asu.edu.eg (M.L.A.)
2. Department of Pharmaceutical Sciences, Pharmacy Program, Batterjee Medical College, North Obhur, P.O. Box 6231, Jeddah 21442, Saudi Arabia
3. Institute of Pharmacy and Molecular Biotechnology, Heidelberg University, Im Neuenheimer Feld 364, 69120 Heidelberg, Germany
* Correspondence: dean@pharma.asu.edu.eg (A.N.B.S.); wink@uni-heidelberg.de (M.W.); Tel.: +20-2-26831231 (A.N.B.S.); +49-6221-54-4880 (M.W.); Fax: +20-2-2405-1107 (A.N.B.S.); +49-6221-54-4884 (M.W.)

Received: 28 August 2019; Accepted: 28 September 2019; Published: 29 September 2019

Abstract: Fungal marine microorganisms are a valuable source of bioactive natural products. Fungal secondary metabolites mainly comprise alkaloids, terpenoids, peptides, polyketides, steroids, and lactones. Proteins and peptides from marine fungi show minimal human toxicity and less adverse effects comparable to synthetic drugs. This review summarizes the chemistry and the biological activities of peptides that were isolated and structurally elucidated from marine fungi. Relevant fungal genera including *Acremonium*, *Ascotricha*, *Aspergillus*, *Asteromyces*, *Ceratodictyon*, *Clonostachys*, *Emericella*, *Exserohilum*, *Microsporum*, *Metarrhizium*, *Penicillium*, *Scytalidium*, *Simplicillium*, *Stachylidium*, *Talaromyces*, *Trichoderma*, as well as *Zygosporium* were extensively reviewed. About 131 peptides were reported from these 17 genera and their structures were unambiguously determined using 1D and 2D NMR (one and two dimensional nuclear magnetic resonance) techniques in addition to HRMS (high resolution mass spectrometry). Marfey and Mosher reactions were used to confirm the identity of these compounds. About 53% of the isolated peptides exhibited cytotoxic, antimicrobial, and antiviral activity, meanwhile, few of them showed antidiabetic, lipid lowering, and anti-inflammatory activity. However 47% of the isolated peptides showed no activity with respect to the examined biological activity and thus required further in depth biological assessment. In conclusion, when searching for bioactive natural products, it is worth exploring more peptides of fungal origin and assessing their biological activities.

Keywords: biological activity; chemistry; marine derived fungi; peptides

1. Introduction

Hundreds of secondary metabolites obtained from marine fungal strains revealed potent pharmacological and biological activity [1]. These mainly comprise alkaloids, terpenoids, and peptides, in addition to polyketides, steroids, and lactones. Relevant bioactivities include antibacterial, anticancer, anti-inflammatory, and antiviral activity [2]. The great diversity in the structure and function of the metabolites derived from marine organisms is mainly attributed to the extensive variation in the chemical and physical conditions of the environment in which the marine organisms survive [3]. As many marine organisms are sessile, they need chemical protection against predators and pathogens.

Marine microorganisms represented by fungi and bacteria, but also marine invertebrates, are regarded as a valuable source of bioactive compounds. Marine microorganisms have the advantage that they can be cultured and thus offer high reproducibility and an everlasting source of natural products [4]. A considerable number of drugs already exist in the market that are of fungal or bacterial origin such as griseofulvin, fucidin, penicillins, and many ergot alkaloids containing products. However, the number of marine fungal metabolites is still quite small [5].

Besides, a number of marine fungal metabolites are characterized by appropriate oral-bioavailability and suitable physico-chemical properties that meet the criteria of formulating effective pharmaceuticals [1]. Furthermore, most fungal proteins and peptides show minimal human toxicity and less adverse effects compared to drugs of synthetic origin [6].

Regarding the history of bioactive peptide isolation from marine organisms, it is noteworthy to highlight that during the past half century hundreds of peptide antibiotics have been explored. They are classified as synthetic peptides (non-ribosomal) and natural (ribosomal) ones. The former are represented by glycopeptides, gramicidins, bacitracins, and polymyxins as well and they are extensively modified and produced mainly by bacterial strains, meanwhile, the latter are equally produced by all species comprising fungi and bacteria and considered as a primary line of defence elicited by these organisms [7].

However, naturally occurring peptides obtained from marine sources possess strongly modified structures either in its backbone or side chain compared to peptides of human origin that undoubtedly do due to the environmental conditions in which they live. This ultimately makes them good candidates for drug design offering great stability from enzymatic degradation as well as thermal conditions. Most of these peptides are taken from ascidians, sponges, as well as mollusks. Besides, wide array of bioactive peptides are produced as the result of the association that exists between microorganisms and the marine organisms. This symbiosis, in turn, generated biochemical pathways in both the marine organisms and its associated microorganisms with concomitant production of many beneficial pharmaceuticals that are of natural origin [8].

Peptides are generally isolated from the fermented fungal biomass culture media via extraction of the culture media using appropriate solvents, most commonly ethyl acetate, and then subjected to evaporation till dryness under vacuum at 40 °C to a semi solid residue. The obtained residue was subjected to a series of chromatographic fractionation using traditional stationary phases such as silica gel and sephadex as well, with concomitant purification using high performance liquid chromatography (HPLC) to fully purify and isolate individual peptides in their single forms [9].

Structural elucidation and characterization of the isolated peptides are unambiguously determined by spectroscopic analysis comprising 1D and 2D NMR techniques, in addition to mass spectrometry. Their absolute configurations were further ascertained by Marfey's methods, chemical structural modification, as well as Mosher's reaction [10]. In addition, ESIMS (Electrospray Ionization Mass Spectrometry) analyses of the free amino acids obtained by acid hydrolysis, as well as HPLC analysis of Marfey products prepared from the acid hydrolysate are also used for determination of peptides structures. However, the peptide amino acid sequence can be also unambiguously determined by MSn ion-trap ESI mass spectrometry [11].

Thus, in this review we comprehensively explore the chemistry and the biological activity of the peptides that were isolated and structurally elucidated from marine fungi of the genera *Acremonium, Ascotricha, Aspergillus, Asteromyces, Ceratodictyon, Clonostachys, Emericella, Exserohilum, Microsporum, Metarrhizium, Penicillium, Scytalidium, Simplicillium, Stachylidium, Talaromyces, Trichoderma*, and *Zygosporium*. Collection of data was done until July 2019 and classification was performed based upon the fungal genera, which are arranged in an alphabetical order. Additionally, a table summarizing the bioactive peptides isolated from marine associated fungi, their sources, and biological activities was added for better illustration of the collected data.

2. Bioactive Peptides in Particular Fungal Genera

2.1. Acremonium

From a fermenter-culture of *Acremonium persicinum*, three new compounds of cycloheptapeptide skeleton were isolated, namely cordyheptapeptides C–E (**1**–**3**). Only compounds (**1**) and (**3**) showed a substantial cytotoxicity versus MCF-7, SF-268, and NCI-H460 cancer cells displaying IC_{50} values between 2.5 and 12.1 µM [12]. Moreover, two new linear pentadecapeptides (efrapeptins Eα (**4**) and H (**5**)) in addition to known efrapeptin F–G (**6**–**7**) were isolated from an atypical *Acremonium* species. Additionally, RHM1 (**8**), RHM2 (**9**), RHM3 (**10**), and RHM4 (**11**), N-methylated linear octapeptides, were also isolated and structurally elucidated using different spectroscopic techniques from the same species (Figure 1A–C). Promising cytotoxic activity was exhibited by efrapeptins Eα (**4**), F (**6**), and G (**7**) versus H125 cells with an IC_{50} value about 1.3 nM; the latter also showed potent cytotoxic activity versus murine L1210 cells as well as versus HCT-116 with IC_{50} values equal to 0.002 nM. Pronounced antibacterial activity was observed for RHM1 (**8**) as well as for efrapeptin G (**7**) against *Staphylococcus epidermidis* with MIC (Minimum Inhibitory Concentration) values equal to 0.015 and 0.049 µM, respectively [13,14].

2.2. Ascotricha

In depth chemical investigation of the marine fungus *Ascotricha* using different chromatographic techniques resulted in the isolation of 10 compounds that are fully elucidated using various spectroscopic techniques in addition to their physicochemical characteristics. Among them are five peptides namely cyclo (Pro-Ala) (**12**), cyclo (Ile-Leu) (**13**), cyclo (Leu-Pro) (**14**), cyclo (Pro-Gly) (**15**), and cyclo (Pro-Val) (**16**) (Figure 2) that were first to be isolated from genus *Ascotricha* [15].

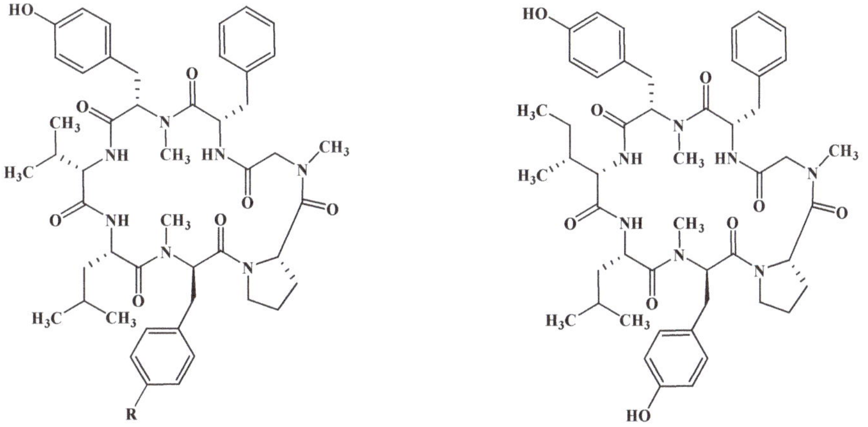

Cordyheptapeptide C (1) R = H
Cordyheptapeptide D (2) R = OH

Cordyheptapeptide E (3)

(**A**)

Figure 1. *Cont.*

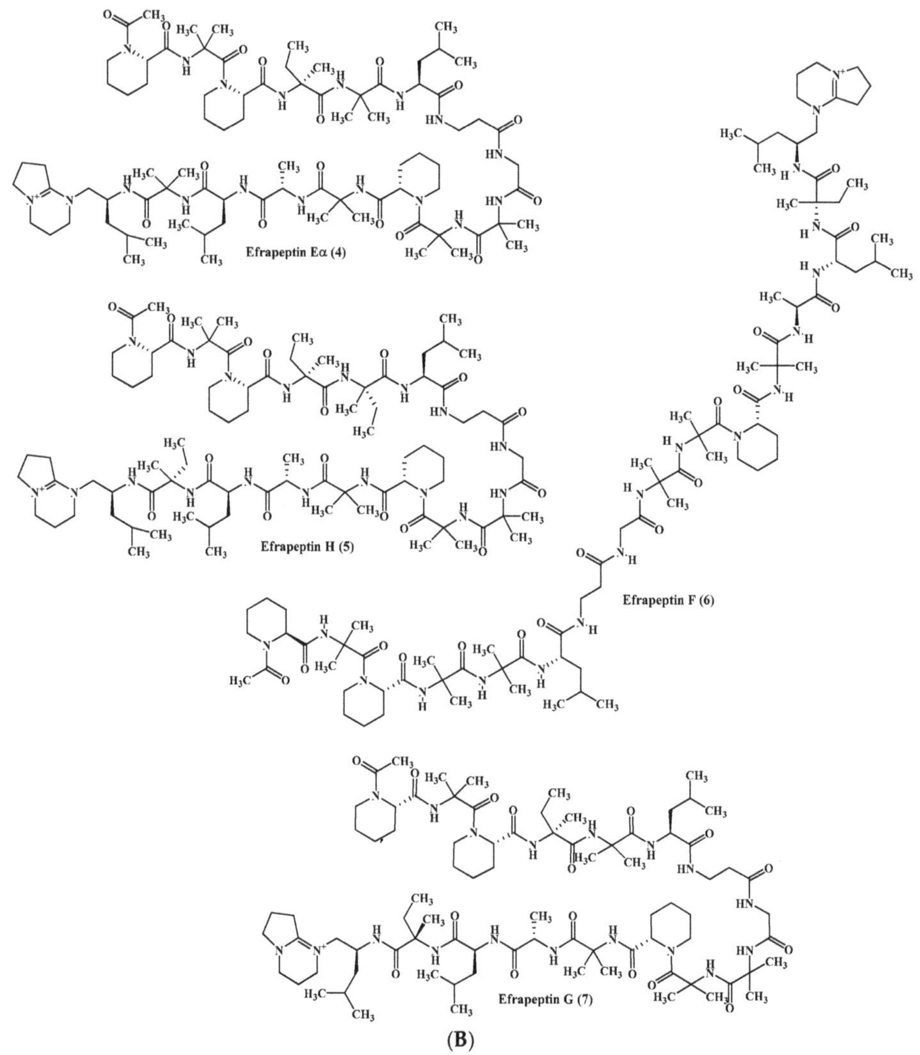

(B)

Figure 1. Cont.

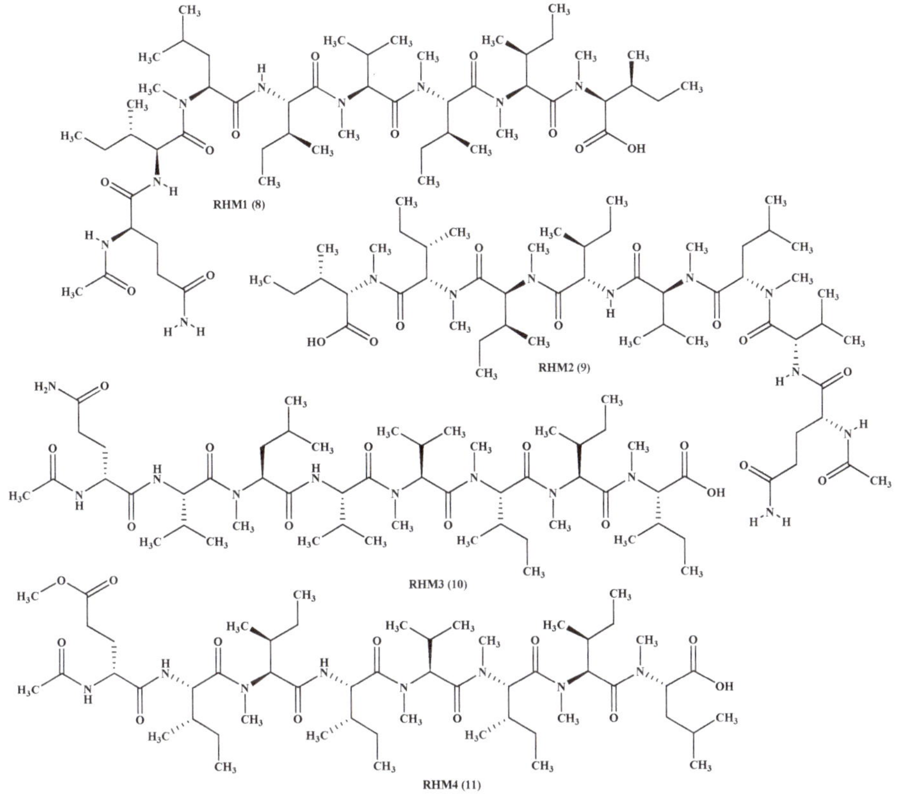

Figure 1. (**A**) Cordyheptapeptides isolated from *Acremonium* species. (**B**) Efrapeptins isolated from *Acremonium* species. (**C**) RHM family isolated from *Acremonium* species.

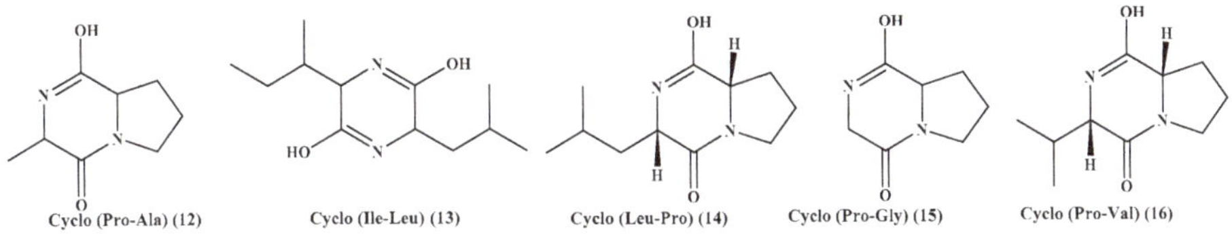

Figure 2. Peptides isolated from *Ascotricha* species.

2.3. Aspergillus

Five new depsipeptides, aspergillicins A–E (**17–21**), were isolated from *Aspergillus carneus* upon comprehensive chemical investigation of a fermenter culture that showed no anti-parasitic activity versus *Haemonchus contortus* in contrast to modest cytotoxic activity with LD_{99} values ranging between 0.03–0.07 µM [11]. Regarding *A. niger*, which was obtained from sediments from the northeast coast of Brazil, then cultured in various growth media, many cyclopeptides were obtained comprising cyclo (L-Pro-L-Phe) (**22**), cyclo (*trans*-4-hydroxy-L-Pro-L-Leu) (**23**), cyclo (L-Pro-L-Leu) (**24**), cyclo (*trans*-4-hydroxy-L-Pro-L-Phe) (**25**), cyclo (L-Pro-L-Val) (**26**), as well as cyclo (L-Pro-L-Tyr) (**27**). The isolated cyclopeptides exhibited no cytotoxic effect against HCT-116 cell line [16]. In addition, other three cyclopeptides namely cyclo-(L-Trp-L-Ile) (**28**), cyclo-(L-Trp-L-Phe) (**29**), and cyclo-(L-Trp-L-Tyr) (**30**) were also reported. The first two cyclopeptides were considered to be plant growth regulators whereas the latter effectively stimulates the differentiation of HT-29 cancer cells. However, neither compounds (**28–30**) showed pronounced antimicrobial activity when tested against either *Staphylococcus aureus*, *Escherichia coli*, *A. niger*, or *Candida albicans* [17]. In addition, two novel hexapeptides were isolated and structurally elucidated from the fungus *A. sclerotiorum*. These hexapeptides were sclerotide A (**31**) and sclerotide B (**32**) which showed modest antifungal activity versus *C. albicans* showing MIC values of 7.0 and 3.5 µM, respectively. Additionally, sclerotide B (**32**) revealed selective activity versus *Pseudomonas aeruginosa* with MIC equals to 35.3 µM, meanwhile, it exerted weak cytotoxic activity versus HL-60 cell line with IC_{50} equal to 56.1 µM [18] (Figure 3A).

One more new cyclic hexapeptide, similanamide (**33**), was isolated from a sponge derived fungus, *A. similanensis*, which displayed weak cytotoxic activity versus MCF-7, A373, and NCI-H460 cancer cells with GI_{50} values equal to 0.2, 0.18, and 0.18 µM, respectively, with no antibacterial activity as the (MIC value was found to be greater 256 µg/mL (0.4 µM)) [19]. Moreover, two new lumazine peptides namely terrelumamides A (**34**) and B (**35**), in addition to two new isomeric modified tripeptides, aspergillamides C (**36**) and D (**37**), and a cyclic tetrapeptide asperterrestide A (**38**) were isolated and unambiguously elucidated from *A. terreus*, which is a marine fungus. Compounds (**34**) and (**35**) displayed a promising improvement in insulin sensitivity as determined by the utilization of mesenchymal cells of a bone marrow origin obtained from human (hBM-MSCs) adopting an adipogenesis model. They exerted their action via increasing the formation of adiponectin during the process of adipogenesis in hBM-MSCs with EC50 values equal to 37.1 and 91.9 µM, for terrelumamides A (**34**) and B (**35**), respectively. It is noteworthy to highlight that the maximum elevation in adiponectin levels via terrelumamide A (**34**) induction was 56.9% comparable to that generated by glibenclamide (the standard anti-hyperglycaemic agent). Meanwhile compound (**38**) showed a potent cytotoxic effect versus U937 and MOLT4 human cancer cell lines with IC50 equal to 6.4 and 6.2 µM, respectively, in addition to a pronounced inhibitory potential versus an influenza virus of H1N1, as well as H3N2 strains with IC50 equal to 15 and 8.1 µM, respectively, that relied upon the presence of a 3-OH-N-CH3-Phe moiety that is rare in nature [20–22]. Besides, other known peptides were isolated from the latter *Aspergillus* species, which are aspergillamide A (**39**) and B (**40**) and cyclo-(L-Pro-L-Phe) (**41**) [21]. *A. unguis* is another marine fungus from which unguisin A (**42**), which is a cyclic peptide, was isolated [23]. In addition, *A. unilateralis* revealed a complex array of secondary metabolites comprising the heterocyclic dipeptides, aspergillazines A–E (**43–47**), which are dipeptides, in addition to trichodermamide A and B (**48–49**) [24] (Figure 3B).

Furthermore, four new compounds, psychrophilins E–H (**50–53**) were isolated from *A. versicolor*, and they are cyclic peptides characterized by the presence of a rare linkage of amide type between anthranilic acid through its carboxylic acid and the indole ring via its nitrogen. Additionally, a new cyclic hexapeptide versicotide C (**54**) was isolated from the same fungus. All the isolated peptides showed no cytotoxicity, however compound (**52**) exhibited a pronounced lipid-reducing activity at approximately 10 µM as determined by oil red O staining assay [25]. Moreover, secondary metabolites isolated from coral derived *A. versicolor* revealed the presence of a new centrosymmetric cyclohexapeptide, namely aspersymmetide A (**55**), in addition to asperphenamate (**56**) which is a known peptide. Noteworthy to mention is that compound (**55**) was the first centrosymmetric cyclohexapeptide to be isolated from fungi, however it showed weak cytotoxicity versus NCI-H292, as well as A431 cell lines, at 10 µM [26]. Besides, two new cyclopentapeptides, namely cotteslosins A (**57**) and B (**58**), were isolated from the same fungus, *A. versicolor*. Cotteslosin A (**57**) displayed weak cytotoxicity versus human melanoma (MM418c5), prostate (DU145), and breast (T47D) cells with EC_{50} values of 0.1, 0.14, and 0.15 µM, respectively [27]. Concerning *A. violaceofuscus*, a sponge associated fungus, three peptides, which are cyclic, were isolated from its ethyl acetate extract and they were first to be isolated in nature. These cyclic peptides are termed, aspochracin-type cyclic tripeptide sclerotiotide L (**59**), diketopiperazine dimer (**60**), in addition to a cyclic tetrapeptide (**61**) where compounds (**60–61**) showed potent anti-inflammatory activity against IL-10 expression of the

(Lipopolysaccharide) LPS-induced THP-1 cells (acute monocytic leukemia cell) as evidenced by its inhibition rates which were estimated to be 84.3 and 78.1%, respectively at 10 µM [28] (Figure 3C).

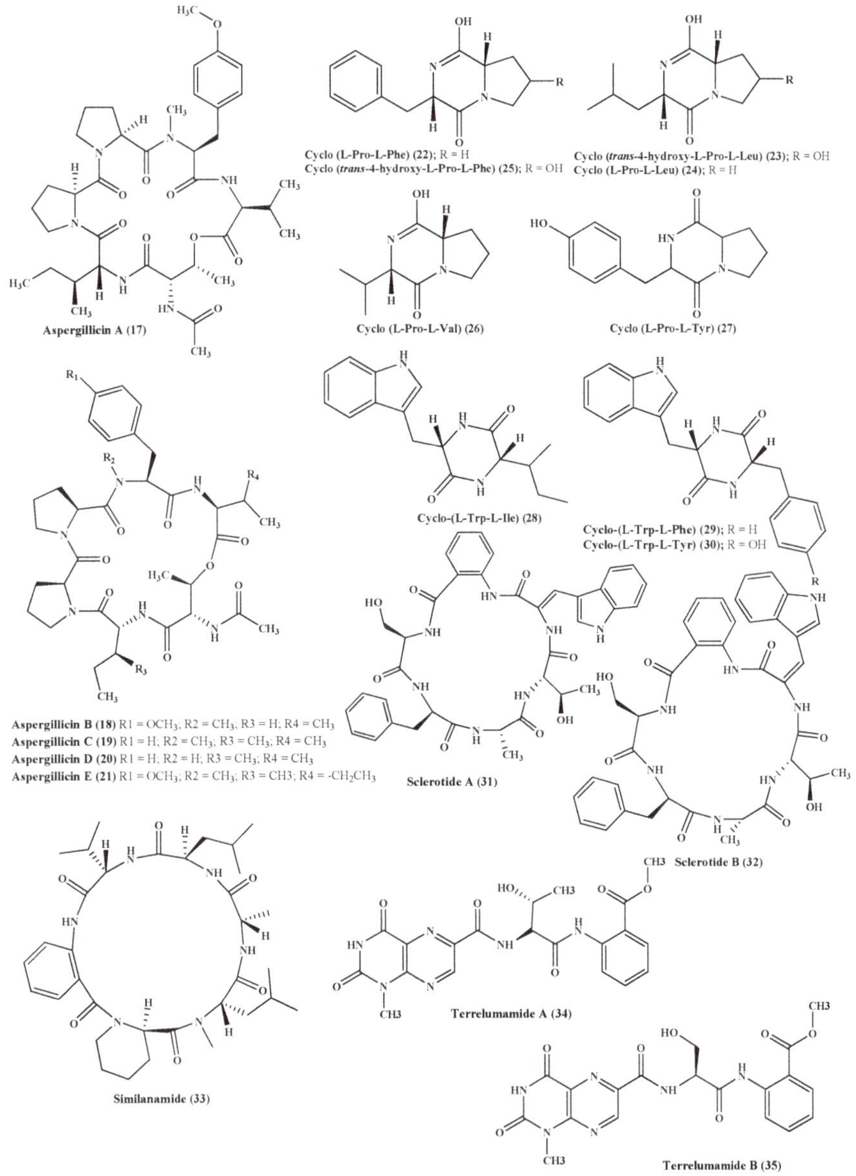

Figure 3. Cont.

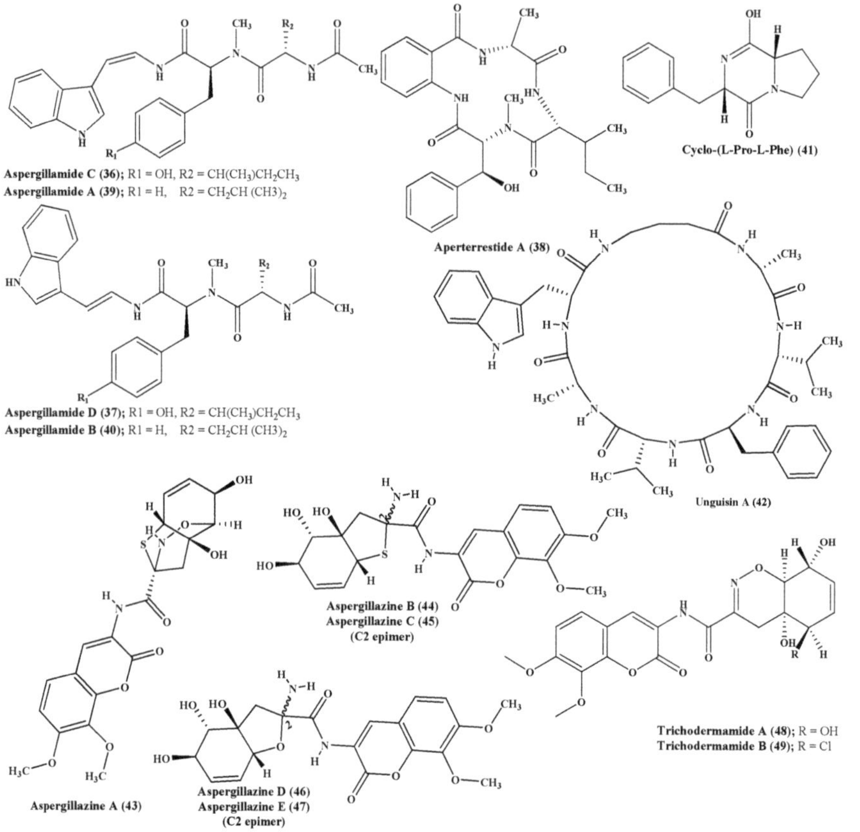

Aspergillamide C (36); R1 = OH, R2 = CH(CH₃)CH₂CH₃
Aspergillamide A (39); R1 = H, R2 = CH₂CH(CH₃)₂

Aperterrestide A (38)

Cyclo-(L-Pro-L-Phe) (41)

Aspergillamide D (37); R1 = OH, R2 = CH(CH₃)CH₂CH₃
Aspergillamide B (40); R1 = H, R2 = CH₂CH(CH₃)₂

Unguisin A (42)

Aspergillazine A (43)

Aspergillazine B (44)
Aspergillazine C (45)
(C2 epimer)

Aspergillazine D (46)
Aspergillazine E (47)
(C2 epimer)

Trichodermamide A (48); R = OH
Trichodermamide B (49); R = Cl

(**B**)

Figure 3. *Cont.*

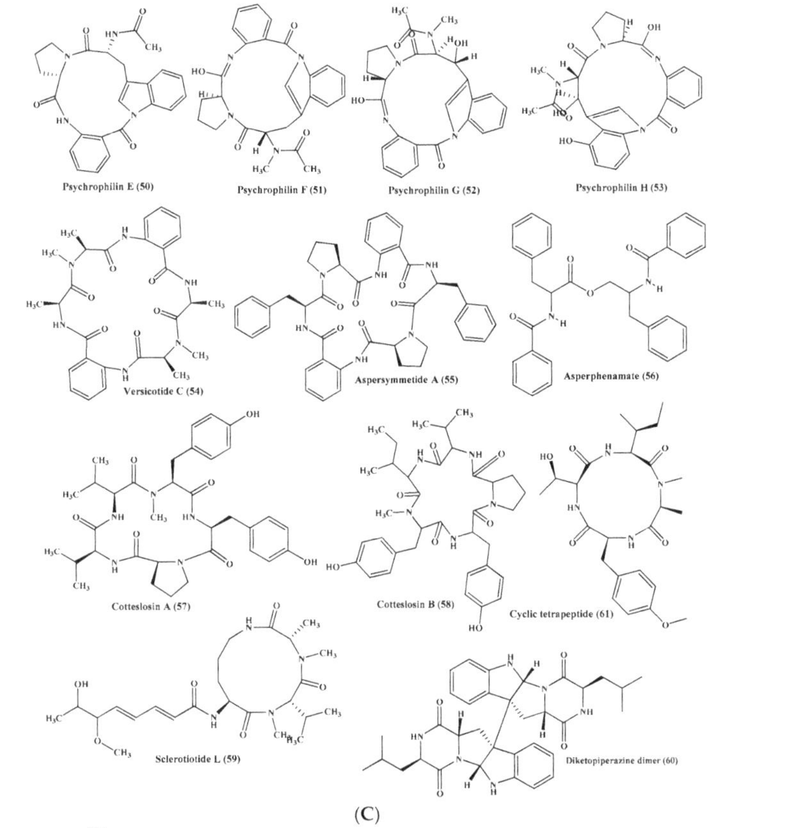

Figure 3. (**A**) Peptides isolated from Aspergillus carneus, A. niger, A. sclerotiorum, and A. terreus. (**B**) Peptides isolated from A. terreus, A. unguis, and A. unilateralis. (**C**) Peptides isolated from A. versicolor and A. violaceofuscus. (**D**) Peptides isolated from miscellaneous *Aspergillus* species.

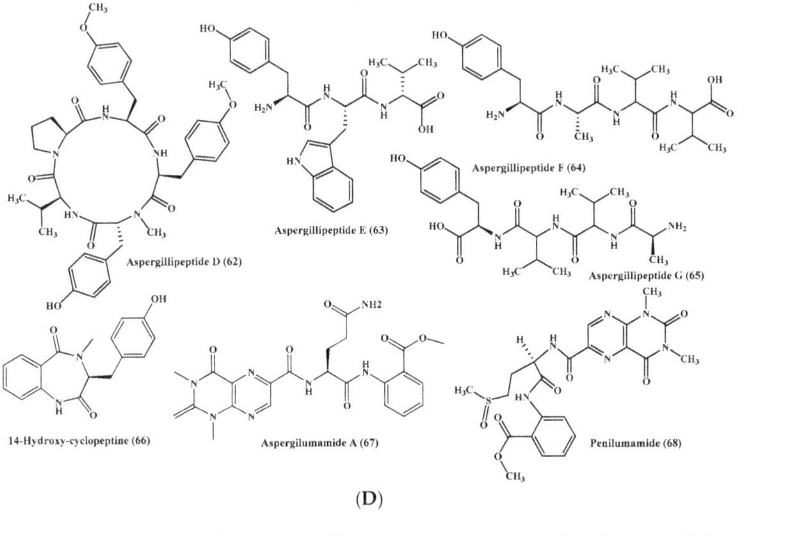

Various peptides were isolated from miscellaneous *Aspergillus* species exemplified by psychrophilin E (**50**), a cyclic tripeptide isolated from two algae associated *Aspergillus* sp whose selectivity inhibited the proliferation of HCT116 (colon) cell line with an IC$_{50}$ value of 28.5 µM comparable to the standard drug cisplatin that showed IC$_{50}$ of 33.4 µM [29]. Additionally, many *Aspergillus* sp. derived peptides displayed antiviral activity such as aspergillipeptides D–G (**62–65**), in which aspergillipeptides D (**62**) and E (**63**) displayed a potent antiviral effect versus herpes simplex virus type 1 (HSV-1) displaying IC$_{50}$ of 9.5 and 19.8 µM, respectively, showing no cytotoxic effect at these concentrations versus Vero cell line, meanwhile aspergillipeptide D (**62**) also exhibited activity versus acyclovir resistant clinical isolates of HSV-1 [30]. Regarding the inhibition of nitric oxide production, it was found that the novel cyclic dipeptide isolated from an *Aspergillus* sp., 14-hydroxy-cyclopeptine (**66**), effectively inhibits nitric oxide production displaying IC$_{50}$ of 0.14 µM in recombinant mouse interferon-γ-activated macrophage-like cell line as well as in a lipopolysaccharide without cytotoxic effect at 0.34 µM [31]. Many other peptides were also isolated from *Aspergillus* sp. derived from *Bruguiera sexangula* var. *rhynchopetala* as aspergilumamide A (**67**) and penilumamide (**68**) [32] (Figure 3D).

2.4. Asteromyces

A new pentapeptide compound, lajollamide A (**69**) was isolated from marine *Asteromyces cruciatus*. This newly isolated peptide showed a weak antimicrobial effect versus Gram-positive bacteria at 100 µM showing 61% and 30% inhibition in bacterial growth for *Bacillus subtilis* and *Staphylococcus epidermidis*, respectively, whereas it showed no inhibition of acetyl cholinesterase activity [33] (Figure 4).

2.5. Ceratodictyon

In depth chemical investigation of the red algae associated fungus, *Ceratodictyon spongiosum*, resulted in the isolation of two new peptides which are dictyonamides A and B (**70–71**). The former displayed a pronounced inhibition on cyclin-dependent kinase 4 with IC$_{50}$ value equals to 0.01 µM however the latter showed no inhibition [34] (Figure 4).

2.6. Clonostachys

Clonostachysins A and B (**72–73**) are two new cyclic peptides isolated from *Clonostachys rogersoniana* that revealed potent inhibitory activity on a dinoflagellate *Prorocentrum micans* at a concentration of 30 µM but revealed no activity to either bacteria or microalgae [35] (Figure 4).

2.7. Emericella

Unguisins A (**42**) and B (**74**) are two cyclic heptapeptides isolated from the fungus *Emericella unguis* [36]. Besides, emericellamides A and B (**75–76**) were also isolated from certain *Emericella* sp. that is co-cultured from *Salinispora arenicola*. Both compounds (**42**) and (**76**) showed encouraging antimicrobial activity against MRSA (methicillin resistant *Staphylococcus aureus* strains) displaying MIC values equal to 3.8 and 6.0 µM, respectively [37] (Figure 4).

2.8. Exserohilum

Rostratins A–D (**77–80**) were first to be isolated from the broth of *Exserohilum rostratum*, a marine associated fungus that showed pronounced cytotoxic activity versus (HCT-116) the human colon carcinoma showing 20, 4.48, 1.6, and 34 nM as IC$_{50}$ values, respectively [38] (Figure 4).

2.9. Microsporum

The marine associated fungus, *Microsporum* cf. *gypseum*, yielded two new peptides microsporins, A and B (**81–82**), which effectively inhibit histone deacetylase with IC$_{50}$ values equal to 0.14 and 0.55 µM against (Histone Deacetylases) HDACs and HDAC8, respectively, in addition to displaying a considerable cytotoxic effect versus human colon adenocarcinoma (HCT-116) with IC$_{50}$ values of 1.17

and 16.5 nM, respectively. Additionally, microsporin A (**81**) displayed notable activity against the 60 cancer cell panel of the National Cancer Institute with mean IC$_{50}$ of 2.7 µM [39] (Figure 4).

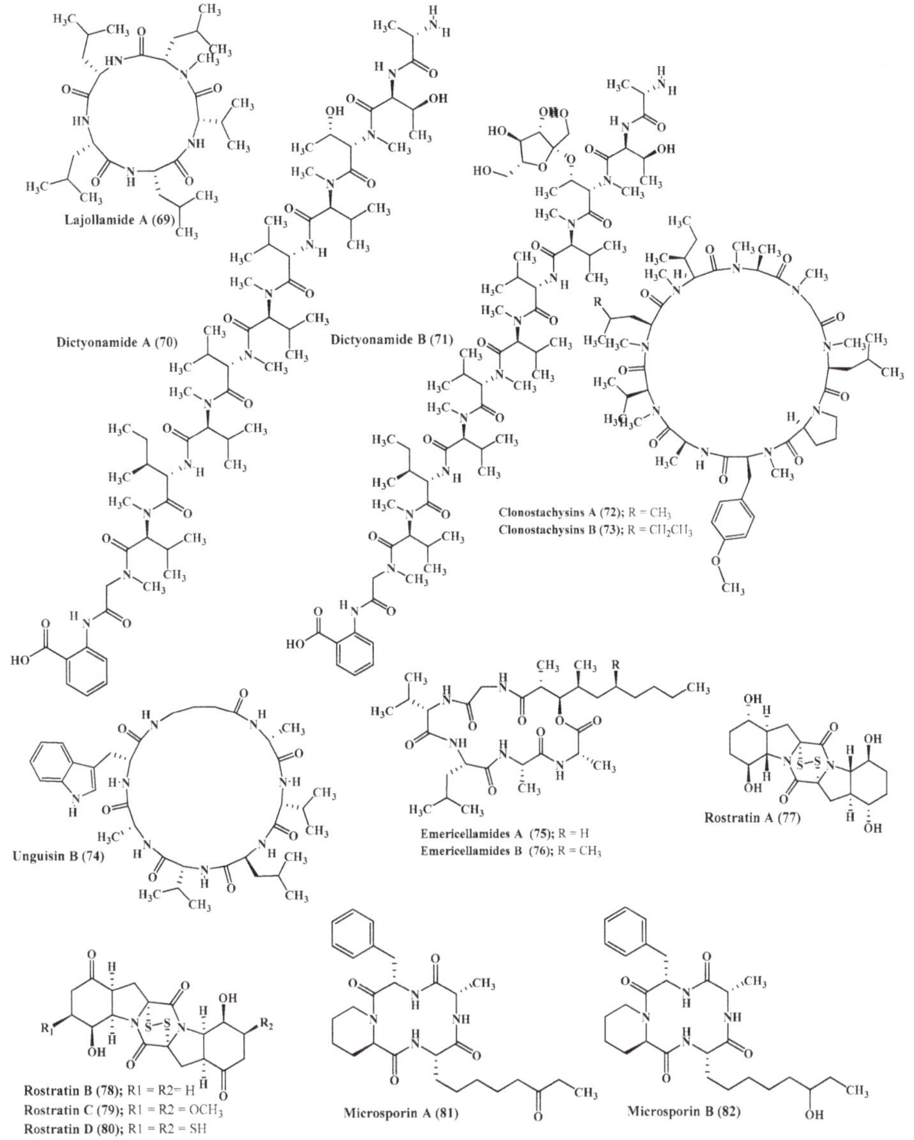

Figure 4. Peptides isolated from Asteromyces, Ceratodictyon, Clonostachys, Emericella, Exserohilum, and Microsporum species.

2.10. Metarrhizium

Destruxin cyclic depsipeptides, including A (**83**) and B (**84**), were reported to be produced by the sponge associated fungus, *Metarrhizium* sp., in addition to efrapeptins Eα (**4**), F (**6**), and G (**7**) [14] (Figure 5).

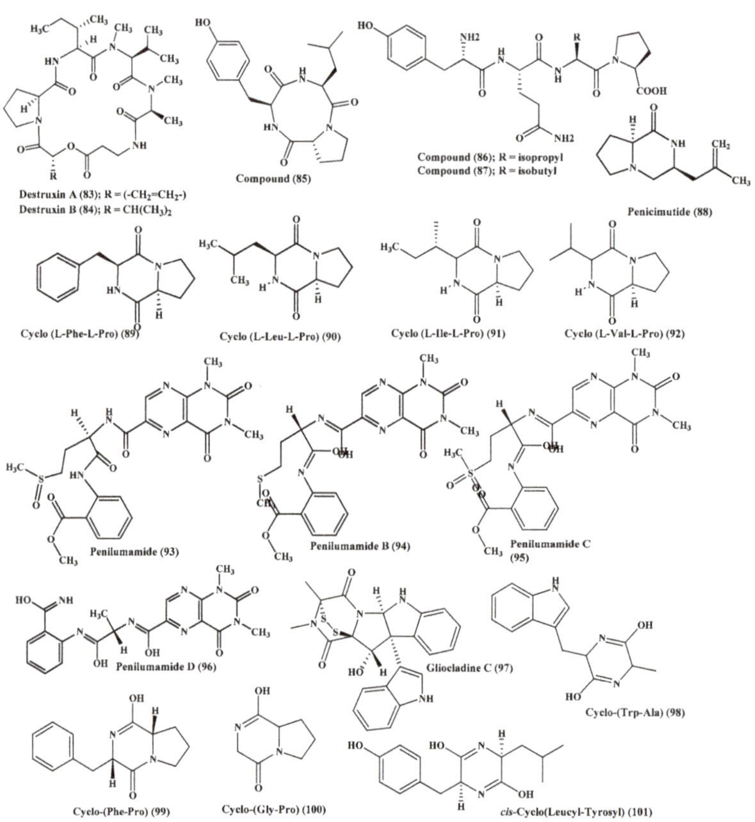

Figure 5. Peptides isolated from *Metarrhizium* and *Penicillium* species.

2.11. Penicillium

Many peptides were isolated from various *Penicillium* species, such as *Penicillium citrinum*, through the stimulation of silent genes using scandium chloride that resulted in the isolation of three new peptide derivatives (85–87). Compound (85) showed potent antibacterial activity against *S. aureus* with MIC value equals to 0.04 µM. However, compounds (86–87) displayed potent cytotoxic activity against MCF-7 and HCT115 cell lines showing IC$_{50}$ equal to 38 and 37 nM, respectively, while compound (85) showed no activity [39]. Furthermore, penicimutide (88), which is a novel dipeptide in a cyclic form in addition to other previously reported dipeptides, namely cyclo (L-Phe-L-Pro) (89), cyclo (L-Leu-L-Pro) (90), cyclo (L-Ile-L-Pro) (91), and cyclo (L-Val-L-Pro) (92) were isolated from *P. purpurogenum*. Penicimutide (88) effectively inhibited growth of HeLa cells showing 39.4% as an inhibition rate at 100 µg/mL (0.5 µM) approaching that of the 5-fluorouracil that showed 41.4% at 100 µg/mL (0.77 µM) [40] (Figure 5).

Besides, penilumamide (93), as well as penilumamides B–D (94–96), were isolated from miscellaneous *Penicillium sp.* [41] in addition to gliocladine C (97), cyclo-(Trp-Ala) (98), cyclo-(Phe-Pro) (99), and cyclo-(Gly-Pro) (100). Compounds (97–100) were assessed for their ability to inhibit HepG2 cells proliferation with different degrees in which gliocladine C (97) effectively inhibited HepG2 cells growth displaying IC$_{50}$ value of 19.6 µM, whereas compounds (98–100) showed no relevant cytotoxic activity [42]. Moreover, *cis*-cyclo (Leucyl-Tyrosyl) (101) isolated from a sponge derived *Penicillium* species showed a significant inhibition to the biofilm formation estimated by 85% which consequently prevents bacterial growth that was further ascertained by a scanning electron microscope [43] (Figure 5).

2.12. Scytalidium

A marine fungus of the genus *Scytalidium* is highly popular for the production of linear, lipophilic peptides, termed the halovirs as halovirs A–E (**102–106**), which showed considerable in vitro antiviral activity against herpes simplex viruses of both type 1 and type 2. Further study on the structure activity relationship between the halovirs and their anti-viral activity showed that the presence of a N^{α}-acyl chain, comprising of at least 14 carbons as well as the Aib-Pro dipeptide, are crucial to preserve the activity. Upon addition of Halovirs A (**102**), B (**103**), and C (**104**) to cells that are exposed to HSV-1 infection for 1 h, they displayed ED_{50} values of 1.1, 3.5, and 2.2 µM, respectively. Meanwhile, halovirs D (**105**) and E (**106**) showed ED_{50} values equal to 2.0 and 3.1 µM, respectively. Besides, halovir A (**102**) effectively prohibits HSV-1 replication showing ED50 value of 0.28 µM adopting the standard plaque reduction assay [44,45] (Figure 6).

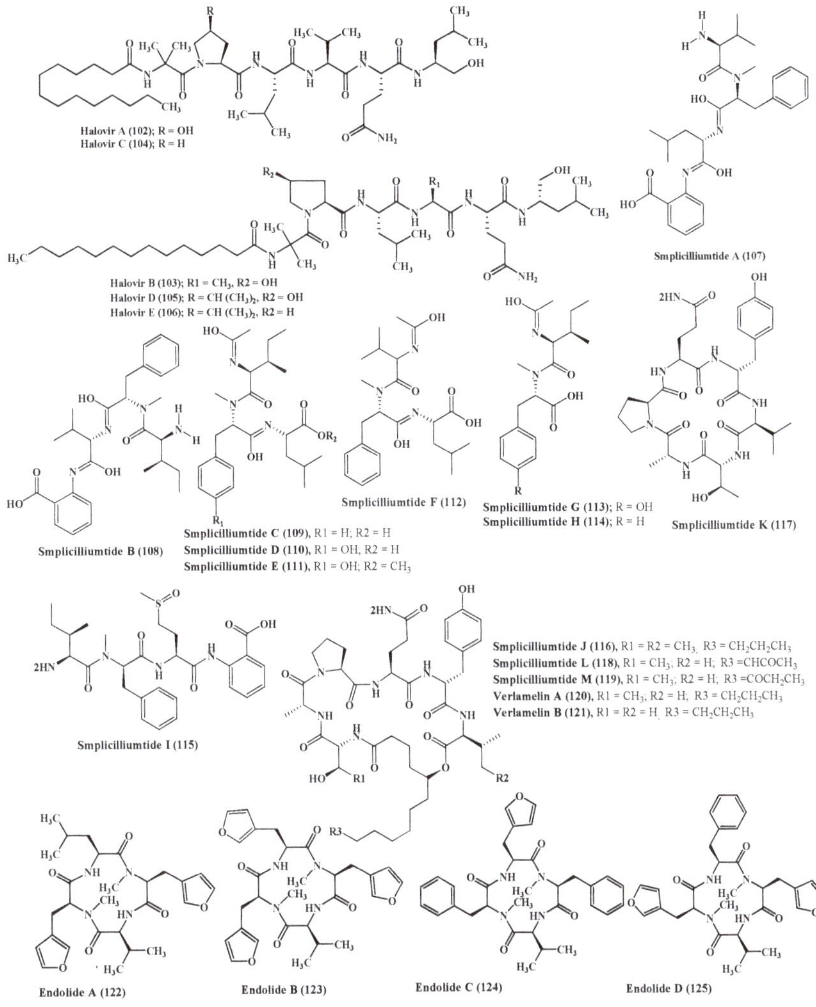

Figure 6. Peptides isolated from *Scytalidium*, *Simplicillium*, and *Stachylidium* species.

2.13. Simplicillium

A series of simplicilliumtide peptides were isolated from the marine fungus *Simplicillium obclavatum* namely; simplicilliumtides A–M (**107–119**) in addition to verlamelins A and B (**120–121**). They showed variable activities including antibacterial, antifungal, antiviral, antifouling, cytotoxic, and acetyl cholinesterase inhibitory activity. Simplicilliumtide D (**110**) displayed a potent antifouling effect versus the larvae of *Bugula neritina* with EC_{50} equal to 0.02 µM and LC_{50}/EC_{50} equal to 100; however, simplicilliumtides A (**107**), E (**111**), G (**113**), and H (**114**) exhibited weak cytotoxic effect against human leukemia HL-60 and K562 cell lines with IC_{50} above 100 µM. In addition, simplicilliumtide J (**116**) exhibited potent antifungal activity versus *Curvularia australiensis* as well as *Aspergillus versicolor* in addition to a potent anti - HSV-1 displaying IC_{50} value of 14.0 µM that could be interpreted in virtue of the presence of lactone linkage and a fatty acid chain moiety [10,46] (Figure 6).

2.14. Stachylidium

Many N-methylated peptides have been isolated from *Stachylidium* sp., a fungus associated with marine sponge, which include endolides A–D (**122–125**) which showed a wide range of biological activities [47]. Endolide A (**122**) revealed potent binding activity to the vasopressin receptor 1A displaying a Ki of 7.04 µM, whereas endolide B (**123**) showed a pronounced binding to serotonin receptor 5HT2b evidenced by its Ki value, which is 0.77 µM [48] (Figure 6).

2.15. Talaromyces

Talarolide A (**126**), in addition to a series of extensively N-methylated linear peptides named talaropeptides A–D (**127–130**), were isolated from *Talaromyces* sp., a fungus derived from a marine tunicate. Biological evaluation of the previously mentioned compounds revealed that compounds (**127–128**) only displayed pronounced antibacterial activity against the growth of *Bacillus subtilis*, a Gram positive bacterium, displaying IC_{50} values of 1.5 and 3.7 µM, respectively. Additionally compound talaropeptide A (**127**) showed a high stability to various rat proteases existing in plasma [49] (Figure 7).

2.16. Trichoderma

Trichoderma strains, derived from marine origin, afforded large amounts peptaibols, which are characterized by being small antimicrobial peptides (AMPs) that are expected to contribute to the antimicrobial defense of *Trichoderma*. *Trichoderma* strains produced 11- and 20-residue peptaibols; optimal yields with 1.4% and 2.3% of the fungal biomass for the 11- and 20-residue, respectively, were obtained on day 9 [50]. Generally, AMPs represent a large group of naturally occurring cationic and amphiphilic short peptides that act as first-line defense for many living organisms and are part of the innate immune system [51]. They act primarily via offering a protection to the host organisms versus the invasion of harmful organisms such as bacteria or fungi [52]. Their mode of action is completely different from traditional antibiotics as they modulate membrane stability and permeability. On the contrary, traditional antibiotics exert their effect mainly by interfering with bacterial metabolism, protein biosynthesis, or cell wall formation. Thus, low cross-resistance and an effective synergism could be achieved between AMPs and traditional antibiotics [53].

2.17. Zygosporium

Zygosporium masonii, a marine fungus that produced a cyclic depsipeptide termed zygosporamide (**131**) showed potent cytotoxic activity in the NCI's 60 cell line panel with median GI_{50} equal to 9.1 µM. However, it revealed a notable selectivity versus the (Central Nervous System) CNS cancer cell SF-268 with GI_{50} equal to 6.5 nM, as well as to the renal cancer cell line RXF 393 showing GI_{50} less than 5.0 nM [54,55] (Figure 7).

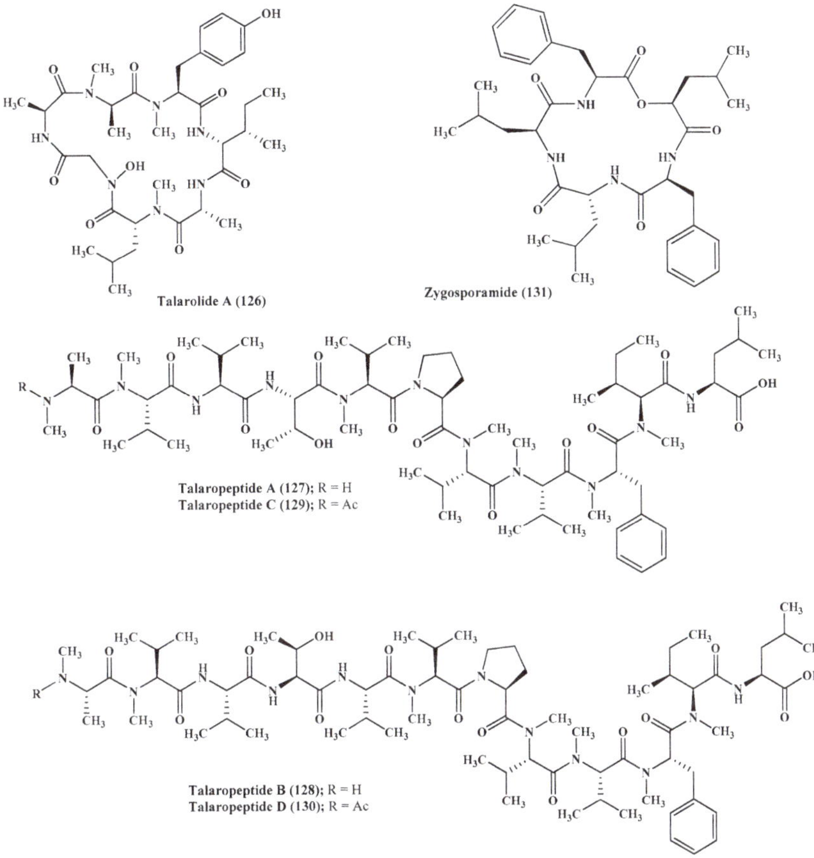

Figure 7. Peptides isolated from *Talaromyces* and *Zygosporium* species.

3. Discussion and General Perspectives

In our analysis we found that 131 peptides from marine sources were isolated from 17 fungal strains. These peptides are either cyclic, composed of two amino acids (dipeptide), as in case of *Ascotricha* up to nine amino acids (nonapeptides) in *Emericella* or linear pentadecapeptide as presented in *Acremonium*. Many depsipeptides (from *Acremonium*, *Metarrhizium*, and *Zygosporium*), peptaibols in *Trichoderma* and N-methylated peptides from *Acremonium*, *Stachylidium*, and *Talaromyces* are also characterized. It is clearly noticed that genus *Aspergillus* was the most extensively studied and it might represent a rich source of peptides with promising biological activity. However, there is no evidence about the chemotaxonomic relation between the production of a certain class of peptides in a specified genus. That could be explained based on the fact that the number of the isolated compounds is not enough to make an in-depth study about this relation. Besides, peptides from marine sources possess strongly modulated structures either in its backbone or side chain comparable to peptides of plant or human origin, which undoubtedly is due to the harsh requirements of the environment in which they live. It worthy to mention that although most of these peptides contain many functional groups, such as carbonyl and amide groups, beside esters as in the case of depsipeptides which gave them the ability to interact with many molecular targets in the cells, most of these peptides are either inactive or showed weak activity. That could be explained by the fact that most of these peptides are weakly soluble in physiological fluids that limit most of their in vivo activity [56].

It was found that about 53% of the isolated peptides exhibited various biological activities represented mainly by cytotoxic, antimicrobial, and antiviral activity, while few of them showed antidiabetic, lipid lowering, and anti-inflammatory activity (Table 1).

Table 1. Bioactive peptides isolated from marine associated fungi, their sources, and biological activities.

Compound	Genus	Biological Activity	Reference
Cordyheptapeptide C (**1**)	*Acremonium*	• Cytotoxic activity versus MCF-7, SF-268 and NCI-H460 cancer cells	[12]
Cordyheptapeptide E (**3**)	*Acremonium*	• Cytotoxic activity versus MCF-7, SF-268 and NCI-H460 cancer cells	[12]
Efrapeptin Eα (**4**)	*Acremonium*	• Cytotoxic activity versus H125 cells	[13,14]
Efrapeptin F (**6**)	*Acremonium*	• Cytotoxic activity versus H125 cells	[13,14]
Efrapeptin G (**7**)	*Acremonium*	• Cytotoxic activity versus H125 and HCT-116 cells • Antibacterial activity versus *Staphylococcus epidermidis*	[13,14]
RHM1 (**8**)	*Acremonium*	• Antibacterial activity versus *Staphylococcus epidermidis*	[13,14]
Aspergillicins A–E (**17–21**)	*Aspergillus*	• Cytotoxic activity	[11]
Cyclo-(L-Trp-L-Tyr) (**30**)	*Aspergillus*	• Cytotoxic activity versus HT-29 cancer cells	[17]
Sclerotide A (**31**)	*Aspergillus*	• Antifungal activity versus *Candida albicans*	[18]
Sclerotide B (**32**)	*Aspergillus*	• Antifungal activity versus *Candida albicans* • Antibacterial activity versus *Pseudomonas aeruginosa* • Weak cytotoxic activity versus HL-60 cell ($IC_{50} > 50$ μM)	[18]
Similanamide (**33**)	*Aspergillus*	• Weak cytotoxic activity versus MCF-7, A373 and NCI-H460 cancer cells ($GI_{50} > 0.15$ μM)	[19]
Terrelumamide A (**34**)	*Aspergillus*	• Improve insulin sensitivity	[20–22]
Terrelumamide B (**35**)	*Aspergillus*	• Improve insulin sensitivity	[20–22]
Compound (**38**)	*Aspergillus*	• Cytotoxic activity versus U937 and MOLT4 human cancer cell lines • Antiviral activity versus influenza virus of H1N1 and H3N2 strains	[20–22].
Psychrophilin E (**50**)	*Aspergillus*	• Cytotoxic activity versus HCT116	[29]

Table 1. Cont.

Compound	Genus	Biological Activity	Reference
Psychrophilin G (**52**)	*Aspergillus*	• Lipid-lowering activity	[25]
Aspersymmetide A (**55**)	*Aspergillus*	• Weak cytotoxic activity versus NCI-H292 as well as A431 cell lines ($IC_{50} > 10$ μM)	[26]
Cotteslosin A (**57**)	*Aspergillus*	• Weak cytotoxic activity versus human melanoma (MM418c5), prostate (DU145) and breast (T47D) cells ($EC_{50} > 0.1$ μM	[27]
Diketopiperazine dimer (**60**)	*Aspergillus*	• Anti-inflammatory activity against IL-10 expression of the LPS-induced THP-1 cells	[28]
Cyclic tetrapeptide (**61**)	*Aspergillus*	• Anti-inflammatory activity against IL-10 expression of the LPS-induced THP-1 cells	[28]
Aspergillipeptid D (**62**)	*Aspergillus*	• Antiviral activity versus herpes simplex virus type 1 (HSV-1) and acyclovir resistant clinical isolates	[30]
Aspergillipeptide E (**63**)	*Aspergillus*	• Antiviral activity versus herpes simplex virus type 1 (HSV-1)	[30]
14-Hydroxy-cyclopeptine (**66**)	*Aspergillus*	• Inhibition of nitric oxide production	[31]
Lajollamide A (**69**)	*Asteromyces*	• Weak antimicrobial activity versus Bacillus subtilis and Staphylococcus epidermidis. • (MIC > 50 μM)	[33]
Dictyonamide A (**70**)	*Ceratodictyon*	• Inhibition on cyclin-dependent kinase 4	[34]
Clonostachysin A (**72**)	*Clonostachys*	• Inhibition of dinoflagellate *Prorocentrum micans*	[35]
Clonostachysin B (**73**)	*Clonostachys*	• Inhibition of dinoflagellate *Prorocentrum micans*	[35]
Unguisin A (**42**)	*Emericella*	• Antimicrobial activity versus MRSA (methicillin resistant *Staphylococcus aureus* strains)	[37]
Emericellamide B (**76**)	*Emericella*	• Antimicrobial activity versus MRSA (methicillin resistant *Staphylococcus aureus* strains)	[37]
Rostratins A–D (**77–80**)	*Exserohilum*	• Cytotoxic activity versus (HCT-116) the human colon carcinoma	[38]
Microsporin A (**81**)	*Microsporum*	• Inhibition of histone deacetylase • Cytotoxic activity versus human colon adenocarcinoma (HCT-116) and the 60 cancer cell panel of the National Cancer Institute	[39]

Table 1. Cont.

Compound	Genus	Biological Activity	Reference
Microsporin B (**82**)	*Microsporum*	• Inhibition of histone deacetylase • Cytotoxic activity versus human colon adenocarcinoma (HCT-116)	[39]
Compound (**85**)	*Penicillium*	• Antibacterial activity versus *S. aureus*	[39]
Compounds (**86–87**)	*Penicillium*	• Cytotoxic activity versus MCF-7 and HCT115 cell lines	[39]
Penicimutide (**88**)	*Penicillium*	• Cytotoxic activity versus HeLa cells	[40]
Gliocladine C (**97**)	*Penicillium*	• Cytotoxic activity versus HepG2 cells	[42]
cis-Cyclo (Leucyl-Tyrosyl) (**101**)	*Penicillium*	• Inhibition to the biofilm formation	[43]
Halovir A (**102**)	*Scytalidium*	• Antiviral activity versus herpes simplex viruses of both type 1 and type 2 and HSV-1	[44,45]
Halovirs B–E (**103–106**)	*Scytalidium*	• Antiviral activity versus herpes simplex viruses of both type 1 and type 2	[44,45]
Simpliciliumtide A (**107**)	*Simplicillium*	• Weak cytotoxic activity versus human leukemia HL-60 and K562 cell line	[10,46]
Simpliciliumtide D (**110**)	*Simplicillium*	• Antifouling effect versus the larvae of *Bugula neritina*	[10,46]
Simpliciliumtides E (**111**), G (**113**), and H (**114**)	*Simplicillium*	• Weak cytotoxic effect versus human leukemia HL-60 and K562 cell line (IC_{50} > 100 µM)	[10,46]
Simpliciliumtide J (**116**)	*Simplicillium*	• Antifungal activity versus Curvularia australiensis and Aspergillus versicolor • Antiviral activity versus HSV-1	[10,46]
Endolide A (**122**)	*Stachylidium*	• Binding activity to the vasopressin receptor 1A	[48]
Endolide B (**123**)	*Stachylidium*	• Binding to serotonin receptor 5HT2b	[48]
Talaropeptide A (**127**)	*Talaromyces*	• Antibacterial activity versus *Bacillus subtilis*	[49]
Talaropeptide B (**128**)	*Talaromyces*	• Antibacterial activity versus *Bacillus subtilis*	[49]
Zygosporamide (**131**)	*Zygosporium*	• Cytotoxic activity versus NCI's 60 cell line panel, CNS cancer cell line SF-268, renal cancer cell line RXF 393	[54,55]

Regarding the cytotoxic effect of the previously mentioned peptides, about 35 bioactive peptides revealed cytotoxic activities against a panel of cancer cells. Twenty five peptides showed potent cytotoxic activity however the other ten peptides exerted weak activity. This was represented by cordyheptapeptides C (**1**) and E (**3**), which exerted notable activity on MCF-7, SF-268, and NCI-H460 cancer cells with IC_{50} ranging between 2.5 and 12.1 µM. Besides, pronounced cytotoxic potential was exerted by efrapeptins Eα (**4**), F (**6**), and G (**7**) against H125 cells with IC_{50} values of about 1.3 nM. Efrapeptin G (**7**) also showed potent cytotoxic activity versus murine cancer cells. Moreover, aspergillicins A–E (**17–21**) exerted substantial activity with LD_{99} values ranging between 0.03 and 0.07 µM. Additionally, effective stimulation to HT-29 cancer cells differentiation was exerted by cyclo-(L-Trp- L-Tyr) (**30**). Furthermore, asperterrestide A (**38**) showed a potent cytotoxic effect versus U937 and MOLT4 human cancer; meanwhile, psychrophilin E (**50**), selectivity prohibited the proliferation of HCT116 (colon) cell line with an IC_{50} value of 28.5 mM. In addition, the cytotoxic effect of dictyonamide A (**70**) can be explained in virtue of its inhibitory effect on cyclin-dependent kinase 4 that showed IC_{50} value equals to 0.01 µM. Rostratins A–D (**77–80**) showed pronounced cytotoxic activity versus (HCT-116) the human colon carcinoma showing 20, 4.48, 1.6, and 34 nM as IC_{50} values, respectively. Moreover, microsporins A and B (**81–82**) exerted an effective cytotoxic effect versus human colon adenocarcinoma (HCT-116). Additionally, *Penicillium citrinum* represents a source of cytotoxic peptides in which compounds (**86–87**) exerted significant cytotoxic activity on MCF-7 and HCT115 cell lines showing IC_{50}s equal to 38 and 37 nM, respectively. Penicimutide (**88**) also showed an effective inhibitory effect on HeLa cells displaying 39.4% as an inhibition rate at 100 µg/mL (0.01 µM) approaching that of the positive control 5-fluorouracil which showed 41.4% at 100 µg/mL. Furthermore, gliocladine C (**97**) effectively inhibited HepG2 cells growth displaying IC_{50} value of 19.6 µM whereas, zygosporamide (**131**) which showed potent cytotoxic activity. Weak cytotoxic activities were exerted by sclerotide A (**31**), sclerotide B (**32**), cotteslosins A (**57**), and B (**58**), in addition to similanamide (**33**) which displayed weak cytotoxic activity versus MCF-7, A373, and NCI-H460 cancer cells. In addition, aspersymmetide A (**55**) showed weak cytotoxicity versus NCI-H292 as well as A431 cell lines at 10 µM; meanwhile, simplicilliumtide A (**107**), E (**111**), G (**113**), and H (**114**) exhibited weak cytotoxic effect versus either human leukemia HL-60 or K562 cell line.

Concerning the antimicrobial and antiviral activities, 23 peptides exerted pronounced activity, among which nine revealed a potent inhibitory effect on bacterial growth, three showed pronounced antifungal activity, whereas eleven exhibited promising antiviral activity. Pronounced antibacterial activity was observed for RHM (**8**) and efrapeptin G (**6**) against *Staphylococcus epidermidis* with MIC values equal to 0.015 and 0.049 µM, respectively. In addition, lajollamide A (**69**) showed a mild antimicrobial effect against Gram-positive bacteria exerting 61% and 30% inhibition in bacterial growth for *Bacillus subtilis* and *Staphylococcus epidermidis* at 100 µM. Besides, unguisin A (**42**) and emericellamide B (**76**) showed considerable antibacterial activity against MRSA (methicillin resistant *Staphylococcus aureus* strains) with MIC values equal to 3.8 and 6.0 µM, respectively, whereas compound (**85**) isolated from *Penicillium citrinum* also showed pronounced antibacterial activity against *S. aureus* displaying 0.04 µM as MIC. However, the effective antimicrobial activity of *cis*-cyclo (Leucyl-Tyrosyl) (**101**) can be explained in virtue of its effective inhibitory effect on bacterial biofilm formation, which is estimated by 85%. Additionally, talaropeptides A–B (**127–128**), showed notable antibacterial activity against the growth of *Bacillus subtilis*, a Gram positive bacterium, displaying IC_{50} values of 1.5 and 3.7 µM, respectively. Noteworthy to highlight is that *Trichoderma* strains afforded large amounts of peptaibols which are characterized by being small antimicrobial peptides (AMPs) that are expected to contribute to the antimicrobial defense of *Trichoderma*. For the antifungal activity, sclerotide A (**31**), sclerotide B (**32**), and simplicilliumtide J (**116**) showed notable antifungal activity.

A considerable number of fungal peptides showed powerful antiviral activity exemplified by asperterrestide A (**38**) which exerted potent potential antiviral activity versus an influenza virus of H1N1 as well as H3N2 strains that could be relied upon the presence of a 3-OH-N-CH3-Phe moiety which is rare in nature. Moreover, aspergillipeptides D–G (**62–65**), showed a pronounced antiviral effect versus herpes simplex virus type 1 (HSV-1) displaying IC_{50} of 9.5 and 19.8 µM, respectively. Halovirs A–E (**102–106**) showed considerable in vitro antiviral activity against herpes simplex viruses of both type 1 and type 2 which is ultimately attributed to the presence of a N^α-acyl chain, comprising of at least 14 carbons as well as the Aib-Pro dipeptide. However, simplicilliumtide J (**116**) exerted a potent anti - HSV-1 displaying IC$_{50}$ value of 14.0 µM which could be interpreted in virtue of the presence of lactone linkage and a fatty acid chain moiety.

The anti-inflammatory activity of some of the isolated peptides can be explained via exerting different mechanisms where compounds (**60–61**) obtained from *Aspergillus* at 10 µM effectively inhibited IL-10 expression of the LPS-induced THP-1 cells showing 84.3% and 78.1% inhibition, respectively. Besides, 14-hydroxy-cyclopeptine (**66**) effectively inhibits nitric oxide production displaying IC$_{50}$ of 0.14 µM in recombinant mouse interferon-γ -activated macrophage-like cell line.

Antidiabetic and lipid lowering activity was also observed for some of the isolated fungal peptides, such as terrelumamides A (**34**) and B (**35**), which displayed a promising improvement in insulin sensitivity as determined by the utilization of mesenchymal cells of a bone marrow origin obtained from human adopting an adipogenesis model. Additionally, psychrophilin G (**52**) exhibited pronounced lipid-reducing activity.

Additionally, miscellaneous activities were reported for the isolated bioactive peptides in which Simplicilliumtide D (**110**) displayed a potent antifouling effect versus the larvae of *Bugula neritina*. Moreover, endolide A (**122**) revealed potent binding activity to the vasopressin receptor 1A displaying a Ki of 7.04 µM whereas endolide B (**123**) showed a pronounced binding to serotonin receptor 5HT2b evidenced by its Ki value which is 0.77 µM. Talaropeptide A (**126**) showed a high stability to various rat proteases existing in plasma, however, microsporins A and B (**81–82**) effectively inhibit histone deacetylase.

Noteworthy to mention is that about 47% of the isolated peptides showed no activity with respect to the examined biological activity and thus required further in depth biological assessment. A pie chart summarizing the percentages of isolated peptides with respect to their biological activity is represented in Figure 8.

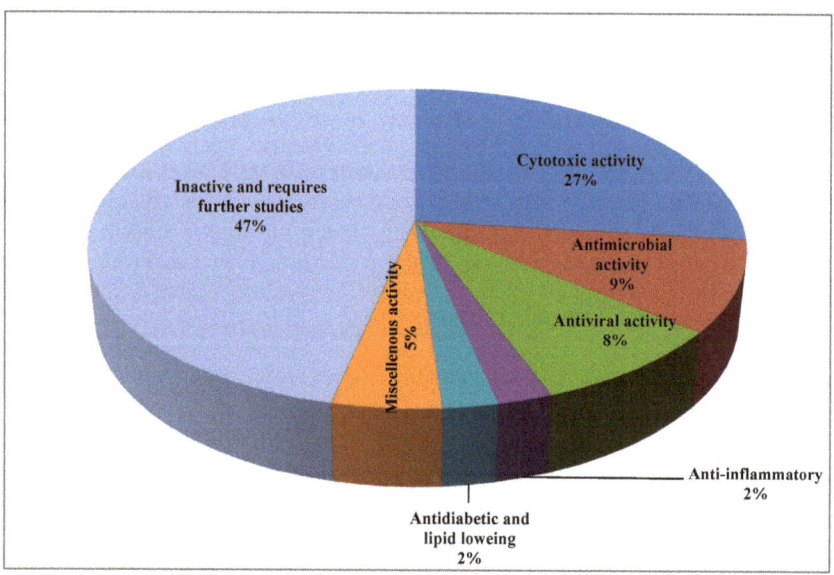

Figure 8. Percentages of isolated peptides with respect to their biological activity represented by a pie chart.

4. Conclusions

Herein, we concluded that about 131 peptides were isolated from marine sources from seventeen fungal strains. Some of them exhibited much biological activity represented mainly by cytotoxic, antimicrobial, and antiviral activity, meanwhile, few of them showed antidiabetic, lipid lowering, and anti-inflammatory activity; however, others should be deeply assessed for their biological potential. Thus, if active natural products are needed for drug development, further investigations of marine fungi are recommended. In addition, it is a challenge to explore more peptides from fungal origin and so it is recommended to confirm their biological activities.

Author Contributions: F.S.Y.; collection of data and writing the manuscript, M.L.A., A.N.B.S. and M.W.; revised the manuscript.

Funding: This research received no external funding.

Acknowledgments: The authors received financial support from the Deutsche Forschungsgemeinschaft and Ruprecht-Karls-Universität Heidelberg within the funding program Open Access Publishing. Also, the authors Fadia S. Youssef and Abdel Nasser B. Singab acknowledge Egyptian Science and Technology Development Funds (STDF) for its financial support through grant No. NCP 25927 entitled "Drug discovery of new anti-infective and anticancer agents from marine organisms and their associated micro-organisms".

Conflicts of Interest: The authors declare no conflict of interest.

References

1. Jin, L.; Quan, C.; Hou, X.; Fan, S. Potential pharmacological resources: Natural bioactive compounds from marine-derived fungi. *Mar. Drugs* **2016**, *14*, 76. [CrossRef] [PubMed]
2. Rateb, M.E.; Ebel, R. Secondary metabolites of fungi from marine habitats. *Nat. Prod. Rep.* **2011**, *28*, 290–344. [CrossRef] [PubMed]
3. Schueffler, A.; Anke, T. Fungal natural products in research and development. *Nat. Prod. Rep.* **2014**, *31*, 1425–1448. [CrossRef] [PubMed]
4. Blunt, J.W.; Copp, B.R.; Keyzers, R.A.; Munro, M.H.; Prinsep, M.R. Marine natural products. *Nat. Prod. Rep.* **2015**, *32*, 116–211. [CrossRef] [PubMed]
5. Blunt, J.W.; Copp, B.R.; Keyzers, R.A.; Munro, M.H.; Prinsep, M.R. Marine natural products. *Nat. Prod. Rep.* **2017**, *34*, 235–294. [CrossRef] [PubMed]
6. Kang, H.K.; Lee, H.H.; Seo, C.H.; Park, Y. Antimicrobial and immunomodulatory properties and applications of marine-derived proteins and peptides. *Mar. Drugs* **2019**, *17*, 350. [CrossRef] [PubMed]
7. Saleem, M.; Ali, M.S.; Hussain, S.; Jabbar, A.; Ashraf, M.; Lee, Y.S. Marine natural products of fungal origin. *Nat. Prod. Rep.* **2007**, *24*, 1142–1152. [CrossRef]
8. Sable, R.; Parajuli, P.; Jois, S. Peptides, peptidomimetics, and polypeptides from marine sources: A wealth of natural sources for pharmaceutical applications. *Mar. Drugs* **2017**, *15*, 124. [CrossRef] [PubMed]
9. Abdel-Wahab, N.M.; Harwoko, H.; Müller, W.E.; Hamacher, A.; Kassack, M.U.; Fouad, M.A.; Kamel, M.S.; Lin, W.; Ebrahim, W.; Liu, Z. Cyclic heptapeptides from the soil-derived fungus Clonostachys rosea. *Bioorg. Med. Chem.* **2019**, *27*, 3954–3959. [CrossRef]
10. Liang, X.; Nong, X.-H.; Huang, Z.-H.; Qi, S.-H. Antifungal and antiviral cyclic peptides from the deep-sea-derived fungus *Simplicillium obclavatum* EIODSF 020. *J. Agric. Food Chem.* **2017**, *65*, 5114–5121. [CrossRef]
11. Capon, R.J.; Skene, C.; Stewart, M.; Ford, J.; Richard, A.; Williams, L.; Lacey, E.; Gill, J.H.; Heiland, K.; Friedel, T. Aspergillicins A–E: Five novel depsipeptides from the marine-derived fungus *Aspergillus carneus*. *Org. Biomol. Chem.* **2003**, *1*, 1856–1862. [CrossRef]
12. Chen, Z.; Song, Y.; Chen, Y.; Huang, H.; Zhang, W.; Ju, J. Cyclic heptapeptides, cordyheptapeptides C–E, from the marine-derived fungus *Acremonium persicinum* SCSIO 115 and their cytotoxic activities. *J. Nat. Prod.* **2012**, *75*, 1215–1219. [CrossRef]
13. Boot, C.M.; Tenney, K.; Valeriote, F.A.; Crews, P. Highly N-methylated linear peptides produced by an atypical sponge-derived *Acremonium* sp. *J. Nat. Prod.* **2006**, *69*, 83–92. [CrossRef]

14. Boot, C.M.; Amagata, T.; Tenney, K.; Compton, J.E.; Pietraszkiewicz, H.; Valeriote, F.A.; Crews, P. Four classes of structurally unusual peptides from two marine-derived fungi: Structures and bioactivities. *Tetrahedron.* **2007**, *63*, 9903–9914. [CrossRef] [PubMed]
15. Xie, L.-R.; Li, D.-Y.; Wang, P.-L.; Hua, H.-M.; Wu, X.; Li, Z.-L. A new 3, 4-seco-lanostane triterpenoid from a marine-derived fungus *Ascotricha* sp. ZJ-M-5. *Acta Pharm. Sin.* **2013**, *48*, 89–93.
16. Uchoa, P.K.S.; Pimenta, A.T.; Braz-Filho, R.; de Oliveira, M.d.C.F.; Saraiva, N.N.; Rodrigues, B.S.; Pfenning, L.H.; Abreu, L.M.; Wilke, D.V.; Florêncio, K.G. New cytotoxic furan from the marine sediment-derived fungi *Aspergillus niger*. *Nat. Prod. Rep.* **2017**, *31*, 2599–2603. [CrossRef] [PubMed]
17. Zhang, Y.; Li, X.-M.; Feng, Y.; Wang, B.-G. Phenethyl-α-pyrone derivatives and cyclodipeptides from a marine algous endophytic fungus *Aspergillus niger* EN–13. *Nat. Prod. Rep.* **2010**, *24*, 1036–1043. [CrossRef] [PubMed]
18. Zheng, J.; Zhu, H.; Hong, K.; Wang, Y.; Liu, P.; Wang, X.; Peng, X.; Zhu, W. Novel cyclic hexapeptides from marine-derived fungus, *Aspergillus sclerotiorum* PT06-1. *Org. Lett.* **2009**, *11*, 5262–5265. [CrossRef] [PubMed]
19. Prompanya, C.; Fernandes, C.; Cravo, S.; Pinto, M.; Dethoup, T.; Silva, A.; Kijjoa, A. A new cyclic hexapeptide and a new isocoumarin derivative from the marine sponge-associated fungus *Aspergillus similanensis* KUFA 0013. *Mar. Drugs* **2015**, *13*, 1432–1450. [CrossRef] [PubMed]
20. You, M.; Liao, L.; Hong, S.; Park, W.; Kwon, D.; Lee, J.; Noh, M.; Oh, D.-C.; Oh, K.-B.; Shin, J. Lumazine peptides from the marine-derived fungus *Aspergillus terreus*. *Mar. Drugs* **2015**, *13*, 1290–1303. [CrossRef] [PubMed]
21. Luo, X.-W.; Lin, Y.; Lu, Y.-J.; Zhou, X.-F.; Liu, Y.-H. Peptides and polyketides isolated from the marine sponge-derived fungus *Aspergillus terreus* SCSIO 41008. *Chin. J. Nat. Med.* **2019**, *17*, 149–154. [CrossRef]
22. He, F.; Bao, J.; Zhang, X.-Y.; Tu, Z.-C.; Shi, Y.-M.; Qi, S.-H. Asperterrestide A, a cytotoxic cyclic tetrapeptide from the marine-derived fungus *Aspergillus terreus* SCSGAF0162. *J. Nat. Prod.* **2013**, *76*, 1182–1186. [CrossRef] [PubMed]
23. Yang, W.-C.; Bao, H.-Y.; Liu, Y.-Y.; Nie, Y.-Y.; Yang, J.-M.; Hong, P.-Z.; Zhang, Y. Depsidone Derivatives and a cyclopeptide produced by marine fungus *Aspergillus unguis* under chemical induction and by its plasma induced mutant. *Molecules* **2018**, *23*, 2245. [CrossRef] [PubMed]
24. Capon, R.J.; Ratnayake, R.; Stewart, M.; Lacey, E.; Tennant, S.; Gill, J.H. Aspergillazines A–E: Novel heterocyclic dipeptides from an Australian strain of *Aspergillus unilateralis*. *Org. Biomol. Chem.* **2005**, *3*, 123–129. [CrossRef]
25. Peng, J.; Gao, H.; Zhang, X.; Wang, S.; Wu, C.; Gu, Q.; Guo, P.; Zhu, T.; Li, D. Psychrophilins E–H and versicotide C, cyclic peptides from the marine-derived fungus *Aspergillus versicolor* ZLN-60. *J. Nat. Prod.* **2014**, *77*, 2218–2223. [CrossRef] [PubMed]
26. Hou, X.-M.; Zhang, Y.-H.; Hai, Y.; Zheng, J.-Y.; Gu, Y.-C.; Wang, C.-Y.; Shao, C.-L. Aspersymmetide A, a new centrosymmetric cyclohexapeptide from the marine-derived fungus *Aspergillus versicolor*. *Mar. Drugs* **2017**, *15*, 363. [CrossRef] [PubMed]
27. Fremlin, L.J.; Piggott, A.M.; Lacey, E.; Capon, R.J. Cottoquinazoline A and cotteslosins A and B, metabolites from an Australian marine-derived strain of *Aspergillus versicolor*. *J. Nat. Prod.* **2009**, *72*, 666–670. [CrossRef] [PubMed]
28. Liu, J.; Gu, B.; Yang, L.; Yang, F.; Lin, H. New anti-inflammatory cyclopeptides from a sponge-derived fungus *Aspergillus violaceofuscus*. *Front. Chem.* **2018**, *6*, 226. [CrossRef] [PubMed]
29. Ebada, S.S.; Fischer, T.; Hamacher, A.; Du, F.-Y.; Roth, Y.O.; Kassack, M.U.; Wang, B.-G.; Roth, E.H. Psychrophilin E, a new cyclotripeptide, from co-fermentation of two marine alga-derived fungi of the genus Aspergillus. *Nat. Prod. Res.* **2014**, *28*, 776–781. [CrossRef]
30. Ma, X.; Nong, X.-H.; Ren, Z.; Wang, J.; Liang, X.; Wang, L.; Qi, S.-H. Antiviral peptides from marine gorgonian-derived fungus Aspergillus sp. SCSIO 41501. *Tetrahedron Lett.* **2017**, *58*, 1151–1155. [CrossRef]
31. Zhou, X.; Fang, P.; Tang, J.; Wu, Z.; Li, X.; Li, S.; Wang, Y.; Liu, G.; He, Z.; Gou, D. A novel cyclic dipeptide from deep marine-derived fungus Aspergillus sp. SCSIOW2. *Nat. Prod. Res.* **2016**, *30*, 52–57. [CrossRef]
32. Zheng, C.J.; Wu, L.Y.; Li, X.B.; Song, X.M.; Niu, Z.G.; Song, X.P.; Chen, G.Y.; Wang, C.Y. Structure and Absolute Configuration of Aspergilumamide A, a novel lumazine peptide from the mangrove-derived fungus Aspergillus sp. *Helv. Chim. Acta.* **2015**, *98*, 368–373. [CrossRef]
33. Gulder, T.; Hong, H.; Correa, J.; Egereva, E.; Wiese, J.; Imhoff, J.; Gross, H. Isolation, structure elucidation and total synthesis of lajollamide A from the marine fungus *Asteromyces cruciatus*. *Mar. Drugs* **2012**, *10*, 2912–2935. [CrossRef]

34. Komatsu, K.; Shigemori, H.; Kobayashi, J.i. Dictyonamides A and B, new peptides from marine-derived fungus. *J. Org. Chem.* **2001**, *66*, 6189–6192. [CrossRef]
35. Adachi, K.; Kanoh, K.; Wisespongp, P.; Nishijima, M.; Shizuri, Y. Clonostachysins A and B, new anti-dinoflagellate cyclic peptides from a marine-derived fungus. *J. Antibiot.* **2005**, *58*, 145. [CrossRef]
36. Malmstrøm, J. Unguisins A and B: New cyclic peptides from the marine-derived fungus *Emericella unguis*. *J. Nat. Prod.* **1999**, *62*, 787–789. [CrossRef]
37. Oh, D.-C.; Kauffman, C.A.; Jensen, P.R.; Fenical, W. Induced production of emericellamides A and B from the marine-derived fungus *Emericella* sp. in competing co-culture. *J. Nat. Prod.* **2007**, *70*, 515–520. [CrossRef] [PubMed]
38. Tan, R.X.; Jensen, P.R.; Williams, P.G.; Fenical, W. Isolation and structure assignments of rostratins A–D, cytotoxic disulfides produced by the marine-derived fungus *Exserohilum r ostratum*. *J. Nat. Prod.* **2004**, *67*, 1374–1382. [CrossRef] [PubMed]
39. Gu, W.; Cueto, M.; Jensen, P.R.; Fenical, W.; Silverman, R.B. Microsporins A and B: New histone deacetylase inhibitors from the marine-derived fungus *Microsporum* cf. *gypseum* and the solid-phase synthesis of microsporin A. *Tetrahedron* **2007**, *63*, 6535–6541. [CrossRef]
40. Wang, N.; Cui, C.-B.; Li, C.-W. A new cyclic dipeptide penicimutide: The activated production of cyclic dipeptides by introduction of neomycin-resistance in the marine-derived fungus *Penicillium purpurogenum* G59. *Arch. Pharm. Res.* **2016**, *39*, 762–770. [CrossRef] [PubMed]
41. Meyer, S.W.; Mordhorst, T.F.; Lee, C.; Jensen, P.R.; Fenical, W.; Köck, M. Penilumamide, a novel lumazine peptide isolated from the marine-derived fungus, *Penicillium* sp. CNL-338. *Org. Biomol. Chem.* **2010**, *8*, 2158–2163. [CrossRef] [PubMed]
42. Hong, R.; Yang, Y. Antitumor metabolites from marine sediment derived *Penicillium* sp. WF-06. *World Notes Antibiots* **2011**, *2*.
43. Scopel, M.; Abraham, W.-R.; Henriques, A.T.; Macedo, A.J. Dipeptide cis-cyclo (Leucyl-Tyrosyl) produced by sponge associated Penicillium sp. F37 inhibits biofilm formation of the pathogenic Staphylococcus epidermidis. *Bioorg. Med. Chem. Lett.* **2013**, *23*, 624–626. [CrossRef]
44. Rowley, D.C.; Kelly, S.; Jensen, P.; Fenical, W. Synthesis and structure–activity relationships of the halovirs, antiviral natural products from a marine-derived fungus. *Bioorg. Med. Chem.* **2004**, *12*, 4929–4936. [CrossRef] [PubMed]
45. Rowley, D.C.; Kelly, S.; Kauffman, C.A.; Jensen, P.R.; Fenical, W. Halovirs A–E, new antiviral agents from a marine-derived fungus of the genus *Scytalidium*. *Bioorg. Med. Chem.* **2003**, *11*, 4263–4274. [CrossRef]
46. Liang, X.; Zhang, X.-Y.; Nong, X.-H.; Wang, J.; Huang, Z.-H.; Qi, S.-H. Eight linear peptides from the deep-sea-derived fungus *Simplicillium obclavatum* EIODSF 020. *Tetrahedron* **2016**, *72*, 3092–3097. [CrossRef]
47. El Maddah, F.; Kehraus, S.; Nazir, M.; Almeida, C.; König, G.M. Insights into the biosynthetic origin of 3-(3-furyl) alanine in *Stachylidium* sp. 293 K04 tetrapeptides. *J. Nat. Prod.* **2016**, *79*, 2838–2845. [CrossRef] [PubMed]
48. Almeida, C.; Maddah, F.E.; Kehraus, S.; Schnakenburg, G.; König, G.M. Endolides A and B, vasopressin and serotonin-receptor interacting N-methylated peptides from the sponge-derived fungus *Stachylidium* sp. *Organic letters.* **2016**, *18*, 528–531. [CrossRef]
49. Dewapriya, P.; Khalil, Z.G.; Prasad, P.; Salim, A.A.; Cruz-Morales, P.; Marcellin, E.; Capon, R.J. Talaropeptides AD: Structure and biosynthesis of extensively N-methylated linear peptides from an Australian marine tunicate-derived *Talaromyces* sp. *Front. Chem.* **2018**, *6*, 394. [CrossRef] [PubMed]
50. Van Bohemen, A.-I.; Zalouk-Vergnoux, A.; Poirier, L.; Phuong, N.N.; Inguimbert, N.; Salah, K.B.H.; Ruiz, N.; Pouchus, Y.F. Development and validation of LC–MS methods for peptaibol quantification in fungal extracts according to their lengths. *J. Chromatogr. B* **2016**, *1009*, 25–33. [CrossRef] [PubMed]
51. Herbel, V.; Wink, M. Mode of action and membrane specificity of the antimicrobial peptide snakin-2. *PeerJ* **2016**, *4*, e1987. [CrossRef] [PubMed]
52. Herbel, V.; Schäfer, H.; Wink, M. Recombinant production of snakin-2 (an antimicrobial peptide from tomato) in *E. coli* and analysis of its bioactivity. *Molecules* **2015**, *20*, 14889–14901. [CrossRef] [PubMed]
53. Fan, X.; Schäfer, H.; Reichling, J.; Wink, M. Bactericidal properties of the antimicrobial peptide Ib-AMP4 from *Impatiens balsamina* produced as a recombinant fusion-protein in *Escherichia coli*. *Biotechnol. J.* **2013**, *8*, 1213–1220.

54. Torres-García, C.; Pulido, D.; Albericio, F.; Royo, M.; Nicolás, E. Triazene as a powerful tool for solid-phase derivatization of phenylalanine containing peptides: *Zygosporamide* analogues as a proof of concept. *J. Org. Chem.* **2014**, *79*, 11409–11415. [CrossRef] [PubMed]
55. Oh, D.-C.; Jensen, P.R.; Fenical, W. Zygosporamide, a cytotoxic cyclic depsipeptide from the marine-derived fungus Zygosporium masonii. *Tetrahedron Lett.* **2006**, *47*, 8625–8628. [CrossRef]
56. Fosgerau, K.; Hoffmann, T. Peptide therapeutics: Current status and future directions. *Drug Discov. Today.* **2015**, *20*, 122–128. [CrossRef]

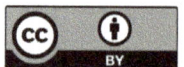

© 2019 by the authors. Licensee MDPI, Basel, Switzerland. This article is an open access article distributed under the terms and conditions of the Creative Commons Attribution (CC BY) license (http://creativecommons.org/licenses/by/4.0/).

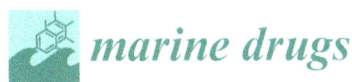

Article

Proteomic Analysis of the Venom of Jellyfishes *Rhopilema esculentum* and *Sanderia malayensis*

Thomas C. N. Leung [1,†], Zhe Qu [2,†], Wenyan Nong [2], Jerome H. L. Hui [2,*] and Sai Ming Ngai [1,*]

1. State Key Laboratory of Agrobiotechnology, School of Life Sciences, The Chinese University of Hong Kong, Hong Kong, China; chunningtleung@cuhk.edu.hk
2. Simon F.S. Li Marine Science Laboratory, State Key Laboratory of Agrobiotechnology, School of Life Sciences, The Chinese University of Hong Kong, Hong Kong, China; quzhe@cuhk.edu.hk (Z.Q.); nongwenyan@cuhk.edu.hk (W.N.)
* Correspondence: jeromehui@cuhk.edu.hk (J.H.L.H.); smngai@cuhk.edu.hk (S.M.N.)
† Contributed equally.

Received: 27 November 2020; Accepted: 17 December 2020; Published: 18 December 2020

Abstract: Venomics, the study of biological venoms, could potentially provide a new source of therapeutic compounds, yet information on the venoms from marine organisms, including cnidarians (sea anemones, corals, and jellyfish), is limited. This study identified the putative toxins of two species of jellyfish—edible jellyfish *Rhopilema esculentum* Kishinouye, 1891, also known as flame jellyfish, and Amuska jellyfish *Sanderia malayensis* Goette, 1886. Utilizing nano-flow liquid chromatography tandem mass spectrometry (nLC–MS/MS), 3000 proteins were identified from the nematocysts in each of the above two jellyfish species. Forty and fifty-one putative toxins were identified in *R. esculentum* and *S. malayensis*, respectively, which were further classified into eight toxin families according to their predicted functions. Amongst the identified putative toxins, hemostasis-impairing toxins and proteases were found to be the most dominant members (>60%). The present study demonstrates the first proteomes of nematocysts from two jellyfish species with economic and environmental importance, and expands the foundation and understanding of cnidarian toxins.

Keywords: jellyfish; *Rhopilema esculentum*; *Sanderia malayensis*; proteome; venom; toxin

---

1. Introduction

Phylum Cnidaria Hatschek, 1888, is one of the most ancient phyla that can be traced back to Cambrian [1]. This phylum is divided into five classes: Anthozoa Ehrenberg, 1834 (corals and sea anemones), Cubozoa Werner, 1973 (box jellyfish), Hydrozoa Owen, 1843, Scyphozoa Götte, 1887 (true jellyfish), and Staurozoa Marques & Collins, 2004 (stalked jellyfish) [2]. Approximately 12,000 extant species are known from freshwater and marine habitats worldwide, from shallow coastal waters to the deep seas [3,4]. Cnidarians are characterized by the presence of nematocytes, which constitute an important specialized cell type that assists prey capture and predator deterrence. Each nematocyte houses a unique organelle called the nematocyst. This Golgi apparatus-derived organelle consists of a capsule containing an inverted tubule immersed in a mixture of venomous substances [5]. Upon mechanical or chemical stimulation, the tubule everts and injects a venomous mixture into the prey or predator. Jellyfish possess nematocytes mainly on the tentacles [6]. The composition of the venom inside the nematocyst varies between different jellyfish species and may be a mixture of proteinaceous and non-proteinaceous toxins with hemolytic, neurotoxic, cytotoxic, and dermonecrotic activities [6]. Depending on the composition of the venom, the symptoms of jellyfish envenomation vary from species to species, ranging from mild local symptoms such as pruritus, pain, and burning sensation to serious manifestations, including hypotension, cardiac failure, respiratory distress, pulmonary edema, and even death [6–9].

Despite the potential hazard to health, evidence is accumulating for jellyfish venoms as promising sources of therapeutic agents. For example, peptide fractions of *Chrysaora quinquecirrha* Desor, 1848, venom have shown anticancer activities in an Ehrlich ascites carcinoma (EAC) tumor mouse model [10]. Similarly, *Nemopilema nomurai* Kishinouye, 1922, crude venom also exhibits anticancer activities in the HepG2 liver cancer cell line and HepG2 xenograft mouse models [11]. Furthermore, the crude venom of *Pelagia noctiluca* Forsskal, 1775, and its peptide fractions not only demonstrate anticancer activities in several cancer cell lines, but also show anti-inflammatory activities [12]. The protein components of *P. noctiluca* venom also exhibit analgesic functions in mouse models, and it has also been suggested that *P. noctiluca* venom is a promising source of neuroprotective drugs due to its plasma antibutyrylcholinestrasic activities [13]. However, the individual components that exhibit the therapeutic functions are not well characterized because the compositions of jellyfish venoms are not well studied, considering that of the 7235 animal toxins and venom proteins recorded in the Tox-Prot database, only six are derived from jellyfish (as of October 2020 [14]). This knowledge gap greatly hinders the discovery of potential drug candidates in jellyfish venom.

Recently, our group reported high-quality de novo reference genomes and transcriptomes for the edible jellyfish *Rhopilema esculentum* and the Amuska jellyfish *Sanderia malayensis*, as well as their transcriptomes [15]. Herein, we extend this study to identify the putative toxins in these two jellyfish species at the protein level. In this work, the venoms were enriched by isolating the nematocytes using the density gradient centrifugation technique. The nematocyte proteomes were determined by nano-flow liquid chromatography tandem mass spectrometry (nLC–MS/MS) and the putative toxins were identified by subsequent bioinformatic analysis.

This study provides the first insights into the venom proteomes of *R. esculentum* and *S. malayensis*, not only facilitating the screening, isolation, and characterization of their novel therapeutic compounds, but also providing clues to the evolutionary and ecological role of these toxins.

2. Results

2.1. Transcriptome and Protein Database Construction

Next-generation sequencing (NGS) was used to construct the *R. esculentum* appendages and the *S. malayensis* tentacle transcriptome followed by gene model predictions using funannotate [15]. Based on the results of transcriptomic analysis, the *R. esculentum* and *S. malayensis* protein databases were generated with 18,923 and 26,914 protein sequences, respectively. Gene Ontology (GO) analysis was performed by the eggNOG-mapper [16] and annotations were assigned to three primary GO domains: biological process (BP), cellular component (CC), and molecular function (MF). In total, 8786 (46.43%) *R. esculentum* proteins and 9138 (33.95%) *S. malayensis* proteins were successfully annotated with 143,350 and 153,009 GO terms, respectively (Table 1 and Figure 1A,B). In addition, 4187 and 4485 enzymes were identified in *R. esculentum* and *S. malayensis*, respectively, classified according to their Enzyme Commission (EC) number. The proportional distributions of the enzymes in both species were similar, which were dominated by transferases and hydrolases (Table 1 and Figure 2). Furthermore, to identify and annotate the putative toxins, the protein sequences generated were run against the UniProt animal venom proteins and toxins database (Tox-Prot) using BLASTp [17]. Protein sequences with an e-value of $<1.0 \times 10^{-5}$ to entries in the database were used as input into "ToxClassifier" to exclude non-toxic homologs [18]. A total of 190 and 186 putative toxins were found in *R. esculentum* and *S. malayensis*, respectively. The toxin profiles of both species were similar in which the toxins could be classified into eight toxin families: hemostasis-impairing toxins, proteases, phospholipases, neurotoxins, cysteine-rich proteins, protease inhibitors, pore-forming toxins, and other toxins (Tables S1 and S2).

Table 1. Description of the analysis of the protein databases generated from the *R. esculentum* and *S. malayensis* transcriptomes.

	R. esculentum	*S. malayensis*
Proteins sequences	18,923	26,914
Proteins sequences annotated with GO terms	8786	9138
GO terms	143,350	153,009
Biological process GO terms	80,786	24,533
Molecular function GO terms	22,970	41,992
Cellular component GO terms	39,612	86,484
Enzymes	4187	4485
Putative toxins	190	186

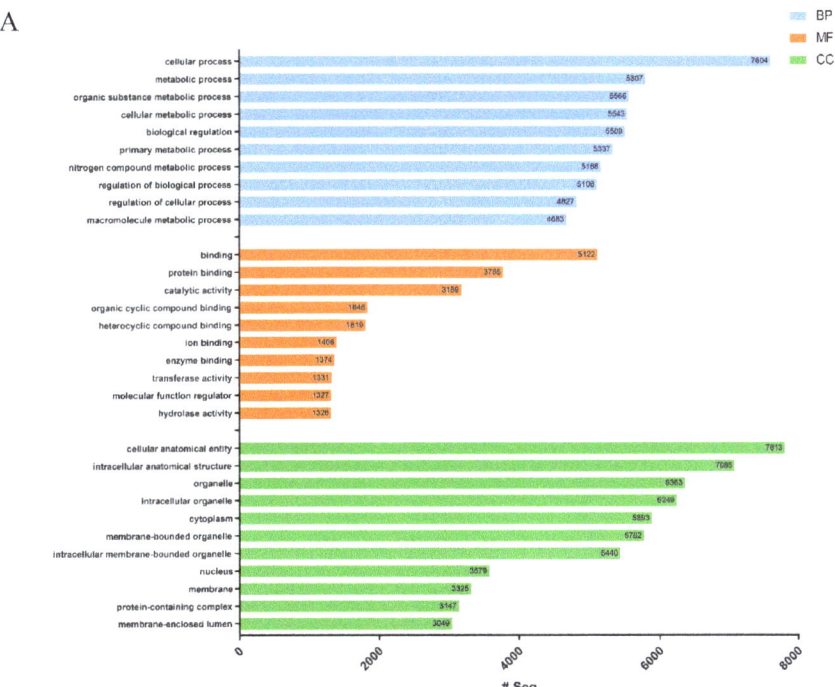

Figure 1. *Cont.*

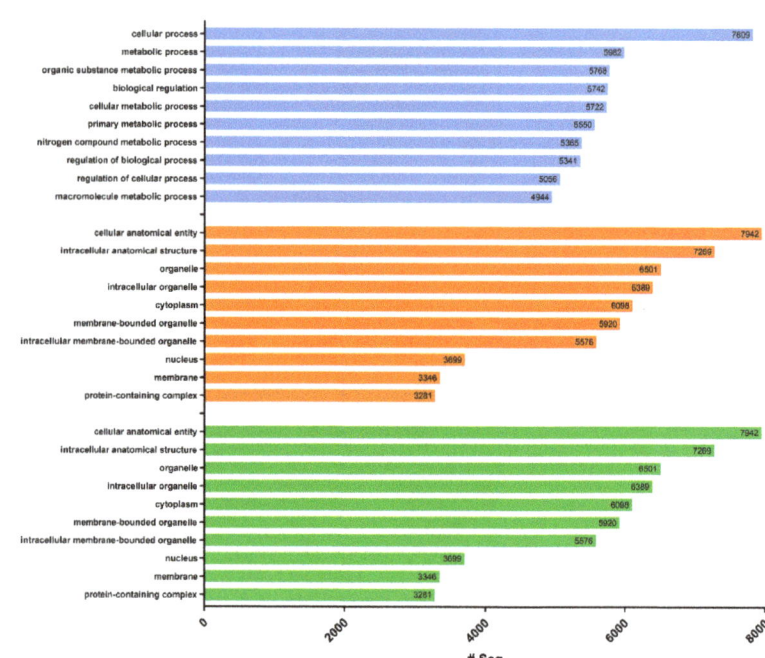

Figure 1. The 10 most represented Gene Oncology (GO) terms of the (**A**) *Rhopilema esculentum* and (**B**) *Sanderia malayensis* protein databases in the three domains of biological process (BP), molecular function (MF), and cellular component (CC) are presented.

2.2. Identification of R. esculentum and S. malayensis Nematocyst Proteins by nano-LC-ESI MS/MS

The nematocysts from *R. esculentum* and *S. malayensis* were purified and their protein profiles were revealed by proteomic analysis. A total of 3083 and 3559 proteins were identified in *R. esculentum* and *S. malayensis*, respectively (Tables S3 and S4), including 40 *R. esculentum* and 51 *S. malayensis* putative toxins. According to their predicted biological function, these toxins were classified into the eight toxin families (Table 2, Tables S5 and S6). The proportional distributions of these toxin families were also similar between the two species (Figure 3). Hemostasis-impairing toxins comprised the most abundant class of identified toxins, representing 32.5% and 39.2% of the *R. esculentum* and *S. malayensis* toxins, respectively, most of which were homologous to ryncolin, a family of proteinaceous toxins originally described from *Cerberus rynchops*. This family also includes a variety of C-type lectins (i.e., C-type lectin, C-type lectin lectoxin-Lio2, and galactose-specific lectin nattectin). In addition, other toxins such as prothrombin activator, coagulation factor V, coagulation factor X, and snaclec bothrojaracin subunit homologs were also identified in the proteome of both species.

Proteases comprised the second most predominant toxin family in both *R. esculentum* and *S. malayensis* proteome, accounting for 27.5% and 21.5% of the *R. esculentum* and *S. malayensis* putative toxins, respectively. Among this family, metalloproteinases were the most abundant. In the *R. esculentum* toxin proteome, three out of the seven metalloproteinases found were homologous to zinc metalloproteinase-disintegrin proteins. Meanwhile, a further two were neprilysin-1 homologs, another two were homologs of astacin-like metalloproteases. In the *S. malayensis* toxins, nine metalloproteinases were found, four of which were zinc metalloproteinase-disintegrin proteins. Four astacin-like metalloproteases and one neprilysin-1 were also detected.

Besides these two major classes of toxins, the *R. esculentum* and *S. malayensis* venoms also exhibited similar proportional distributions of other toxins. Meanwhile, L-amino-acid oxidase, acetylcholinesterase, and venom acid phosphatase were only found in *S. malayensis* venom, and U-actitoxin-Avd3j and calglandulin were only detected in *R. esculentum* venom.

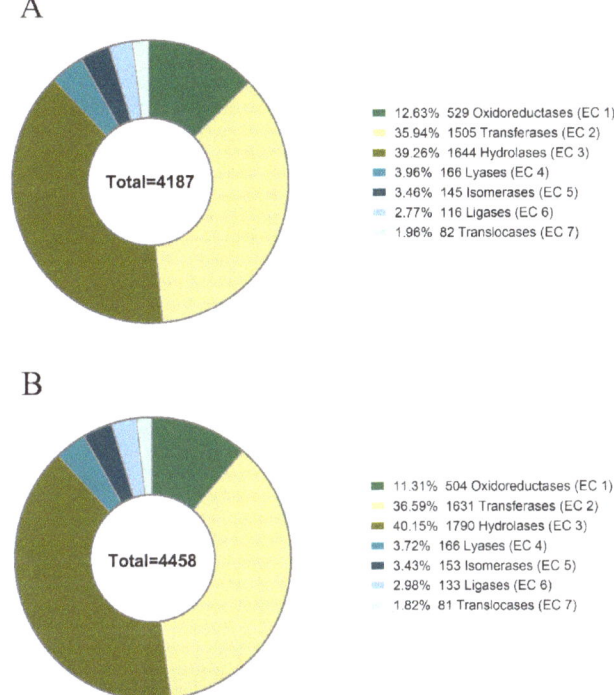

Figure 2. Distribution of the enzyme predicted by eggNOG-mapper in the protein databases of the (**A**) *R. esculentum* and (**B**) *S. malayensis* jellyfishes.

Table 2. Toxin families identified in each jellyfish species.

Toxin Family	R. esculentum		S. malayensis	
	UniProt Accession	Description	UniProt Accession	Description
Hemostasis-impairing toxins				
	A7X3Z7	C-type lectin lectoxin-Lio2 (CTL)	C6JUN9	C-type lectin (CTL)
	Q593B6	Coagulation factor V (cleaved into coagulation factor V heavy chain and coagulation factor V light chain)	Q593B6	Coagulation factor V (cleaved into coagulation factor V heavy chain and coagulation factor V light chain)
	Q66S03	Galactose-specific lectin nattectin (CTL)	Q4QXT9	Coagulation factor X (EC 3.4.21.6) (cleaved into factor X light chain, factor X heavy chain, and activated factor Xa heavy chain)
	D8VNS8	Ryncolin-2	Q66S03	Galactose-specific lectin nattectin (CTL)
	D8VNT0	Ryncolin-4	D8VNS8	Ryncolin-2
	P22030	Snaclec botrocetin subunit beta (platelet coagglutinin)	D8VNT0	Ryncolin-4
	Q7SZN0	Venom prothrombin activator pseutarin-C non-catalytic subunit (PCNS) (vPA) (venom coagulation factor Va-like protein) (cleaved into pseutarin-C non-catalytic subunit heavy chain and pseutarin-C non-catalytic subunit light chain)	Q56EB0	Snaclec bothrojaracin subunit beta (BJC subunit beta)
	A6MFK7	Venom prothrombin activator vestarin-D1 (vPA) (EC 3.4.21.6) (venom coagulation factor Xa-like protease) (cleaved into vestarin-D1 light chain and vestarin-D1 heavy chain)	Q58L90	Venom prothrombin activator omicarin-C non-catalytic subunit (vPA) (venom coagulation factor Va-like protein) (cleaved into omicarin-C non-catalytic subunit heavy chain and omicarin-C non-catalytic subunit light chain)
			Q58L91	Venom prothrombin activator oscutarin-C non-catalytic subunit (vPA) (venom coagulation factor Va-like protein) (cleaved into oscutarin-C non-catalytic subunit heavy chain and oscutarin-C non-catalytic subunit light chain)
			Q7SZN0	Venom prothrombin activator pseutarin-C non-catalytic subunit (PCNS) (vPA) (venom coagulation factor Va-like protein) (cleaved into pseutarin-C non-catalytic subunit heavy chain and pseutarin-C non-catalytic subunit light chain)
			A6MFK8	Venom prothrombin activator vestarin-D2 (vPA) (EC 3.4.21.6) (venom coagulation factor Xa-like protease) (cleaved into vestarin-D2 light chain and vestarin-D2 heavy chain)
Proteases				
	C9D7R2	Astacin-like metalloprotease toxin 2 (EC 3.4.24.-) (Loxosceles astacin-like protease 2) (LALP2)	A0FKN6	Astacin-like metalloprotease toxin 1 (EC 3.4.24.-) (Loxosceles astacin-like protease 1) (LALP1)
	Q76B45	Blarina toxin (BLTX) (EC 3.4.21.-)	P0DM62	Astacin-like metalloprotease toxin 5 (EC 3.4.24.-) (Loxosceles astacin-like protease 5) (LALP5) (Fragment)
	K7Z9Q9	Nematocyst-expressed protein 6 (NEP-6) (EC 3.4.24.-) (astacin-like metalloprotease toxin)	Q76B45	Blarina toxin (BLTX) (EC 3.4.21.-)
	W4VS99	Neprilysin-1 (EC 3.4.24.-)	K7Z9Q9	Nematocyst-expressed protein 6 (NEP-6) (EC 3.4.24.-) (astacin-like metalloprotease toxin)
	B2D0J4	Venom dipeptidyl peptidase 4 (allergen C) (venom dipeptidyl peptidase IV) (EC 3.4.14.5) (allergen Api m 5)	W4VS99	Neprilysin-1 (EC 3.4.24.-)
	Q7M413	Venom protease (EC 3.4.21.-) (allergen Bom p 4)	B2D0J4	Venom dipeptidyl peptidase 4 (allergen C) (venom dipeptidyl peptidase IV) (EC 3.4.14.5) (allergen Api m 5)
	C9WMM5	Venom serine carboxypeptidase (EC 3.4.16.5) (allergen Api m 9)	O73795	Zinc metalloproteinase/disintegrin (cleaved into snake venom metalloproteinase Mt-b (SVMP) (EC 3.4.24.-) and disintegrin
	J3S830	Zinc metalloproteinase-disintegrin-like 3a (EC 3.4.24.-) (snake venom metalloproteinase) (SVMP)	P20164	Zinc metalloproteinase-disintegrin-like HR1b (EC 3.4.24.-) (snake venom metalloproteinase) (SVMP) (trimerelysin I) (trimerelysin-1) (cleaved into disintegrin-like 1b)

Table 2. Cont.

Toxin Family	R. esculentum		S. malayensis	
	UniProt Accession	Description	UniProt Accession	Description
	F8RKW0	Zinc metalloproteinase-disintegrin-like MTP8 (EC 3.4.24.-) (snake venom metalloproteinase) (SVMP)	A8QL59	Zinc metalloproteinase-disintegrin-like NaMP (EC 3.4.24.-) (snake venom metalloproteinase) (SVMP)
	Q2LD49	Zinc metalloproteinase-disintegrin-like TSV-DM (EC 3.4.24.-) (snake venom metalloproteinase) (SVMP)		
Phospholipase				
	P80003	Acidic phospholipase A2 PA4 (PLA2) (EC 3.1.1.4) (phosphatidylcholine 2-acylhydrolase) (cleaved into acidic phospholipase A2 PA2)	P80003	Acidic phospholipase A2 PA4 (PLA2) (EC 3.1.1.4) (phosphatidylcholine 2-acylhydrolase) (cleaved into acidic phospholipase A2 PA2)
	P16354	Phospholipase A2 isozymes PA3A/PA3B/PA5 (PLA2) (EC 3.1.1.4) (phosphatidylcholine 2-acylhydrolase)	I7CQA7	Phospholipase A2 (EC 3.1.1.4) (phosphatidylcholine 2-acylhydrolase)
			P16354	Phospholipase A2 isozymes PA3A/PA3B/PA5 (PLA2) (EC 3.1.1.4) (phosphatidylcholine 2-acylhydrolase)
Protease inhibitors				
	B1PIJ3	Cystatin-1 (cystatin JZTX-75)	J3RYX9	Cystatin-1
	P0C8W3	Kunitz-type serine protease inhibitor Hg1 (delta-KTx 1.1)	Q6T269	Kunitz-type serine protease inhibitor bitisilin-3 (two-Kunitz protease inhibitor) (fragment)
			W4VSH9	Kunitz-type U19-barytoxin-Tl1a (U19-BATX-Tl1a) (Kunitz-type serine protease inhibitor Kunitz-1)
Pore-forming toxins				
	Q91453	Stonustoxin subunit beta (SNTX subunit beta) (DELTA-synanceitoxin-Sh1b) (DELTA-SYTX-Sh1b) (trachynilysin subunit beta) (TLY subunit beta)	A0Z5K4	Neoverrucotoxin subunit beta (NeoVTX subunit beta)
Cysteine-rich proteins				
	Q3SB07	Cysteine-rich venom protein pseudechetoxin-like (CRVP)	A6MFK9	Cysteine-rich venom protein (CRVP) (cysteine-rich secretory protein) (CRISP)
	Q8AVA3	Cysteine-rich venom protein pseudecin (CRVP Pdc)	P81656	Venom allergen 5 (antigen 5) (Ag5) (cysteine-rich venom protein) (CRVP) (allergen Pol d 5)
Neurotoxins				
	Q25338	Delta-latroinsectotoxin-Lt1a (delta-LIT-Lt1a) (delta-latroinsectotoxin) (delta-LIT)	G0LXV8	Alpha-latrotoxin-Lh1a (Alpha-LITX-Lh1a) (alpha-latrotoxin) (fragment)
Other toxins				
	Q8AY75	Calglandulin	Q92035	Acetylcholinesterase (BfAChE) (EC 3.1.1.7)
	A7ISW2	Glutaminyl-peptide cyclotransferase (EC 2.3.2.5) (glutaminyl cyclase) (QC) (glutaminyl-tRNA cyclotransferase)	A7ISW1	Glutaminyl-peptide cyclotransferase (EC 2.3.2.5) (glutaminyl cyclase) (QC) (glutaminyl-tRNA cyclotransferase)
	Q75WF2	Plancitoxin-1 (EC 3.1.22.1) (plancitoxin I) (plan-I) (cleaved into plancitoxin-1 subunit alpha and plancitoxin-1 subunit beta)	J3S820	Hyaluronidase (EC 3.2.1.35) (hyaluronoglucosaminidase) (venom-spreading factor)
	J3S9D9	Reticulocalbin-2 (taipoxin-associated calcium-binding protein 49 homolog)	A8QL51	L-amino-acid oxidase (Bm-LAAO) (LAO) (EC 1.4.3.2)
	M5B4R7	Translationally controlled tumor protein homolog (GTx-TCTP1)	Q75WF2	Plancitoxin-1 (EC 3.1.22.1) (plancitoxin I) (plan-I) (cleaved into plancitoxin-1 subunit alpha and plancitoxin-1 subunit beta)
	P0DN11	U-actitoxin-Avd3j (U-AITX-Avd3j) (AsKC7)	J3S9D9	Reticulocalbin-2 (taipoxin-associated calcium-binding protein 49 homolog)
			M5B4R7	Translationally controlled tumor protein homolog (GTx-TCTP1)
			Q5BLY5	Venom acid phosphatase Acph-1 (EC 3.1.3.2) (allergen Api m 3)

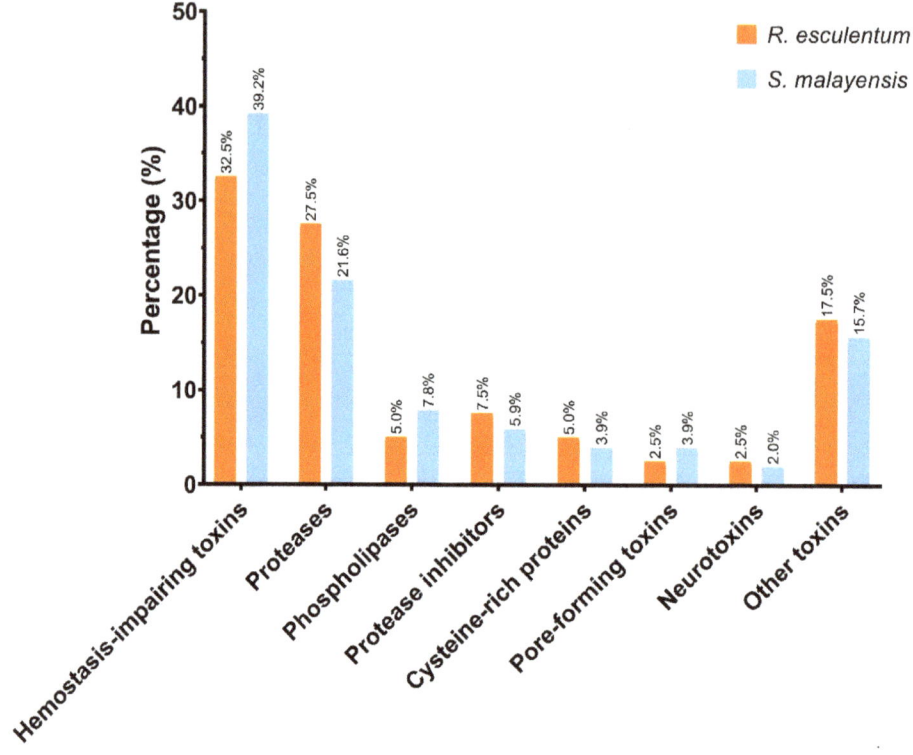

Figure 3. Graphical overview of the distribution of the toxin families identified in the *R. esculentum* and *S. malayensis* proteomes.

2.3. Functional Analysis of the Putative Toxins

A total of 282 and 408 GO terms were assigned to 20 (50%) *R. esculentum* and 27 (54.9%) *S. malayensis* putative toxins, respectively (Tables S3 and S4). The 10 most represented GO terms in the three domains of biological process (BP), cellular component (CC), and molecular function (MF) are shown in Figure 4. Furthermore, the presence of signal peptides was predicted by SignalP, showing that 52.5% and 29.4% of the *R. esculentum* and *S. malayensis* putative toxins contain secretory signal peptides, respectively. Moreover, DeepLoc analysis indicated that 52.5% and 54.9% of the putative toxins were located in the extracellular region. Taken together, there 75% of the putative toxins in *R. esculentum* and 62.7% in *S. malayensis* were predicted as extracellular proteins (by SignalP and/or DeepLoc). Additionally, 16 and 20 enzymes were identified in the *R. esculentum* and *S. malayensis* putative toxins. In both species, hydrolase (EC 3) was the predominant enzyme (13 and 16 of *R. esculentum* and *S. malayensis* putative toxins, respectively; Figure 5A,C), the majority of which was comprised by esterase (EC3.1) and peptidase (EC 3.4) (Figure 5B,D).

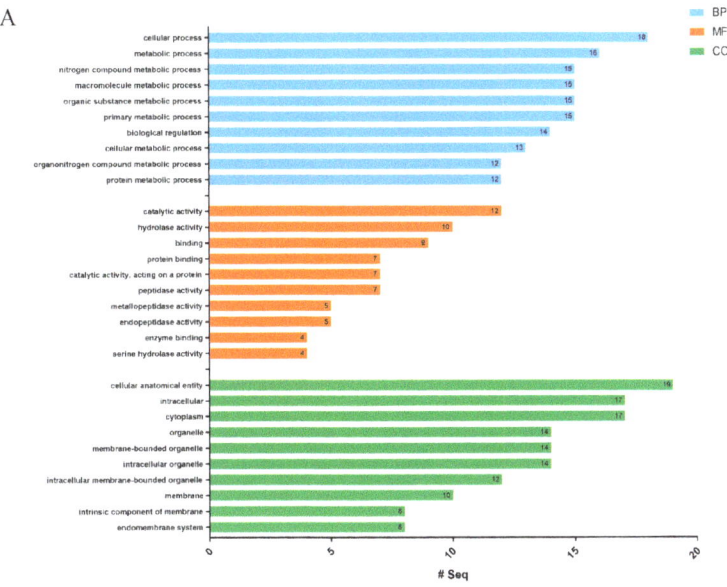

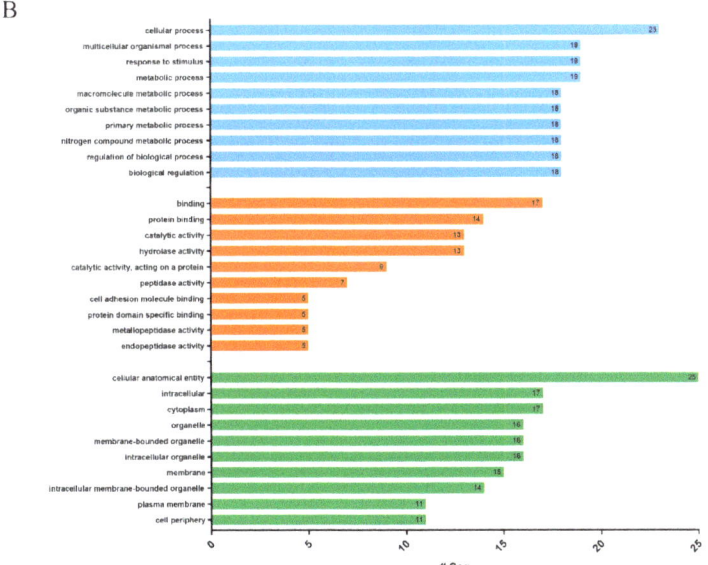

Figure 4. The 10 most represented GO terms of the (**A**) *R. esculentum* and (**B**) *S. malayensis* potential toxins in the three domains of biological process (BP), molecular function (MF), and cellular component (CC) are presented.

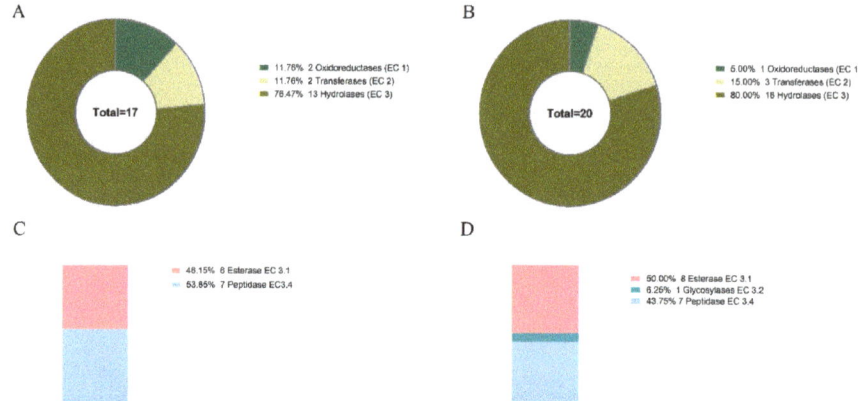

Figure 5. Distribution of the enzymes predicted by eggNOG-mapper in the putative toxins of (**A**) *R. esculentum* and (**B**) *S. malayensis* and the proportional distribution of the hydrolase subclass in (**C**) *R. esculentum* and (**D**) *S. malayensis*.

2.4. InterProScan Analysis

The protein domains of the putative toxins were annotated by InterProScan. A total of 47 and 55 protein domains were assigned to the *R. esculentum* and *S. malayensis* putative toxins, respectively (Tables S7 and S8). The top ten most represented domains are shown in Figure 6. In general, the results agreed with the BLASTp-ToxClassifier results. Two domains related to hemostasis were found, namely, fibrinogen, alpha/beta/gamma chain, C-terminal globular domain, and coagulation factor 5/8 C-terminal domain, the former being highly represented in both species. Although there were no predominant single protease-related domains, a variety of protease-related domains (peptidase M12B, peptidase M12A, astacin-like metallopeptidase domain, serine proteases/trypsin domain, and disintegrin domain) were found. Furthermore, the domains related to cysteine-rich proteins (CAP domain and SCP domain), the C-type lectin-like domain, and the phospholipase A2 domain were screened in both species. In addition, the ShKT domain and the Kunitz domain, the protein domains with high potential therapeutic value, were also detected in the putative toxins of both species. A total of three and six ShKT domain-containing proteins were identified in the *R. esculentum* and *S. malayensis* putative toxins, respectively, most (seven out of nine) of which were protease-type toxins. In these ShKT domain-containing proteases, the ShKT domain is either associated with the trypsin domain or the peptidase_M12A domain (a metalloproteases domain). Although the sequence of the ShKT domain found in trypsin was slightly different form that of metalloproteases, both of them were characterized by the typical pattern of six cysteines, except the second ShKT domain of Sma_022066-T1 (Sma_022066-T1_M12_ShKT_2), which lacked the fifth cysteine residue of the motif (Figure 7A,B). Furthermore, a total of five Kunitz domains were detected in four protease inhibitor-type putative toxins, with Sma_015170-T1 containing two domains. Most of the detected Kunitz domains displayed the conserved motif of C-8X-C-15X-C-4X-YGGC-12X-C-3X-C. The only exception was the Kunitz domains of Sma_021821-T1, which deviated from the conserved architecture by a Y31F substitution (Figure 7C).

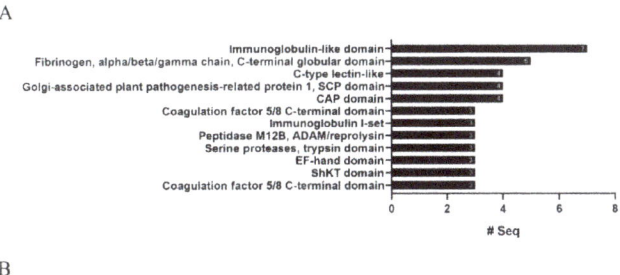

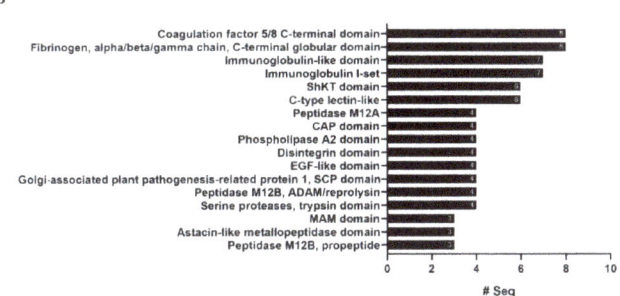

Figure 6. The highly represented protein domains of the (**A**) *R. esculentum* and (**B**) *S. malayensis* putative toxins. The number of proteins that contain the protein domain is labeled at the end of the column.

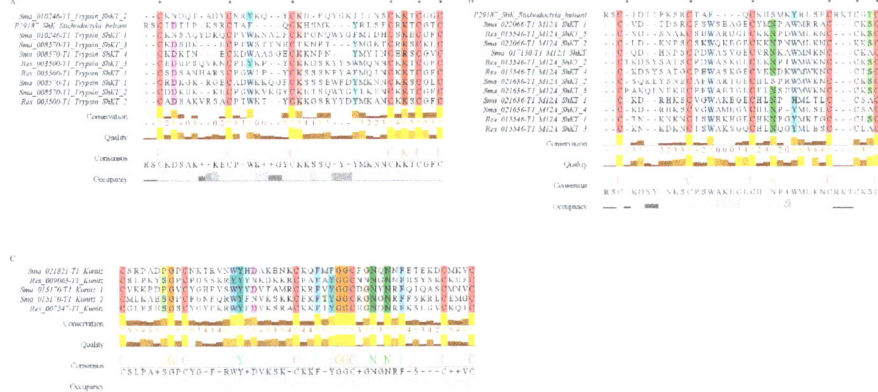

Figure 7. (**A**) Multiple sequence alignment of the ShKT domains from the trypsin toxins and the full length of Kappa-stichotoxin-She3a (ShK) from Sun anemone *Stichodactyla helianthus* (UniProt accession: P29187). (**B**) Multiple sequence alignment of the ShKT domains from the metalloproteases toxins and the full length of ShK (UniProt accession: P29187). (**C**) Multiple sequence alignment of the Kunitz domains. The conserved cysteine residue ShKT domains are labeled by an asterisk; the sequence consensus is indicated by the logo under the alignment.

3. Discussion

Animal venoms comprise a mixture of bioactive molecules that include different types of toxic proteins. Most of these proteinaceous toxins arise from gene duplication and contain a non-toxic physiological function [19,20]. Owing to this nature of proteinaceous toxins, it is difficult to distinguish between toxic proteins and their non-toxic homologs using BLAST alone. Therefore, most studies based on identifying toxic proteins apply different manual filters to filter out the non-toxic homologs, which may lead to problems in verifying the results. In this study, the protein sequences obtained from proteomic analysis were compared against the UniProt animal venom proteins and toxins database (Tox-Prot) using BLASTp. After that, ToxClassifier, a machine learning model, was used to differentiate toxins from other proteins having non-toxic physiological functions [18]. By using this approach, 190 and 186 putative toxins were predicted from R. esculentum and S. malayensis transcriptomic data, respectively (Table 1). Furthermore, 40 R. esculentum and 51 S. malayensis putative toxins were identified at the protein level (Table 2).

Hemostasis-impairing toxins were the most predominant toxin family of both the R. esculentum and S. malayensis venom proteomes. Most of the toxins in this family share sequence similarity with ryncolins, a group of hemostasis-impairing toxins originally described from C. rynchops [21]. Ryncolin genes [22], transcripts, and proteins [23–26] have also been found in other species of jellyfish, but their functions are not well-characterized. C-type lectins, another major group of hemostasis-impairing toxins, are commonly found in the venoms of a wide variety of animals [27–30], including several jellyfish species: Pacific sea nettle Chrysaora fuscescens [31], Lion's mane jellyfish Cyanea capillata, Nomura's jellyfish N. nomurai [26], and cannonball jellyfish Stomolophus meleagris [23]. C-type lectins are calcium-dependent carbohydrate-binding proteins that exhibit pro/anticoagulant, and pro/antithrombotic activities. This type of toxin is also involved in pain and itch sensitization through Toll-like receptors [32]. Therefore, the C-type lectins in R. esculentum and S. malayensis venom might explain the pruritus and pain caused by the sting.

The prediction of eggNOG-mapper revealed that protease was the most abundant enzyme in the venoms of both species (Figure 5). Consistent with the prediction, 11 proteases were identified as putative toxins in both the R. esculentum and S. malayensis venoms, which comprise the second most abundant class of toxins. In the venoms of both species, metalloproteases were the predominant proteases. Mainly, they were homologous to zinc metalloproteinase-disintegrin-like and astacin-like metalloprotease, which were also identified in the proteome of the venom of other cnidarians, including Lion's mane jellyfish C. capillata [26], sea wasp Chironex fleckeri [33], Pacific sea nettle C. fuscescens [31], ghost jellyfish Cyanea nozakii [34], Cyanea sp. [25], Nomura's jellyfish N. nomurai [24,26], cannonball jellyfish S. Meleagris [23], and starlet sea anemone Nematostella vectensis [35]. It has been suggested that metalloprotease induces protease-mediated tissue damage by the degradation of the extracellular matrix, which eventually results in necrosis, edema, and hemorrhage [36]. Correspondingly, the skin and tissue necrosis caused by S. malayensis envenomation [9] are most likely associated with the highly represented metalloproteases in its venom. In addition, our results are also in agreement with another study, which demonstrated significant metalloprotease activity in R. esculentum venom [36].

Other than metalloproteases, several serine proteases and serine carboxypeptidases were also identified in the venom proteomes. The presence of proteases has also been reported in the venom of several jellyfish species [24–26,31,33]. The functional role of proteases in jellyfish venom is not well understood; while based on observations in other venomous animals, we suggest that the proteases in the venom may be responsible for promoting the spreading and activation of other toxins [37,38].

In addition to these two predominated toxin families, other toxins were also identified. Phospholipases, for example, were identified in the venom proteomes of both species, all of which were phospholipases A2 (PLA2s) with two and four copies of PLA2s in R. esculentum and S. malayensis venom, respectively. PLA2s has also been found in the venom of various other jellyfish species [23–26,31,33,34,39,40], and the PLA2 activity has been detected in the oral arm of R. esculentum [41]. PLA2s are considered hemolysin in jellyfish venom [42]; thus, we suspect that the presence of PLA2s in R. esculentum venom might be associated with its hemolytic activities reported previously [43]. Meanwhile, more experiments are required to investigate whether S. malayensis also exhibits PLA2-induced hemolytic activity. In addition, the homologs of reticulocalbin, the mediators of PLA2 toxins [44,45], were detected in the venom of both species. This finding implies that PLA2s play an important role in R. esculentum and S. malayensis envenomation.

Proteases inhibitors, another group of toxins commonly found in jellyfish venom [24–26,31,34,46], were also found in the proteomes of R. esculentum and S. malayensis venom. In our proteomic study, four Kunitz-type serine protease inhibitors were found, two in R. esculentum and another two in S. malayensis venom, characterized by the conserved motif of C-8X-C-15X-C-4X-YGGC-12X-C-3X-C (Figure 7C). Kunitz-type serine protease inhibitors inhibit proteases, which cause inflammation and interferes with blood coagulation [47]. It has also been suggested that the protease inhibitors also play an auxiliary role in envenomation by maintaining the integrity of the proteinaceous toxins [42]. Moreover, in sea anemones and scorpions, Kunitz-type serine protease inhibitors exhibit an ion channel-blocking function, which might result in paralysis [47]. Further investigation is required to clarify the functions of the protease inhibitors in jellyfish venom.

Other toxins rarely reported in jellyfish venom were also identified in this study. A venom acid phosphatase was identified in the S. malayensis venom proteome. This type of toxin is commonly found in honeybees and weever fish, which can induce allergic reaction through the induction of histamine release [48]. To the best of our knowledge, the venom acid phosphatase protein has not been identified in jellyfish venom proteome before. Furthermore, some lethally pore-forming toxins were found in the venom of both species. Three stonustoxins (SNTXs) were identified: One SNTX subunit beta homolog (a hemolysin from estuarine stonefish) and two neoverrucotoxin subunit beta homologs (a hemolysin from reef stonefish) detected in R. esculentum and S. malayensis venom, respectively. SNTXs show hemolytic and hypotensive activity in stonefish venom [49,50]; however, the function of these toxins in jellyfish venom remains to be tested.

In terms of the discovery of novel therapeutic compounds, our data suggest that R. esculentum and S. malayensis venoms might be a potential source for drug screening. Our InterProScan results have identified two protein domains with potential therapeutic value, namely, the ShKT domain and the Kunitz domain. The ShKT domain is one of the best-studied protein domains with high therapeutic potential. ShKT is a potent potassium ion channel blocker with high affinity for KV1.3 channels [51]; this channel is essential for effector memory T (TEM) cell activation, which is a hallmark of autoimmune diseases [52,53]. Therefore, KV1.3 is considered a promising target of autoimmune disease treatment. Several modified ShKT peptides with increased selectivity of KV1.3 have been synthetized as potential drugs for treating autoimmune diseases [54–58]. Among them, dalazatide has completed clinical phase 1b [52]. Moreover, Kunitz domain-containing proteases inhibitors were also found in the venoms of both species, which could be considered potential sources of therapeutic compounds. A previous study demonstrated that the potassium ion channel blockade function of Kunitz domain-containing peptides grants them the potential application as neuroprotective drugs [59]. In addition, Kunitz domain-containing proteins also show therapeutic potential in the treatment of cancer [60] and hereditary angioedema [61], attributed to their protease inhibition ability.

The putative toxins identified in this study were predicted based on the toxins recorded in the Tox-Prot database. Further investigations will be needed to confirm the toxicities of these putative toxins and to elucidate their role in envenomation. Regardless, this work revealed that R. esculentum and S. malayensis nematocysts contain various putative toxins with a high diversity of biological functions. Moreover, our study provides valuable information for the screening of novel therapeutic compounds and an enriched jellyfish toxin database.

4. Materials and Methods

4.1. Jellyfish Collection

Specimens of R. esculentum and S. malayensis were wild-caught and obtained from a local supplier in Hong Kong. S. malayensis was also provided by the Ocean Park Hong Kong. Medusae of both species were cultured in circulating artificial seawater (salinity 30 ppt) at room temperature at the Chinese University of Hong Kong. Individuals of R. esculentum were fed once per week with newly hatched *Artemia* and were starved for at least two days prior to sampling. Individuals of *S. malayensis* were not fed for several days after arrival in the laboratory before sampling.

4.2. Sample Preparation for Proteomic Analysis

Nematocysts were isolated according to methods described in previous studies [26,31]. Protein was extracted from the cleaned nematocysts by dissolving in lysis buffer (6 M urea, 2 M thiourea, and 1 mM dithiothreitol (DTT)). After removing the insoluble impurities by centrifugation at 21,000× g, the protein samples were then alkylated with 5 mM of iodoacetamide for 30 min in the dark at room temperature and digested in 1/20 sequencing-grade trypsin (Promega) overnight at 37 °C. The digested peptides were fractionated into four fractions with increasing acetonitrile (ACN) concentrations (7.5%, 12.5%, 17.5%, and 50%) using a high-pH reversed-phase fractionation kit (Thermo Fisher Scientific, Waltham, MA, USA). The fractions were dried in a SpeedVac and resuspended in 5% formic acid (*v/v*) and 5% ACN (*v/v*). Then, 1 μg of peptides was subjected to nano-flow liquid chromatography separation using a Dionex UltiMate 3000 RSLC nano-system. The sample was separated using a 25-cm-long, 75 μm internal diameter C18 column. The peptides were eluted from the column at a constant flow rate of 0.3 μl/min with a linear gradient from 2% to 35% of ACN over 120 min. The eluted peptides were analyzed by an Orbitrap Fusion Lumos Tribrid mass spectrometer (Thermo Fisher Scientific). MS and MS/MS scans were acquired in the Orbitrap with a mass resolution of 60,000 and 15,000, respectively. MS scan range was from 375 to 1500 *m/z* with an automatic gain control (AGC) target 4e5, and the maximum injection time was 50 ms. The AGC target and the maximum injection time for MS/MS were 5e4 and 250 ms, respectively. The higher-energy collisional dissociation (HCD) mode was used as the fragmentation mode with 30% collision energy. The precursor isolation windows were set to 1.6 *m/z*.

4.3. Spectral Searches and Bioinformatics Analysis

Data were analyzed by Proteome Discoverer version 2.3 with SEQUEST as a search engine. The searching parameters were as follows: oxidation of methionine (+15.9949 Da) and carbamidomethylation of cysteine (+57.0215 Da) was set as the dynamic modification; precursor ion mass tolerance, 10 ppm; fragment ion mass tolerance, 0.02 Da. The data were searched against the translated protein sequences from our constructed transcriptome database obtained previously [15]. The protein level false discovery rate was estimated by Percolator at an experimental q-value (exp. q-value) threshold of 0.05. To identify the putative toxins, the proteins sequences were run against the UniProt animal toxin and venom database to identify toxin contents using BLASTp (e-value of $<1.0 \times 10^{-5}$) [17]. Then, BLASTp annotation was validated by ToxClassifier to exclude the proteins with non-toxic physiological functions [18]. GO annotations were done by eggNOG-mapper using the default setting [16]. The signal peptides and subcellular localization were predicted by SignalP-5.0 [62] and DeepLoc-1.0 [63], respectively. The protein domains were screened by InterProScan (5.47–82.0) [46].

Supplementary Materials: The following are available online at http://www.mdpi.com/1660-3397/18/12/655/s1: Table S1. Putative toxins of the *R. esculentum* protein database; Table S2. Putative toxins of the *S. malayensis* protein database; Table S3. Proteomic analysis results of *R. esculentum*; Table S4. Proteomic analysis results of *S. malayensis*; Table S5. Annotation table for the putative toxins identified in the proteomic analysis for *R. esculentum*; Table S6. Annotation table for the putative toxins identified in the proteomic analysis for *S. malayensis*; Table S7. Protein domains annotated by InterProScan for the *R. esculentum* putative toxins detected by proteomic analysis; Table S8. Protein domains annotated by InterProScan for the *S. malayensis* putative toxins detected by proteomic analysis.

Author Contributions: Conceptualization, J.H.L.H. and S.M.N.; investigation, T.C.N.L., Z.Q., and W.N.; methodology, T.C.N.L. and Z.Q.; writing—original draft, T.C.N.L.; writing—review and editing, T.C.N.L., Z.Q., W.N., J.H.L.H., and S.M.N. All authors have read and agreed to the published version of the manuscript.

Funding: This research was funded by the TUYF Charitable Trust (grant number: 6903956), UGC The Eighth Matching Grant Scheme (MG8) (grant number: 8509100), and the Innovation Technology Fund of the Innovation Technology Commission: Funding Support to State Key Laboratory of Agrobiotechnology.

Acknowledgments: The authors would like to thank the Aquarium Department of the Ocean Park Hong Kong and other local companies for the specimens.

Conflicts of Interest: The authors declare no conflict of interest.

References

1. Hagadorn, J.W.; Dott, R.H.; Damrow, D. Stranded on a Late Cambrian shoreline: Medusae from central Wisconsin. *Geology* **2002**, *30*, 147–150. [CrossRef]
2. Kayal, E.; Roure, B.; Philippe, H.; Collins, A.G.; Lavrov, D.V. Cnidarian phylogenetic relationships as revealed by mitogenomics. *BMC Evol. Biol.* **2013**, *13*, 5. [CrossRef] [PubMed]
3. Shostak, S. Cnidaria (Coelenterates). In *Encyclopedia of Life Sciences*; John Wiley & Sons, Ltd.: Chichester, UK, 2005.
4. WoRMS—World Register of Marine Species. Available online: http://www.marinespecies.org/aphia.php?p=browser&accepted=1&id[]=2#focus (accessed on 20 October 2020).
5. Beckmann, A.; Özbek, S. The Nematocyst: A molecular map of the Cnidarian stinging organelle. *Int. J. Dev. Biol.* **2012**, *56*, 577–582. [CrossRef] [PubMed]
6. Santhanam, R. Venomology of Marine Cnidarians. In *Biology and Ecology of Venomous Marine Cnidarians*; Springer Singapore: Singapore, 2020; pp. 287–320, ISBN 9789811516030.0.
7. Remigante, A.; Costa, R.; Morabito, R.; LaSpada, G.; Marino, A.; Dossena, S. Impact of scyphozoan venoms on human health and current first aid options for stings. *Toxins* **2018**, *10*, 133. [CrossRef]
8. Kawahara, M.; Uye, S.; Burnett, J.; Mianzan, H. Stings of edible jellyfish (Rhopilema hispidum, Rhopilema esculentum and Nemopilema nomurai) in Japanese waters. *Toxicon* **2006**, *48*, 713–716. [CrossRef]
9. Fenner, P.J. Venomous jellyfish of the world. *S. Pac. Underw. Med. Soc. J.* **2005**, *35*, 131–138.
10. Balamurugan, E.; Reddy, B.V.; Menon, V.P. Antitumor and antioxidant role of Chrysaora quinquecirrha (sea nettle) nematocyst venom peptide against ehrlich ascites carcinoma in Swiss Albino mice. *Mol. Cell. Biochem.* **2010**, *338*, 69–76. [CrossRef]
11. Lee, H.; Bae, S.K.; Kim, M.; Pyo, M.J.; Kim, M.; Yang, S.; Won, C.K.; Yoon, W.D.; Han, C.H.; Kang, C.; et al. Anticancer Effect of Nemopilema nomurai Jellyfish Venom on HepG2 Cells and a Tumor Xenograft Animal Model. *Evid. Based Complement. Altern. Med.* **2017**, *2017*, 2752716. [CrossRef]
12. Ayed, Y.; Sghaier, R.M.; Laouini, D.; Bacha, H. Evaluation of anti-proliferative and anti-inflammatory activities of Pelagia noctiluca venom in Lipopolysaccharide/Interferon-γ stimulated RAW264.7 macrophages. *Biomed. Pharmacother.* **2016**, *84*, 1986–1991. [CrossRef]
13. Ayed, Y.; Dellai, A.; Mansour, H.B.; Bacha, H.; Abid, S. Analgesic and antibutyrylcholinestrasic activities of the venom prepared from the Mediterranean jellyfish Pelagia noctiluca (Forsskal, 1775). *Ann. Clin. Microbiol. Antimicrob.* **2012**, *11*, 15. [CrossRef]
14. Taxonomy: "Metazoa [33208]" (Keyword: Toxin OR Annotation: (Type: "Tissue Specificity" Venom)) and Reviewed: Yes. Available online: https://www.uniprot.org/uniprot/?query=taxonomy%3A%22Metazoa+%5B33208%5D%22+AND+%28keyword%3Atoxin++OR+annotation%3A%28type%3A%22tissue+specificity%22+AND+venom%29%29+AND+reviewed%3Ayes (accessed on 28 October 2020).
15. Nong, W.; Cao, J.; Li, Y.; Qu, Z.; Sun, J.; Swale, T.; Yip, H.Y.; Qian, P.Y.; Qiu, J.W.; Kwan, H.S.; et al. Jellyfish genomes reveal distinct homeobox gene clusters and conservation of small RNA processing. *Nat. Commun.* **2020**, *11*, 3151. [CrossRef] [PubMed]
16. Huerta-Cepas, J.; Szklarczyk, D.; Heller, D.; Hernández-Plaza, A.; Forslund, S.K.; Cook, H.; Mende, D.R.; Letunic, I.; Rattei, T.; Jensen, L.J.; et al. eggNOG 5.0: A hierarchical, functionally and phylogenetically annotated orthology resource based on 5090 organisms and 2502 viruses. *Nucleic Acids Res.* **2018**, *47*, 309–314. [CrossRef] [PubMed]
17. Jungo, F.; Bougueleret, L.; Xenarios, I.; Poux, S. The UniProtKB/Swiss-Prot Tox-Prot program: A central hub of integrated venom protein data. *Toxicon* **2012**, *60*, 551–557. [CrossRef] [PubMed]
18. Gacesa, R.; Barlow, D.J.; Long, P.F. Machine learning can differentiate venom toxins from other proteins having non-toxic physiological functions. *PeerJ Comput. Sci.* **2016**, *2016*, e90. [CrossRef]
19. Negi, S.S.; Schein, C.H.; Ladics, G.S.; Mirsky, H.; Chang, P.; Rascle, J.B.; Kough, J.; Sterck, L.; Papineni, S.; Jez, J.M.; et al. Functional classification of protein toxins as a basis for bioinformatic screening. *Sci. Rep.* **2017**, *7*, 13940. [CrossRef]

20. Hargreaves, A.D.; Swain, M.T.; Hegarty, M.J.; Logan, D.W.; Mulley, J.F. Restriction and recruitment-gene duplication and the origin and evolution of snake venom toxins. *Genome Biol. Evol.* **2014**, *6*, 2088–2095. [CrossRef] [PubMed]
21. Ompraba, G.; Chapeaurouge, A.; Doley, R.; Devi, K.R.; Padmanaban, P.; Venkatraman, C.; Velmurugan, D.; Lin, Q.; Kini, R.M. Identification of a novel family of snake venom proteins veficolins from cerberus rynchops using a venom gland transcriptomics and proteomics approach. *J. Proteome Res.* **2010**, *9*, 1882–1893. [CrossRef]
22. Li, Y.; Gao, L.; Pan, Y.; Tian, M.; Li, Y.; He, C.; Dong, Y.; Sun, Y.; Zhou, Z. Chromosome-level reference genome of the jellyfish Rhopilema esculentum. *GigaScience* **2020**, *9*, giaa036. [CrossRef]
23. Li, R.; Yu, H.; Xue, W.; Yue, Y.; Liu, S.; Xing, R.; Li, P. Jellyfish venomics and venom gland transcriptomics analysis of Stomolophus meleagris to reveal the toxins associated with sting. *J. Proteom.* **2014**, *106*, 17–29. [CrossRef]
24. Choudhary, I.; Hwang, D.H.; Lee, H.; Yoon, W.D.; Chae, J.; Han, C.H.; Yum, S.; Kang, C.; Kim, E. Proteomic analysis of novel components of nemopilema nomurai jellyfish venom: Deciphering the mode of action. *Toxins* **2019**, *11*, 153. [CrossRef]
25. Liang, H.; Jiang, G.; Wang, T.; Zhang, J.; Liu, W.; Xu, Z.; Zhang, J.; Xiao, L. An integrated transcriptomic and proteomic analysis reveals toxin arsenal of a novel Antarctic jellyfish Cyanea sp. *J. Proteom.* **2019**, *208*, 103483. [CrossRef]
26. Wang, C.; Wang, B.; Wang, B.; Wang, Q.; Liu, G.; Wang, T.; He, Q.; Zhang, L. Unique Diversity of Sting-Related Toxins Based on Transcriptomic and Proteomic Analysis of the Jellyfish Cyanea capillata and Nemopilema nomurai (Cnidaria: Scyphozoa). *J. Proteome Res.* **2019**, *18*, 436–448. [CrossRef]
27. Gutiérrez, J.M.; Sanz, L.; Escolano, J.; Fernández, J.; Lomonte, B.; Angulo, Y.; Rucavado, A.; Warrell, D.A.; Calvete, J.J. Snake venomics of the lesser antillean pit vipers bothrops caribbaeus and Bothrops lanceolatus: Correlation with toxicological activities and immunoreactivity of a heterologous antivenom. *J. Proteome Res.* **2008**, *7*, 4396–4408. [CrossRef]
28. Öhler, M.; Georgieva, D.; Seifert, J.; VonBergen, M.; Arni, R.K.; Genov, N.; Betzel, C. The venomics of bothrops alternatus is a pool of acidic proteins with predominant hemorrhagic and coagulopathic activities. *J. Proteome Res.* **2010**, *9*, 2422–2437. [CrossRef]
29. Valenzuela, J.G.; Garfield, M.; Rowton, E.D.; Pham, V.M. Identification of the most abundant secreted proteins from the salivary glands of the sand fly Lutzomyia longipalpis, vector of Leishmania chagasi. *J. Exp. Biol.* **2004**, *207*, 3717–3729. [CrossRef]
30. Magalhães, G.S.; Junqueira-de-Azevedo, I.L.M.; Lopes-Ferreira, M.; Lorenzini, D.M.; Ho, P.L.; Moura-da-Silva, A.M. Transcriptome analysis of expressed sequence tags from the venom glands of the fish Thalassophryne nattereri. *Biochimie* **2006**, *88*, 693–699. [CrossRef]
31. Ponce, D.; Brinkman, D.L.; Potriquet, J.; Mulvenna, J. Tentacle transcriptome and venom proteome of the pacific sea nettle, Chrysaora fuscescens (Cnidaria: Scyphozoa). *Toxins* **2016**, *8*, 102. [CrossRef]
32. Ishikawa, A.; Miyake, Y.; Kobayashi, K.; Murata, Y.; Iizasa, S.; Iizasa, E.; Yamasaki, S.; Hirakawa, N.; Hara, H.; Yoshida, H.; et al. Essential roles of C-type lectin Mincle in induction of neuropathic pain in mice. *Sci. Rep.* **2019**, *9*, 872. [CrossRef]
33. Brinkman, D.L.; Jia, X.; Potriquet, J.; Kumar, D.; Dash, D.; Kvaskoff, D.; Mulvenna, J. Transcriptome and venom proteome of the box jellyfish Chironex fleckeri. *BMC Genom.* **2011**. [CrossRef]
34. Li, R.; Yu, H.; Yue, Y.; Liu, S.; Xing, R.; Chen, X.; Li, P. Combined proteomics and transcriptomics identifies sting-related toxins of jellyfish Cyanea nozakii. *J. Proteom.* **2016**, *148*, 57–64. [CrossRef]
35. Moran, Y.; Praher, D.; Schlesinger, A.; Ayalon, A.; Tal, Y.; Technau, U. Analysis of Soluble Protein Contents from the Nematocysts of a Model Sea Anemone Sheds Light on Venom Evolution. *Mar. Biotechnol.* **2013**, *15*, 329–339. [CrossRef]
36. Lee, H.; Jung, E.; Kang, C.; Yoon, W.D.; Kim, J.S.; Kim, E. Scyphozoan jellyfish venom metalloproteinases and their role in the cytotoxicity. *Toxicon* **2011**, *58*, 277–284. [CrossRef]
37. Almeida, F.M.; Pimenta, A.M.C.; DeFigueiredo, S.G.; Santoro, M.M.; Martin-Eauclaire, M.F.; Diniz, C.R.; DeLima, M.E. Enzymes with gelatinolytic activity can be found in Tityus bahiensis and Tityus serrulatus venoms. *Toxicon* **2002**, *40*, 1041–1045. [CrossRef]
38. Serrano, S.M.T.; Maroun, R.C. Snake venom serine proteinases: Sequence homology vs. substrate specificity, a paradox to be solved. *Toxicon* **2005**, *45*, 1115–1132. [CrossRef]
39. Li, A.; Yu, H.; Li, R.; Liu, S.; Xing, R.; Li, P. Inhibitory Effect of Metalloproteinase Inhibitors on Skin Cell Inflammation Induced by Jellyfish Nemopilema nomurai Nematocyst Venom. *Toxins* **2019**, *11*, 156. [CrossRef]

40. Kim, H.M.; Weber, J.A.; Lee, N.; Park, S.G.; Cho, Y.S.; Bhak, Y.; Lee, N.; Jeon, Y.; Jeon, S.; Luria, V.; et al. The genome of the giant Nomura's jellyfish sheds light on the early evolution of active predation. *BMC Biol.* **2019**, *17*, 28. [CrossRef]
41. Zhu, S.; Ye, M.; Xu, J.; Guo, C.; Zheng, H.; Hu, J.; Chen, J.; Wang, Y.; Xu, S.; Yan, X. Lipid Profile in Different Parts of Edible Jellyfish Rhopilema esculentum. *J. Agric. Food Chem.* **2015**, *63*, 8283–8291. [CrossRef]
42. Liu, G.; Zhou, Y.; Liu, D.; Wang, Q.; Ruan, Z.; He, Q.; Zhang, L. Global transcriptome analysis of the tentacle of the Jellyfish Cyanea capillata using deep sequencing and expressed sequence tags: Insight into the toxin-and degenerative disease-related transcripts. *PLoS ONE* **2015**, *10*, e0142680. [CrossRef]
43. Yu, H.; Li, C.; Li, R.; Xing, R.; Liu, S.; Li, P. Factors influencing hemolytic activity of venom from the jellyfish Rhopilema esculentum Kishinouye. *Food Chem. Toxicol.* **2007**, *45*, 1173–1178. [CrossRef]
44. Hseu, M.-J.; Yen, C.-H.; Tzeng, M.-C. Crocalbin: A new calcium-binding protein that is also a binding protein for crotoxin, a neurotoxic phospholipase A 2. *FEBS Lett.* **1999**, *445*, 440–444. [CrossRef]
45. Dodds, D.; Schlimgen, A.K.; Lu, S.-Y.; Perin, M.S. Novel Reticular Calcium Binding Protein Is Purified on Taipoxin Columns. *J. Neurochem.* **2002**, *64*, 2339–2344. [CrossRef]
46. Jones, P.; Binns, D.; Chang, H.-Y.; Fraser, M.; Li, W.; Mcanulla, C.; Mcwilliam, H.; Maslen, J.; Mitchell, A.; Nuka, G.; et al. InterProScan 5: Genome-scale protein function classification. *Bioinformatics* **2014**, *30*, 1236–1240. [CrossRef]
47. Mourão, C.B.F.; Schwartz, E.F. Protease inhibitors from marine venomous animals and their counterparts in terrestrial venomous animals. *Mar. Drugs* **2013**, *11*, 2069–2112. [CrossRef]
48. Gorman, L.M.; Judge, S.J.; Fezai, M.; Jemaà, M.; Harris, J.B.; Caldwell, G.S. The venoms of the lesser (Echiichthys vipera) and greater (Trachinus draco) weever fish—A review. *Toxicon X* **2020**, *6*, 100025. [CrossRef]
49. Sung, J.M.L.; Low, K.S.Y.; Khoo, H.E. Characterization of the mechanism underlying stonustoxin-mediated relaxant response in the rat aorta in vitro. *Biochem. Pharmacol.* **2002**, *63*, 1113–1118. [CrossRef]
50. Yew, W.S.; Khoo, H.E. The role of tryptophan residues in the hemolytic activity of stonustoxin, a lethal factor from stonefish (*Synanceja horrida*) venom. *Biochimie* **2000**, *82*, 251–257. [CrossRef]
51. Pennington, M.W.; Byrnes, M.E.; Zaydenberg, I.; Khaytin, I.; de Chastonay, J.; Krafte, D.S.; Hill, R.; Mahnir, V.M.; Volberg, W.A.; Gorczyca, W. Chemical synthesis and characterization of ShK toxin: A potent potassium channel inhibitor from a sea anemone. *Int. J. Pept. Protein Res.* **1995**, *46*, 354–358. [CrossRef]
52. Chandy, K.G.; Norton, R.S. Peptide blockers of Kv1.3 channels in T cells as therapeutics for autoimmune disease. *Curr. Opin. Chem. Biol.* **2017**, *38*, 97–107. [CrossRef]
53. Beeton, C.; Wulff, H.; Standifer, N.E.; Azam, P.; Mullen, K.M.; Pennington, M.W.; Kolski-Andreaco, A.; Wei, E.; Grino, A.; Counts, D.R.; et al. Kv1.3 channels are a therapeutic target for T cell-mediated autoimmune diseases. *Proc. Natl. Acad. Sci. USA* **2006**, *103*, 17414–17419. [CrossRef]
54. Tarcha, E.J.; Chi, V.; Muñoz-Elías, E.J.; Bailey, D.; Londono, L.M.; Upadhyay, S.K.; Norton, K.; Banks, A.; Tjong, I.; Nguyen, H.; et al. Durable pharmacological responses from the peptide ShK-186, a specific Kv1.3 channel inhibitor that suppresses T cell mediators of autoimmune disease. *J. Pharmacol. Exp. Ther.* **2012**, *342*, 642–653. [CrossRef]
55. Pennington, M.W.; Chang, S.C.; Chauhan, S.; Huq, R.; Tajhya, R.B.; Chhabra, S.; Norton, R.S.; Beeton, C. Development of highly selective Kv1.3-blocking peptides based on the sea anemone peptide ShK. *Mar. Drugs* **2015**, *13*, 529–542. [CrossRef]
56. Pennington, M.W.; Harunur Rashid, M.; Tajhya, R.B.; Beeton, C.; Kuyucak, S.; Norton, R.S. A C-terminally amidated analogue of ShK is a potent and selective blocker of the voltage-gated potassium channel Kv1.3. *FEBS Lett.* **2012**, *586*, 3996–4001. [CrossRef]
57. Chang, S.C.; Huq, R.; Chhabra, S.; Beeton, C.; Pennington, M.W.; Smith, B.J.; Norton, R.S. N-terminally extended analogues of the K+ channel toxin from Stichodactyla helianthus as potent and selective blockers of the voltage-gated potassium channel Kv1.3. *FEBS J.* **2015**, *282*, 2247–2259. [CrossRef]
58. Pennington, M.W.; Beeton, C.; Galea, C.A.; Smith, B.J.; Chi, V.; Monaghan, K.P.; Garcia, A.; Rangaraju, S.; Giuffrida, A.; Plank, D.; et al. Engineering a stable and selective peptide blocker of the Kv1.3 channel in T lymphocytes. *Mol. Pharmacol.* **2009**, *75*, 762–773. [CrossRef]
59. Liao, Q.; Li, S.; Siu, S.W.I.; Yang, B.; Huang, C.; Chan, J.Y.W.; Morlighem, J.É.R.L.; Wong, C.T.T.; Rádis-Baptista, G.; Lee, S.M.Y. Novel Kunitz-like Peptides Discovered in the Zoanthid Palythoa caribaeorum through Transcriptome Sequencing. *J. Proteome Res.* **2018**, *17*, 891–902. [CrossRef]
60. Ranasinghe, S.L.; Rivera, V.; Boyle, G.M.; McManus, D.P. Kunitz type protease inhibitor from the canine tapeworm as a potential therapeutic for melanoma. *Sci. Rep.* **2019**, *9*, 16207. [CrossRef]

61. Farkas, H.; Varga, L. Ecallantide is a novel treatment for attacks of hereditary angioedema due to C1 inhibitor deficiency. *Clin. Cosmet. Investig. Dermatol.* **2011**, *4*, 61. [CrossRef]
62. Almagro Armenteros, J.J.; Tsirigos, K.D.; Sønderby, C.K.; Petersen, T.N.; Winther, O.; Brunak, S.; von Heijne, G.; Nielsen, H. SignalP 5.0 improves signal peptide predictions using deep neural networks. *Nat. Biotechnol.* **2019**, *37*, 420–423. [CrossRef]
63. Almagro Armenteros, J.J.; Sønderby, C.K.; Sønderby, S.K.; Nielsen, H.; Winther, O. DeepLoc: Prediction of protein subcellular localization using deep learning. *Bioinformatics* **2017**, *33*, 3387–3395. [CrossRef]

Publisher's Note: MDPI stays neutral with regard to jurisdictional claims in published maps and institutional affiliations.

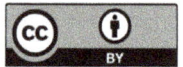

© 2020 by the authors. Licensee MDPI, Basel, Switzerland. This article is an open access article distributed under the terms and conditions of the Creative Commons Attribution (CC BY) license (http://creativecommons.org/licenses/by/4.0/).

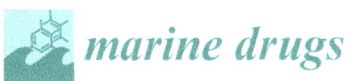

Review

Marine Antitumor Peptide Dolastatin 10: Biological Activity, Structural Modification and Synthetic Chemistry

Gang Gao [1,2], Yanbing Wang [3], Huiming Hua [2], Dahong Li [2] and Chunlan Tang [1,*]

[1] School of Medicine, Ningbo University, 818 Fenghua Road, Ningbo 315211, China; gaogang9213@163.com
[2] Key Laboratory of Structure-Based Drug Design & Discovery, Ministry of Education, and School of Traditional Chinese Materia Medica, Shenyang Pharmaceutical University, 103 Wenhua Road, Shenyang 110016, China; huimhua@163.com (H.H.); lidahong0203@163.com (D.L.)
[3] School of Life Science and Biopharmaceutics, Shenyang Pharmaceutical University, 103 Wenhua Road, Shenyang 110016, China; wangyanbing96@163.com
* Correspondence: tangchunlan@nbu.edu.cn

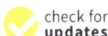

Citation: Gao, G.; Wang, Y.; Hua, H.; Li, D.; Tang, C. Marine Antitumor Peptide Dolastatin 10: Biological Activity, Structural Modification and Synthetic Chemistry. *Mar. Drugs* **2021**, *19*, 363. https://doi.org/10.3390/md19070363

Academic Editor: Tatiana V. Ovchinnikova

Received: 27 May 2021
Accepted: 20 June 2021
Published: 24 June 2021

Publisher's Note: MDPI stays neutral with regard to jurisdictional claims in published maps and institutional affiliations.

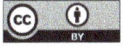

Copyright: © 2021 by the authors. Licensee MDPI, Basel, Switzerland. This article is an open access article distributed under the terms and conditions of the Creative Commons Attribution (CC BY) license (https://creativecommons.org/licenses/by/4.0/).

Abstract: Dolastatin 10 (Dol-10), a leading marine pentapeptide isolated from the Indian Ocean mollusk *Dolabella auricularia*, contains three unique amino acid residues. Dol-10 can effectively induce apoptosis of lung cancer cells and other tumor cells at nanomolar concentration, and it has been developed into commercial drugs for treating some specific lymphomas, so it has received wide attention in recent years. In vitro experiments showed that Dol-10 and its derivatives were highly lethal to common tumor cells, such as L1210 leukemia cells (IC_{50} = 0.03 nM), small cell lung cancer NCI-H69 cells (IC_{50} = 0.059 nM), and human prostate cancer DU-145 cells (IC_{50} = 0.5 nM), etc. With the rise of antibody-drug conjugates (ADCs), milestone progress was made in clinical research based on Dol-10. A variety of ADCs constructed by combining MMAE or MMAF (Dol-10 derivatives) with a specific antibody not only ensured the antitumor activity of the drugs themself but also improved their tumor targeting and reduced the systemic toxicity. They are currently undergoing clinical trials or have been approved for marketing, such as Adcetris®, which had been approved for the treatment of anaplastic large T-cell systemic malignant lymphoma and Hodgkin lymphoma. Dol-10, as one of the most medically valuable natural compounds discovered up to now, has brought unprecedented hope for tumor treatment. It is particularly noteworthy that, by modifying the chemical structure of Dol-10 and combining with the application of ADCs technology, Dol-10 as a new drug candidate still has great potential for development. In this review, the biological activity and chemical work of Dol-10 in the advance of antitumor drugs in the last 35 years will be summarized, which will provide the support for pharmaceutical researchers interested in leading exploration of antitumor marine peptides.

Keywords: marine peptide; dolastatin 10; antitumor; lead exploration

1. Introduction

The living environment of marine organisms is different from that of terrestrial creatures, and the peptide secondary metabolites of the former have special structures and provide bioactive components distinct from the latter [1–3]. Since the beginning of the 21st century, the potential of unique marine natural products as candidate drugs has been widely recognized, and significant advancement has been seen in the clinical research of marine-derived medicines [4–13]. After decades of exploration, a series of antitumor polypeptides with high biological activity have been isolated from various marine organisms, such as hemiasterlins, cryptophycins, vitilevuamide, diazonamide, etc. [14,15]. Structures of these polypeptides are dissimilar from that of terrestrial plant peptides (mainly glycopeptides). Marine peptides are rich in hydroxy acids, thiophenols, and D- and α-amino acids. Some components possess ethylenic bonds and acetylenic bonds, which improve the stability and bioavailability of peptides [16–21]. Compared with traditional small molecule inhibitors, marine peptides present high activity, strong targeting, low toxicity, easy transmembrane absorption, and own a wide range of biological activities, such as antitumor, anti-inflammatory, antivirus, and antiinfection. Currently, an increasing number of candidate drugs derived from marine peptides have entered clinical trials or been approved for marketing [22–28].

The bioactive antitumor components from mollusk Dolabella auricularia, a sea hare that mainly inhabits the Indian Ocean, were first investigated by Pettit and his co-workers. Since 1972, they had gradually discovered 18 short-chain peptide compounds, named as dolastatins 1–18, which contained several unusual amino acids. In the dolastatins family, dolastatin 10 (Dol-10, **1**, Figure 1) had been proved to be one of the most potent antiproliferative active ingredients, and it allowed for prolonging the life span of P388 leukemia mice [21,29–31]. The chemical structures of its constituent subunits were analyzed, and all four subunits, starting from the amino N-terminal of Dol-10, (S)-dolavaline (Dov, **2**, Figure 1), (S)-valine (Val, **3**), (3R,4S,5S)-dolaisoleuine (Dil, **4**), and (2R,3R,4S)-dolaproine (Dap, **5**), were actual amino acid residues, while (S)-dolaphenine (Doe, **6**), a peculiar primary amine possibly stemmed from phenylalanine, worked as carboxyl C-terminal. Even so, researchers were still accustomed to regard Dol-10 as a pentapeptide [32–34].

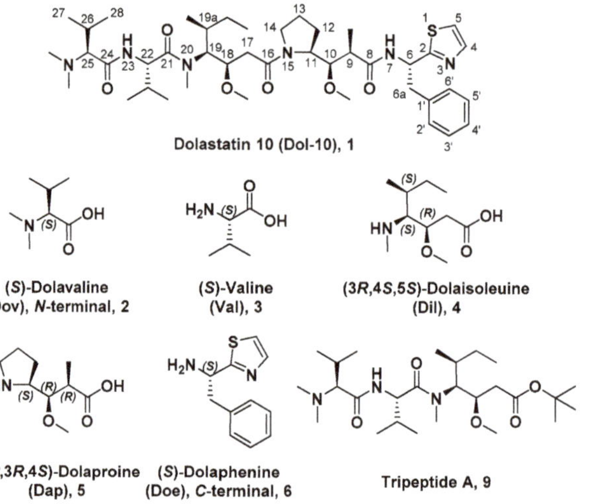

Figure 1. Chemical structures of Dol-10 (**1**), key amino acid components (**2–6**) of Dol-10 were ordered from N-terminal to C-terminal and tripeptide A (**9**).

Excitedly, since Dol-10 was first discovered, its biological activity was more potent than those of most known anticancer drugs (murine PS leukemia cells, ED_{50} = 4.6 × 10^{-5} µg/mL), so it had attracted extensive attention in the field of anticancer research. In in vitro antitumor screening, it was found that Dol-10 had a strong antiproliferation effect on L1210 leukemia cells (IC_{50} = 0.03 nM) [35], non-Hodgkin lymphoma cells [36], B16 melanoma cells, small cell lung cancer NCI-H69 cells (IC_{50} = 0.059 nM) [37], human prostate cancer DU-145 cells (IC_{50} = 0.5 nM) [38], etc. In addition, it had been confirmed that the ability of Dol-10 to induce apoptosis mainly came from its effective inhibition of tubulin polymerization [30,35,39–41]. However, the rare content in organisms brings great obstacles to the enrichment and further biological evaluation of bioactive peptides. Because of the relatively simple chemical structure, scientists prepared a large amount of Dol-10 by chemical synthesis, which laid the foundation for its further development and clinical evaluation [16,21,42]. Due to its adverse effects, such as the most common peripheral neuropathy, Dol-10 was stagnated in phase II clinical trial [43,44]. It is inspiring to know that a lot of synthetic analogs of Dol-10 with potent antitumor activity have been reported. For example, TZT-1027 (Soblidotin) entered the phase I clinical trial, the main toxicity and neutropenia were observed, and the dosage level was insufficient to achieve clinical efficacy [45,46]. MMAE (a Dol-10 derivative, 7, Figure 2) conjugated with the special monoclonal antibody to construct the Adcetris® (Brentuximab vedotin), and Adcetris® was approved by the FDA in 2011 for the treatment of anaplastic large T-cell systemic malignant lymphoma and Hodgkin lymphoma [47].

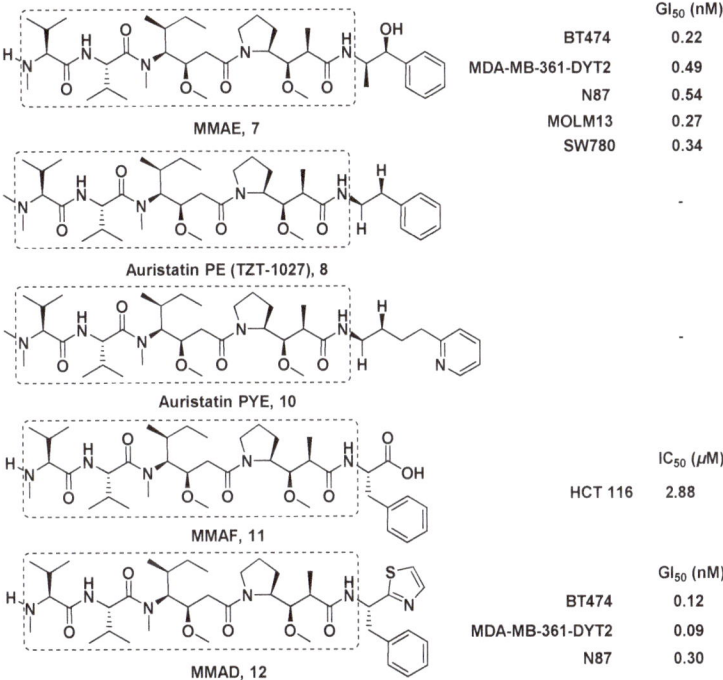

Figure 2. Chemical structures of key auristatin analogs.

Up to now, a large number of research articles have reported on Dol-10 and its derivatives, but to the best of our knowledge, there are few literatures that systematically summarized Dol-10. Therefore, this review will introduce the pharmacological characteristics of Dol-10, the antitumor activity of its structurally modified derivatives, chemical synthesis of Dol-10 and its subunits, and its development and application on the basis of ADCs in detail.

2. Pharmacological Characteristics

The in vitro evaluation of pharmacological activity showed that Dol-10 could cause apoptosis of many tumor cells at nanomolar concentrations, the strong antitumor activity came from the unique mechanism of inducing apoptosis, including interactions with β-tubulin, regulating the expression of special oncoproteins, loss of telomeric repeat sequence of chromosome and provoking chromosome aberrations. In the application of Dol-10 in various tumor treatment (Table 1), the therapeutic activity in clinical trials was obviously inferior to that, in preclinical trials, and the reason remained uncertain. Since accumulated retention in cells and high affinity binding with tubulin might affect the therapeutic effect of Dol-10, it was speculated that the administration scheme would interfere with the clinical evaluation results, and infusion administration was superior to bolus administration [48,49]. Furthermore, to provide reasonable guidance for clinical application, and ensure the safety and effectiveness of chemotherapy, the pharmacokinetics, pharmacodynamics, toxicity, and drug resistance of Dol-10 had also been explored in preclinical and phase I clinical trial. All of the above investigations will be elaborated through the following sections.

Table 1. Therapeutic use and evaluation of Dol-10 in various antitumor research.

Therapeutic Use	Development State	Evaluation Outcome *	Reference
Anti-lymphoma	Preclinical	++	[36,49–51]
Anti-lung cancer	Preclinical	++	[37]
Anti-ovarian carcinoma	Phase II	+	[48]
Anti-prostate cancer	Preclinical, phase II	++, + (respectively)	[36,52]
Anti-soft tissue sarcoma	Phase II	-	[53]
Anti-breast cancer	Phase II	-	[54]
Anti-hepatobiliary pancreatic carcinoma	Phase II	-	[55]

*-, almost no objective curative effect and toxic symptoms were observed; +, positive; ++, strongly positive.

2.1. Antitumor Effects

2.1.1. Anti-Lymphoma Effect

Lymphoma is a malignant tumor originated from the lymphohematopoietic system, and it is also a disease that threatens human life. Fortunately, Dol-10 had significant antiproliferative activity in four diverse human lymphoma cell lines (DB, HT, RL, and SR), which was about 3–4 logarithms stronger than vincristine. The inhibitory effect of tumor cells could be reversed by removing the agent within the first 4 h of treatment [50]. Maki et al. confirmed that Dol-10 would effectively trigger the apoptosis of non-Hodgkin lymphoma cells [36]. In the model of human diffuse large cell lymphoma cell line (WSU-DLCL 2), the antitumor activity of Dol-10 was not obvious at concentrations less than 500 pg/mL, but auristatin PE (TZT-1027, 8, a typical derivative of Dol-10, Figure 2) possessed the remarkable antiproliferative ability at concentrations as low as 10 pg/mL, and the administration concentration was allowed to be 10-fold higher than that of Dol-10 [51]. The uptake and efflux of Dol-10 and vinblastine in human Burkitt lymphoma CA46 cells were studied by radioactive labeling. It was found that the tight binding of Dol-10 with tubulin not only prolonged intracellular residence time, but also determined the preferential activity. In addition, in clinical application, the best way to administer Dol-10 might be infusion rather than bolus injection [49].

2.1.2. Anti-Small Cell Lung Cancer Effect

Overexpression of Bcl-2 is common in small cell lung cancer (SCLC), and Dol-10 has the ability of inducing Bcl-2 phosphorylation to induce apoptosis in SCLC cell lines and xenografts. In the related efficacy evaluation, the standardized MTT assay was employed to estimate the growth inhibitory efficiency in vitro, and the in vivo activity was evaluated based on SCID mice subcutaneous and metastatic SCLC xenoplantation models. The results showed that the growth of four SCLC cell lines (NCI-H69, NCI-H82, NCI-H446, and NCI-H510) was strongly inhibited through Bcl-2 phosphorylation triggered by Dol-10 (IC_{50} = 0.032–0.184 nM) [37].

2.1.3. Anti-Ovarian Carcinoma Effect

In order to evaluate the therapeutic efficacy of Dol-10 on relapsed platinum-sensitive ovarian carcinoma, the patients were injected with 400 µg/m² of Dol-10 intravenously every three weeks, and the tumor status was measured 1–2 cycles after administration. Under the limited level of toxicity, the drug was only effective for some patients, which indicated that Dol-10 needed further improvement for the treatment of platinum-sensitive recurrent ovarian cancer [48].

2.1.4. Anti-Prostate Cancer Effect

In the tissue culture and athymic nude mice experiment, the growth of human prostate cancer DU-145 cells was completely inhibited by 1 nM Dol-10 (IC_{50} = 0.5 nM) [36]. In the phase II clinical trial of patients with hormone refractory prostate cancer, Dol-10 showed excellent tolerance, especially among the elderly pre-treatment population, but the clinical efficiency as a single drug was seriously insufficient [52].

2.1.5. Anti-Soft Tissue Sarcoma Effect

In the phase II trials of Dol-10, the therapeutic activity of this microtubule inhibitor to recurrent or metastatic soft tissue sarcoma was verified by Mehren et al. During the course of treatment, no patient got obvious improvement, but one died of respiratory failure, which indicated that Dol-10 was not warranted for further research on the chemotherapy for advanced or metastatic soft tissue sarcoma [53].

2.1.6. Anti-Breast Cancer Effect

Dol-10 was also applied as the first-line or second-line chemotherapy for advanced breast cancer, and the results showed that the marine polypeptide had no significant activity. In addition, the drug was found to have hematological toxicity in an acceptable range. It was speculated that a large dose of Dol-10 might overcome its drug resistance and induce effective antitumor activity [54].

2.1.7. Anti-Hepatobiliary Pancreatic Carcinoma Effect

With the aim of characterizing the efficacy and toxicity of Dol-10 for patients with advanced hepatobiliary cancer and pancreatic cancer, Kindler et al. performed two parallel phase II trials. Patients with metastatic pancreatic cancer, liver cancer, cholangiocarcinoma, or gallbladder cancer and had not received corresponding chemotherapy before, were eligible for the trials. The results showed that the toxicity of Dol-10 was tolerable, but there was no obvious therapeutic effect [55].

2.2. Mechanisms of Inducing Apoptosis
2.2.1. Interactions with β-tubulin

Spindle microtubule was one of the key proteins affecting cell proliferation, which was composed of α- and β-tubulin (Figure 3). At the late stage of cells division, spindle microtubules pulled sister chromatids from the equatorial plane to the poles of the spindle. After mitosis, spindle microtubules were depolymerized [32,35,41]. Hence, if the equilibrium (polymerization and depolymerization) of tubulin-microtubule is broken, the mitosis would stagnate in the G_2/M phase, which further inhibits the growth or induces apoptosis of tumor cells [56–60].

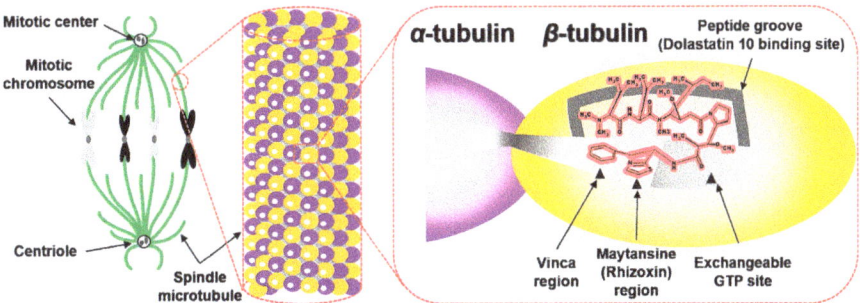

Figure 3. The graphical model of spindle microtubules in the mitosis and binding relationship of between ligands and β-tubulin.

Dol-10, interfered with tubulin-microtubule balance, had potential to be developed as a new antimitotic drug. It was generally believed that the binding sites (more than one) of Dol-10 (Figure 3) located in the β-tubulin subunits in the central part of spindle microtubules [58,61,62], and there was no interaction between α-tubulin and Dol-10 [63]. The combination of Dol-10 and β-tubulin would trigger a series of activities related to apoptosis. For example, microtubule assembly, tubulin-dependent GTP hydrolysis and β^s cross-linking were all inhibited, but microtubule depolymerization was enhanced [33,64]. In addition, a schematic model of the relationship between binding sites of Dol-10, vinca, maytansine/rhizoxin, and exchangeable GTP site on β-tubulin was proposed (Figure 3). Tripeptide A (**4**, Figure 1) was a tripeptide residue at the N-terminal of Dol-10 and located in a hydrophobic pocket or groove which was part of the binding site of Dol-10 but had little or no overlap with the other three binding sites. Therefore, it was speculated that the other two residues at the C-terminal of the Dol-10 would hinder the binding of vinca alkaloids and GTP exchange in space. The accuracy and rationality of the above model were confirmed in a series of experiments [65–68]. As the noncompetitive inhibitor of vinca alkaloids, Dol-10 targeted vinblastine, maytansine/rhizoxin binding domain in β-tubulin to realize the microtubule inhibition activity. Later work verified that tripeptide A (**4**) inhibited tubulin polymerization but hardly disturbed the binding of vincristine to tubulin and GTP exchange [33,62,64,69]. In addition, the β^s cross-link between the sulfur atom of cysteine 12 of β-tubulin and thiazole portion of Dol-10 interfered with the binding of Dol-10 to β-tubulin. Auristatin PE, the equivalent analog of Dol-10 lacking thiazole ring, failed to establish this cross-link. Model research also confirmed that the binding site of Dol-10 (possibly containing cysteine 12) was adjacent to the exchangeable GTP site [63,70].

2.2.2. Regulating the Expression of Bcl-2, c-myc, and p53

Oncoproteins, such as coding products of oncogenes Bcl-2, c-*myc*, and tumor suppressor gene p53, are the critical functional proteins in the apoptosis signal pathway. It is significant to further mediate cell proliferation and apoptosis by regulating the expression of oncoproteins. Dol-10 down-regulated or inhibited the expression of anti-apoptotic Bcl-2 protein and promoted the overexpression of c-*myc* or p53, which as the initial signal of reactivating apoptosis pathway would further induce apoptosis of tumor cells (Figure 4) [36,37,71]. Bcl-2 phosphorylation and apoptosis induced by Dol-10 were discussed by Haldar et al. in 1998. In the G_2/M phase of the cell cycle, it was observed by site-directed mutagenesis that several serine residues (in charge of drug-induced phosphorylation of Bcl-2) on Bcl-2 protein were translated and then induced to phosphorylation by Dol-10, which led to apoptosis of malignant tumor cells [72].

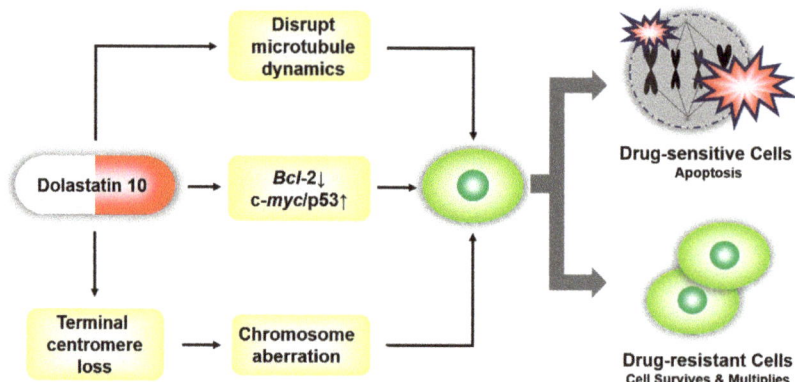

Figure 4. Dol-10-mediated reactivation of the apoptosis pathway in tumor cells. Drug-sensitive tumor cells were arrested at the G2/M phase of the cell cycle, and then apoptosis occurred. Resistance to Dol-10 led to the survival of drug-resistant cells.

2.2.3. The Loss of Telomeric Repeats and Induction of Chromosome Aberrations

In addition to the inhibition of microtubule aggregation and induction of Bcl-2 phosphorylation, the mechanism of inducing apoptosis mediated by loss of telomere repeats sequence and chromosomal aberrations had also aroused researchers' interest. The efficacy of Dol-10 on chromosome morphology, telomere association, polyploid induction and apoptosis of K1735 clone X-21 were identified based on the mouse metastatic melanoma cell line model. The investigation suggested that the loss of telomere repeats promoted the formation of telomeric associations, multicentric chromosomes and ring configurations, and led to chromosome aberration, which eventually contributed to cell death induced by Dol-10 (Figure 4) [73–75].

2.3. Pharmacokinetics and Pharmacodynamics

From preclinical research to the clinical trial, it was necessary to study the pharmacokinetics and pharmacodynamics of Dol-10 in detail, especially to measure the maximum tolerated dose (MTD), so as to achieve the maximum therapeutic activity, reduce the adverse reactions and ensure that each patient receives the best dose of treatment. An assay based on HPLC/ESI-MS was employed to characterize the clinical pharmacokinetics and pharmacodynamics of Dol-10. Preliminary examination showed that the three-compartment model was the optimum approach to describe the distribution and elimination of Dol-10, and $t_{1/2\alpha}$, $t_{1/2\beta}$, and $t_{1/2\gamma}$ were 0.087 h, 0.69 h, and 8.0 h, respectively. At MTD level (about 300 µg/m^2), 33% of the treated patients with advanced solid tumors had granulocytopenia (the dose-limiting toxicity), but it was well-tolerated, and some patients with stable tumor growth had no objective reaction to the drug. Pharmacokinetic analysis revealed that the drug distribution was rapid, but the process of plasma elimination was relatively slow (with a $t_{1/2z}$ of 5.3 h). The change of Dol-10 concentration with time was closely related to the decrease of white blood cell count [44,76–78]. Given all that, Dol-10 showed good preclinical characteristics and can be used for further clinical research.

2.4. Toxicity

According to the results of preclinical toxicology research, it is of great significance to predict the dose-limiting toxicity of the safe initial dose to human body for clinical guidance. The treatment of Dol-10 for advanced or metastatic soft tissue sarcoma triggered hematological and vascular toxicity, but there was no apparent gastrointestinal, liver or kidney toxicity [53]. The preclinical toxicity evaluation on this cytotoxic peptide had proved that the transient reversible toxicity symptoms were mainly concentrated in bone marrow of ordinary mammals. In this animal experiment, granulocytopenia and bone marrow toxicity were dose-limited, and the Dol-10 MTD of dogs and humans was equivalent (about 325–455 µg/m^2) [79]. The temporary adverse reactions of Dol-10 to dogs with non-Hodgkin lymphoma included granulocytopenia with dose-limiting toxicity, and this examination predicted that the initial dose of 300 µg/m^2 was suitable for human beings [80]. Since 1990, Dol-10 had successively entered the phase I and II clinical trials, preliminary statistics presented that 40% of patients helped with Dol-10 had moderate peripheral neuropathy [43]. Some patients accompanied by bone marrow suppression and phlebitis, etc. If the patient had potential mental illness, then the side effects would be more obvious [81].

2.5. Drug Resistance

Dol-10 as a new member of multidrug resistance (MDR) phenotype expressed by sublines of murine PC4 and human U-937 leukemia cells, the drug resistance mechanism (Figure 4) and how to ensure the effectiveness and rational application of Dol-10 had attracted widespread concern. In the parallel investigations in a CHO cell line transfected with human *mdr*1 cDNA, Toppmeyer et al. had confirmed the resistance of transfected cells to Dol-10 was originated from the normal expression of P-glycoprotein (P-gp), and this resistance could be reversed by verapamil. The employment of Dol-10 resulted in a decrease in the photoaffinity labeling of P-gp, which further demonstrated the binding of Dol-10 to P-gp. The drug resistance to Dol-10 was at least related to the expression of the *mdr*1 gene and the interaction between Dol-10 and P-gp [82].

3. Medicinal Chemistry

Due to the unexpected results of Dol-10 in phase II clinical trials, researchers turned their attention to its antitumor derivatives. These derivatives mainly focused on *N*-terminal (Dov) and *C*-terminal (Doe) subunits with great potential for drug development. However, there were relatively fewer modifications of central residues Dil, Dap, and Doe [83,84]. Auristatins (Figure 2) based on the bipolar modification of Dol-10 had potent microtubule inhibitory activity and cytotoxicity. Auristatin PE (TZT-1027) and auristatin PYE (**10**, Figure 2) showed remarkable therapeutic effects in clinic. However, due to the complicated chemical structure and low water solubility, the clinical research progress of these drugs was not satisfactory. Later, with the rise of research on ADCs, the application of auristatins as payload provided an excellent platform for the preparation of ADCs. Related ADCs, such as Adcetris®, which successfully went on the market, also made notable progress in clinical trials [85]. Design, synthesis, and structure-activity relationship of various antitumor derivatives classified according to specific modified subunits are detailed as follows.

3.1. Antitumor Derivatives

3.1.1. Doe Unit Modified Derivatives

By replacing Doe residue with Met, Phe, or appropriately modified phenethylamide, the activity of synthesized derivatives in interfering with microtubule assembly, vinblastine, and GTP targeting tubulin and mitosis of various human and mouse cancer cell lines was evaluated. Moreover, it was confirmed that the antitumor ability of some Dol-10 derivatives was equivalent to that of Dol-10 [86]. Auristatin PYE, derived from Doe unit of Dol-10 replaced by pyridine group, interfered with polymerization and stability of microtubules in micromole concentration range, leading to apoptosis and growth inhibition of tumor cells [87]. Auristatin PE (TZT-1027), a Dol-10 derivative synthesized by replacing Doe unit with phenylethylamine, had the same mechanism as Auristatin PYE, expanded the antitumor spectrum of the pentapeptide [88], and exhibited higher in vivo antitumor activity than other anticancer agents, such as paclitaxel, adriamycin, and vincristine, against murine fibrosarcoma Meth A [89,90].

Substituting various functional groups for Doe unit of novel derivatives is also essential to expand the application of Dol-10 analogs in conjugated drugs. A series of Dol-10 derivatives which added a carbonyl functional group to the C-4 of thiazole of Doe unit were synthesized by Yokosaka and co-workers (Scheme 1). In the tumor cell proliferation evaluation, amine, aniline, alcohol, phenol, and thiol derivatives were observed to have extremely strong activity (data shown in Table 2), which were also considered as the versatile payloads of conjugated drugs [91].

Dol-10 derivatives based on substitution of the Doe unit with phosphate, aminoquinoline (AQ) auristatin isomer 2/6-AQ, and emetine were synthesized. The activity of all new auristatins in mouse and human cancer cell lines was evaluated. The results showed that the sodium phosphate derivative so auristatin TP (**24**), auristatin 2-AQ (**25**), auristatin 6-AQ (**26**), and 2-*N'*-(Dov-Val-Dil-Dap)-emetine (**27**) had remarkable growth inhibitory effects (Scheme 2, Table 3) [92,93].

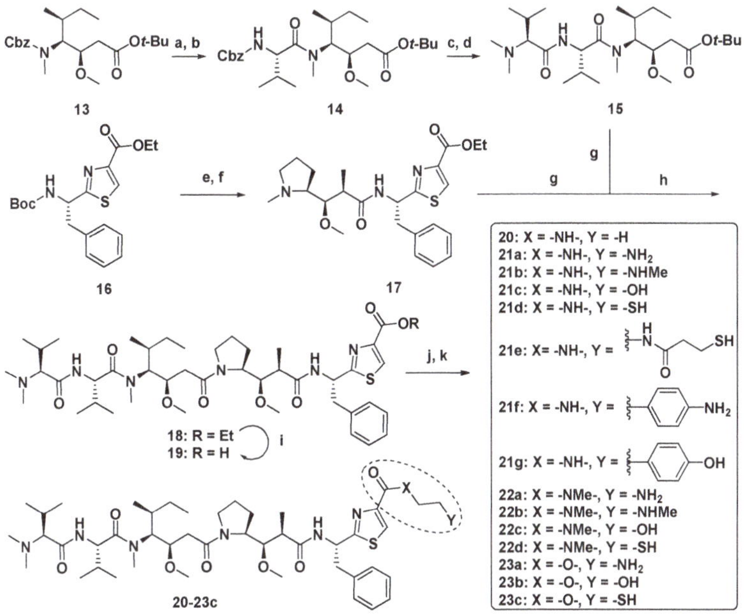

Scheme 1. Synthesis of Dol-10 derivatives with C-terminal modifications. Reagents and conditions: (a) H$_2$, Pd/C, MeOH, 71%; (b) Cbz-Val-OH, COMU, DIPEA, DMF, 97%; (c) H$_2$, Pd/C, MeOH, 93%; (d) Dov-OH, HATU, DIPEA, DMF, 75%; (e) HCl, AcOEt, 99%; (f) Boc-Dap-OH, HATU, DIPEA, DMF, 85%; (g) TFA, CH$_2$Cl$_2$; (h) HATU, DIPEA, DMF, 83%; (i) NaOH, EtOH, quant; (j) amine, HATU, DIPEA, DMF, 43–100% (**17**, **21a–g**, **22a–d**, and **23a**) or alcohol, 2-methyl-6-nitrobenzoic anhydride, Et$_3$N, DMAP, CH$_2$Cl$_2$, 73–92% (**23b–c**); (k) deprotection of protecting groups (Boc: **21a–b**, **22a–b**, **23a**, THP: **23b**, Trt: **21d–e**, **22d**, **23c**) if needed.

Table 2. Structure-activity relationships for Dol-10 derivatives with carbonyl functional group at the C-4 of thiazole of Doe unit.

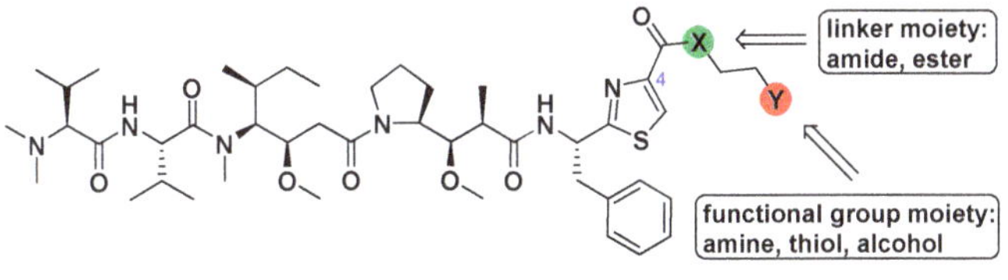

Compound	-X-	-Y	IC$_{50}$ (nM)		
			SKOV-3	A549	L1210
MMAE (7)	-	-	0.66	1.3	2.1
18	-O-	-H	0.024	-	-
20	-NH-	-H	0.55	0.74	6.5
21a	-NH-	-NH$_2$	>10	>10	>50
21b	-NH-	-NHMe	>10	9.9	27
21c	-NH-	-OH	4.7	1.7	28
21d	-NH-	-SH	0.44	1.9	31
21e	-NH-	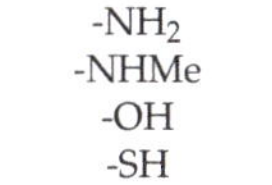 -NH-C(O)-CH$_2$-CH$_2$-SH	>10	>10	>50

Table 2. Cont.

Compound	-X-	-Y	IC$_{50}$ (nM)		
			SKOV-3	A549	L1210
21f	-NH-	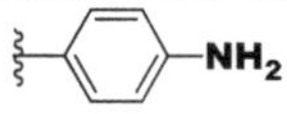 -C$_6$H$_4$-NH$_2$	0.27	1.1	4.1
21g	-NH-	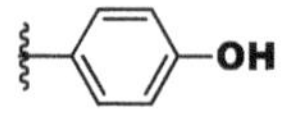 -C$_6$H$_4$-OH	0.37	1.3	5.6
22a	-NMe-	-NH$_2$	0.56	0.81	12
22b	-NMe-	-NHMe	0.19	1.9	14
22c	-NMe-	-OH	1.5	1.6	8.5
22d	-NMe-	-SH	1.1	1.2	7.0
23a	-O-	-NH$_2$	0.85	0.83	29
23b	-O-	-OH	0.086	1.8	4.7
23c	-O-	-SH	0.13	6.9	14

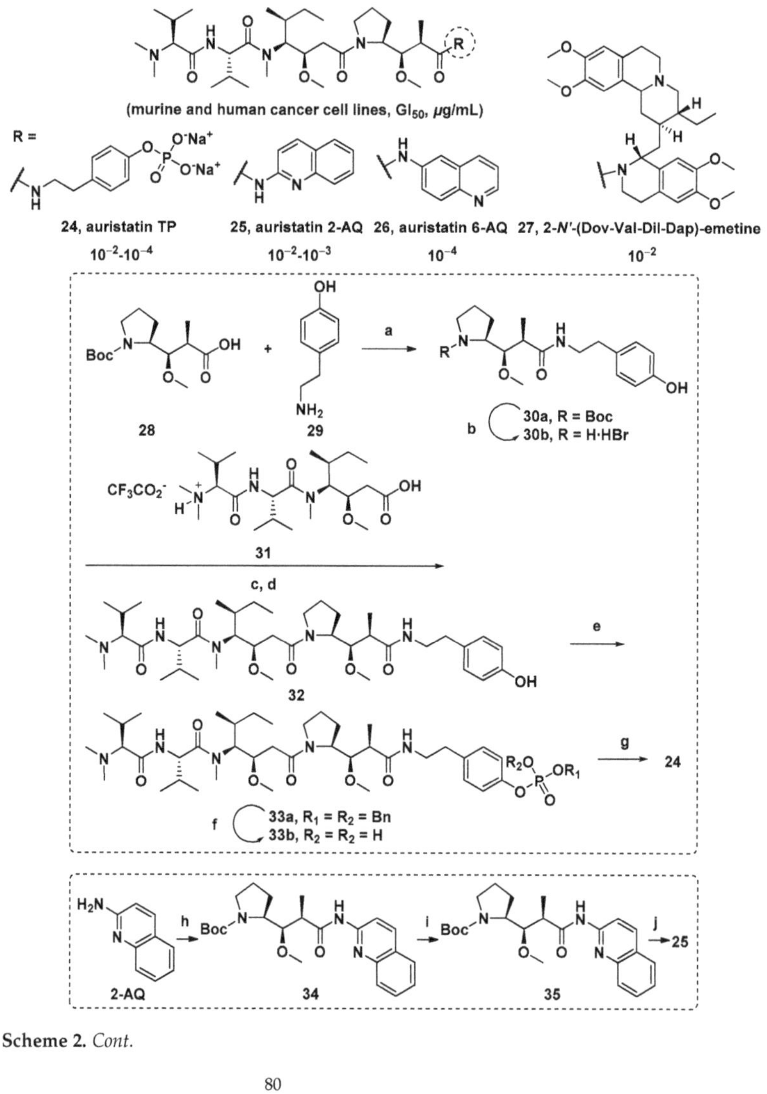

(murine and human cancer cell lines, GI$_{50}$, µg/mL)

24, auristatin TP 10^{-2}-10^{-4}
25, auristatin 2-AQ 10^{-2}-10^{-3}
26, auristatin 6-AQ 10^{-4}
27, 2-N'-(Dov-Val-Dil-Dap)-emetine 10^{-2}

Scheme 2. Cont.

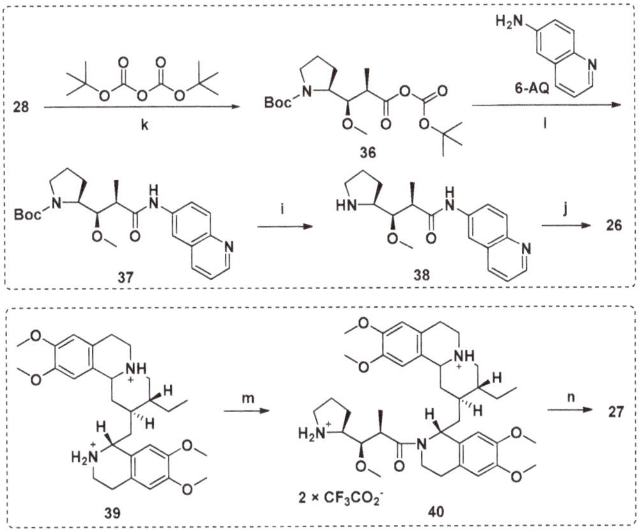

Scheme 2. The chemical structures and synthesis of **24, 25, 26,** and **27**. Reagents and conditions: (a) (1) EDCI, HOBT; (2) DIEA, DMF; (b) TMSBr; (c) EDCI, HOBT; (d) DIEA, DMF; (e) (BnO)$_2$P(O)H, CCl$_4$, DIEA, DMAP; (f) Pd/C, H$_2$; (g) ion exchange; (h) 28, DEPC, TEA; (i) TEA; (j) 32, DEPC, TEA; (k) pyridine; (l) 6-AQ, DEPC, TEA; (m) (1) 28, TEA, HBTU, DMF; (2)TFA, CHCl$_2$; (n) 31, CH$_2$Cl$_2$, DEPC, TEA, 0 °C-r.t.

Table 3. The growth inhibition of **24, 25, 26,** and **27** in murine and human cancer cell lines (ED$_{50}$ (µg/mL) and GI$_{50}$ (nM)) [a].

Compound	Cell Line [b]						
	P388	NCI-H460	KM20L2	DU-145	BXPC-3	MCF-7	SF-268
24	<0.001 (<1.2)	0.00088 (1.05)	0.00061 (0.72)	0.00054 (0.64)	0.046 (54.6)	0.00068 (0.81)	0.00125 (1.48)
25	0.031 (42.8)	0.0160 (22.1)	0.0077 (10.6)	0.023 (31.8)	0.029 (40.1)	0.0046 (6.35)	0.029 (40.1)
26	0.0026 (3.59)	0.00036 (0.50)	0.00025 (0.35)	0.00030 (0.41)	0.00031 (0.43)	0.00014 (0.19)	0.00016 (0.22)
27	- (-)	- (198.0)	- (35.82)	- (12.26)	- (386.5)	- (35.82)	- (30.17)

[a] The nanomolar values in brackets are the cytotoxicity concentrations. [b] The sequence of tumor cell lines: murine lymphocytic leukemia (P388), lung (NCI-H460), colon (KM20L2), prostate (DU-145), pancreas (BXPC-3), breast (MCF-7), and CNS (SF-268).

3.1.2. Dap Unit Modified Derivatives

The introduction of azide functional group into Dap subunit enhanced the cytotoxicity of Dol-10 in vitro, which was observed by Akaiwa et al. Inspired by this modification, azide functional groups were introduced into Val subunit and Dap subunit simultaneously, and Doe subunit were replaced by phenylalanine, thus obtaining Dol-10 analog **41** (Figure 5). Compared with MMAE (**7**), the cytotoxic activity of the analog **41** was more potent (GI$_{50}$ = 0.057 nM). These two azide groups not only had the function of regulating growth inhibition but also served as a connecting link to synthesize the brand-new macrocyclic dolastatin analog (**42**) and as a site of drug linker (**43**) attachment for preparing ADCs. Nevertheless, the activity of the synthesized macrocyclic analog (**42**) was disappointingly weak [83].

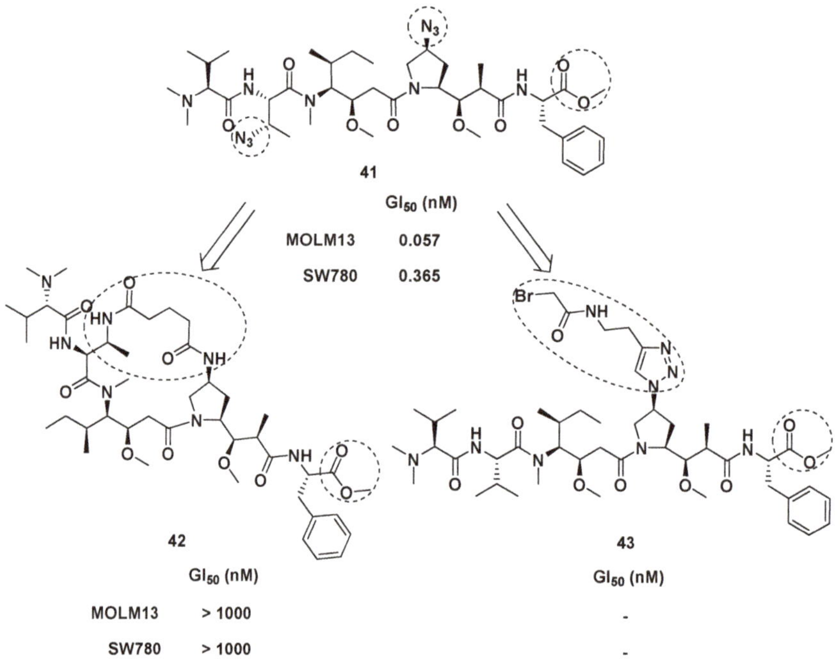

Figure 5. The design and chemical structures of Dol-10 analog (**41**), macrocyclic dolastatin analog (**42**), and drug linker (**43**).

3.1.3. Dil Unit Modified Derivatives

In the cytotoxicity evaluation of P388 lymphocytic leukemia (PS system), (19aR)-isodalastatin 10 (the chiral isomer of Dil unit, **44**, ED$_{50}$ = 4.9 × 10^{-5} μg/mL, Figure 6) had 10-fold stronger inhibitory activity on cell growth than Dol-10 (**1**, ED$_{50}$ = 10^{-4} μg/mL). It had been proved that the antitumor effect was extremely sensitive to the stereochemical modification of the Dil unit (C-18 and C-19). In addition, the general reaction sequence for the synthesis of Dol-10 was also suitable for the total synthesis of 19aR-Dil sequence products (including **44**) [94]. Nie et al. established a diastereoselective method to prepare Dil modified derivatives by SmI$_2$-induced radical addition reaction. These crucial fragments were applied in the divergent synthesis of Dol-10 (**1**), and nine of the analogs of Dol-10 were obtained. It is worth expecting that, if the antitumor activity of these analogs could be evaluated through relevant biological experiments, it would be helpful for the further development of this synthetic strategy in this field [95].

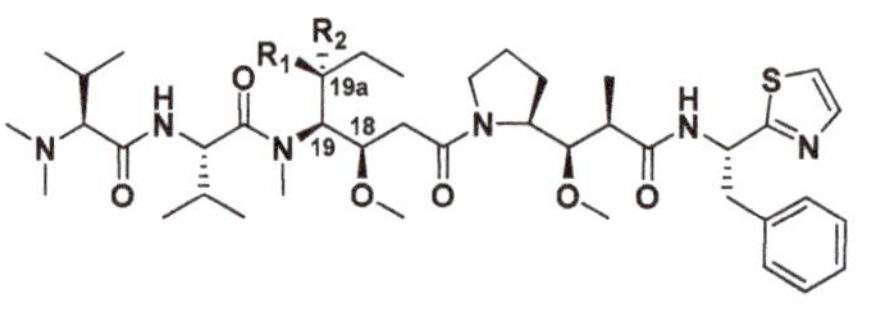

1, R$_1$ = CH$_3$, R$_2$ = H, dolastatin 10, P388 ED$_{50}$ = 10^{-4} μg/mL
44, R$_1$ = H, R$_2$ = CH$_3$, 19aR-isodalastatin 10, P388 ED$_{50}$ = 4.9×10^{-5} μg/mL

Figure 6. Comparison of chemical structures and activity between (19aR)-isodalastatin 10 (**44**) and Dol-10 (**1**).

Both marine peptides Dol-10 and dolastatin 15 (**45**, Figure 7) had an inextricable connection in structure or biological activity spectrum. The synthesis of compounds **46** and **47** was conducted by replacing the MeVal-Pro dipeptide in dolastatin 15 with the central

Dil residue of Dol-10, and vice versa. It was confirmed that both Dil unit and MeVal-Pro dipeptide were essential to cytotoxicity of dolastatins, but the former was superior to the latter in terms of cytotoxicity and inhibition of tubulin polymerization in vitro [96].

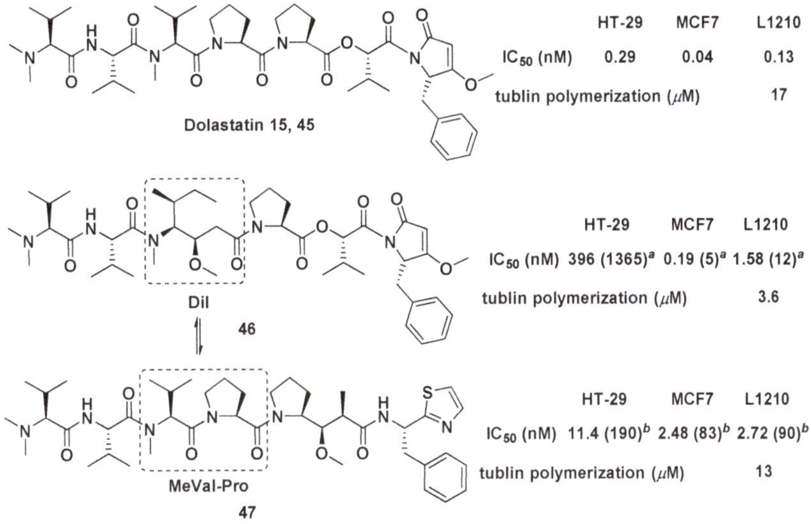

Figure 7. Chemical structures of dolastatin 15 (**45**), **46**, and **47**. Inhibition of cell growth (IC_{50}, nM) of Dol-10: HT-29 (0.06), MCF7 (0.03), and L1210 (0.03); tubulin polymerization of Dol-10 (IC_{50} = 2.2 µM). [a] Ratio IC_{50} (**46**)/IC_{50} (dolastatin 15); [b] Ratio IC_{50} (**47**)/IC_{50} (Dol-10).

3.1.4. Val Unit Modified Derivatives

By introducing heteroatoms to the Val unit, Tessier and co-workers obtained a series of auristatins. Dol-10 analog **48** (Figure 8) with Val and Doe subunits modified by azide and phenylalanine, respectively, had effective cytotoxicity when applied to ADCs. Through activity analysis, it was found that phenylalanine replacing Doe unit was crucial in enhancing the in vitro activity of Val unit modified derivatives. Further work confirmed that the modification of the Val unit also needed to modify the Doe unit into an aromatic structure containing ester or amide [84].

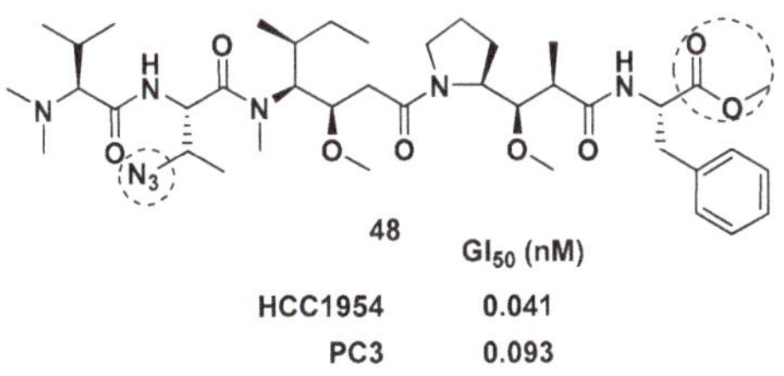

Figure 8. The chemical structure of Val unit modified derivative **48**.

3.1.5. Dov Unit Modified Derivatives

Four Dol-10 analogs of monomethyl auristatin F (MMAF, **11**, Figure 2) modified by N-terminal (Dov unit) were designed and synthesized (Scheme 3). These four analogs were more cytotoxic than MMAF against HCT 116 human colon cancer cells [97].

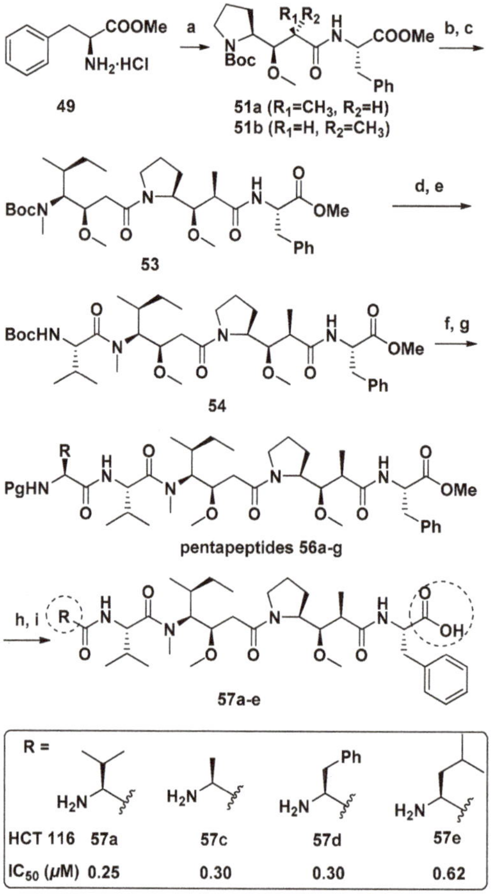

Scheme 3. Synthesis of compounds **57a–e**. Reagents and conditions: (a) DEPC, DIPEA, DMF, **50a** or **50b** (83–90%); (b) TFA, CH$_2$Cl$_2$; (c) DEPC, DIPEA, DMF, **52a** or **52b** (76–85%); (d) TFA, CH$_2$Cl$_2$; (e) Brop, DIPEA, CH$_2$Cl$_2$, N-Boc-L-valine, (71–92%); (f) TFA, CH$_2$Cl$_2$; (g) DEPC, DIPEA, DMF, **55a–g** (please refer to Reference [98]), (46–87%); (h) LiOH·H$_2$O, MeOH/H$_2$O; (i) TFA, CH$_2$Cl$_2$ or Pd/C, H$_2$, MeOH, 82–94%.

Maderna et al. modified the Dov unit of Dol-10 with α,α-disubstituted amino acids and obtained a novel auristatin analog PF-06380101(**62**, Scheme 4). Compared with other existing auristatin analogs, **62** had outstanding curative effect and unique ADME characteristics in analyzing the proliferation of tumor cell. Firstly, the systemic clearance rate, distribution volume and elimination half-life ($t_{1/2}$) of **62** were all in good condition, and no drug accumulation was observed during the interval of drug administration. Furthermore, compared with whole blood, **62** tendentiously distributed in human plasma as a substrate of P-glycoprotein(P-gp). Additionally, if **62** was administered in combination with clinical inhibitors and/or inducers of enzyme CYP3A4, drug-drug interactions might occur, since **62** was mainly metabolized by CYP3A4 [85].

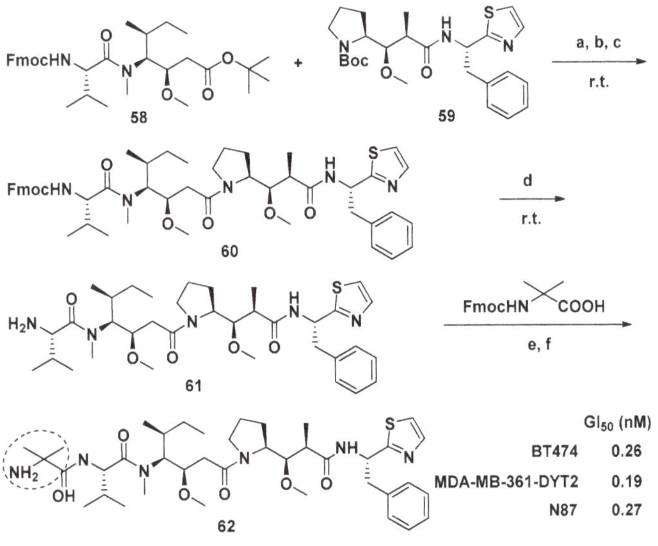

Scheme 4. Synthesis of new auristatin analog **62**. Reagents and conditions: (a) TFA/DCM for **58**; (b) HCl dioxane for **59**; (c) HATU, i-Pr$_2$NEt, DCM, 78%; (d) Et$_2$NH, THF, r.t., 87%. Boc-protected **61** was previously prepared by an alternative method; (e) HATU, Et$_3$N, DMF; (f) Et$_2$NH, THF, yields: 27–67% over two steps. N-Fmoc: protected amine.

With the application of ADCs in cancer treatment, the coupling of Dol-10 derivatives with antibodies had been widely concerned. The hydrophilic Dov unit modified derivatives with maleimide group were synthesized through the polymerization and convergent synthesis (Figure 9). Discrete polyethylene glycols (PEG) with various chain lengths was introduced into the cytotoxic agent (**68**), which was used as drug linkers for synthesizing ADCs to increase hydrophilicity (Scheme 5). In cytotoxicity assay against SK-BR3 and MDA-MB-231 cells, the related ADC based on trastuzumab had excellent target specificity, and their cytotoxicity (EC$_{50}$) was interfered with the length of the PEG linker. The solubility problem of ADCs related to hydrophobic anticancer drugs was also solved, and the natural highly cytotoxic peptide Dol-10 was avoided as starting material [99].

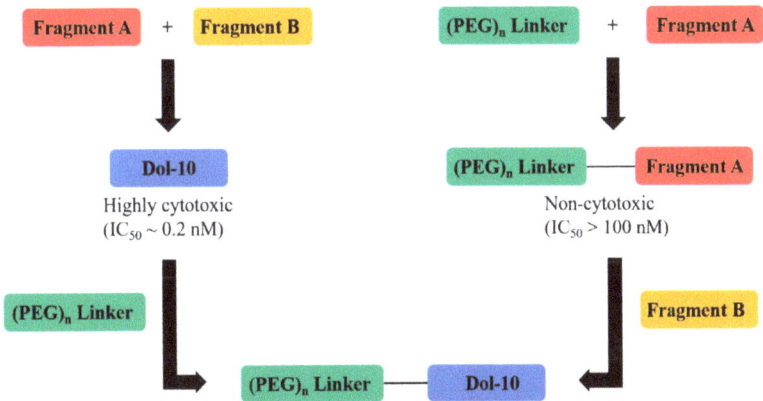

Figure 9. Synthetic plan of cytotoxic Dol-10 derivatives with hydrophilic drug linkers.

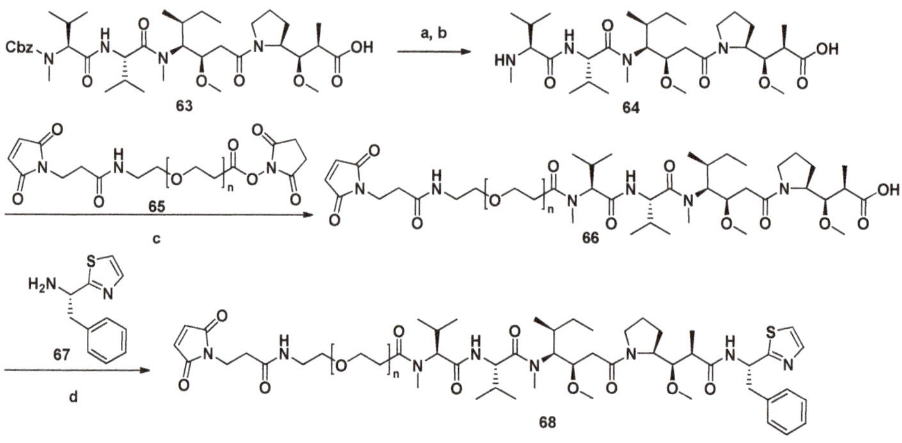

ADC (trastuzumab conjugated 68)	n = 4	n = 6	n = 8	n = 12	n = 24
SK-BR3 EC$_{50}$ (ng/mL)	1.15	< 0.1	< 0.1	< 0.1	8.23
MDA-MB-231 EC$_{50}$ (µg/mL)	> 1000	> 81	> 1000	> 1000	> 1000

Scheme 5. The synthesis of hydrophilic cytotoxic agent (**68**) containing PEG linker. Reagents and conditions: (a) HBr/AcOH; (b) Et$_3$N, r.t.; (c) 1,4-dioxane, 80 °C; (d) DECP/DIPEA, r.t.

Furthermore, some ADCs constructed by combining derivatives modified by Dov unit based on MMAE or MMAF with different antibodies have already entered clinical research or been authorized to market. MEDI-547, for example, was constructed by coupling the cytotoxic drug MMAF with the human anti-EphA2 monoclonal antibody (1C1). In in vitro experiments, MEDI-547 decreased the viability of Hec-1A and Ishikawa cells in endometrial carcinoma cell lines and accelerated their apoptosis. MEDI-547 also induced the degradation of EphA2, effectively inhibited the diffusion of tumor (the inhibition rate was about 85%) and diminished the metastasis rate of tumors. Because of these excellent performances, MEDI-547 was expected to treat patients with insufficient expression of EphA2 in malignant tumor cells. Nevertheless, in the open-label first-in-human examination, it was found that the safety characteristics of MEDI-547 did not allow further clinical research on patients with advanced solid tumors [100–104]. As the most successful representative of ADCs, Adcetris® (also known as SGN-35, **69**, Figure 10), as a cAC10-Val-cit-MMAE conjugate constructed by conjugation of MMAE and anti-CD30 antibody (i.e., cAC10, a specific monoclonal antibody). Adcetris's anti-CD30 antibody binds to CD30 antigen in Hodgkin disease cells and Le^Y antigen in cancer cells, while MMAE, the drug toxin, effectively inhibits mitosis by inhibiting tubulin polymerization. In 2011, Adcetris® (Brentuximab vedotin for injection), jointly developed by Seattle Genetics and Takeda, was first marketed in the United States, and authorized to treat anaplastic large T-cell systemic malignant lymphoma and Hodgkin lymphoma [4,40,47,105–109]. At the beginning of August 2020, Takeda announced that Adcetris® was officially listed in China, which brought new treatment options to patients in need. Up to now, Adcetris® has benefited patients in more than 70 countries around the world, and it is also the most successful ADC in the field of hematology oncology in the world.

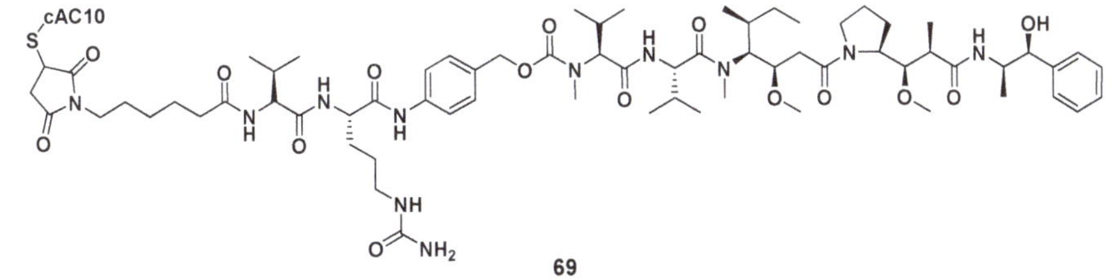

Figure 10. The chemical structure of ADC Adcetris® (69).

3.1.6. Multiunit Modified Derivatives

By systematically modifying each subunit of Dol-10 in turn, a series of analogs with stronger antitumor activity than Dol-10 (Scheme 6) were developed by Miyazaki and co-workers. On the basis of P388 leukemia model in mice, the influences of subunit deletion and the change of functional group of each subunit were analyzed. The investigation had confirmed that derivatives **73**, **77**, **81**, and **85** modified by four different units had significant inhibitory effects on tumors in vivo (Table 4). Particularly, compound **85** lacking thiazole group of Doe unit was more effective than the parent compound **1** and was applied as a new candidate for antitumor agent [110].

The antiproliferative activities of Dol-10 (**1**), its homologues trisnordolastatin 10 (**86**), 9-*epi*-trisnordolastatin 10 (**87**), and their synthetic intermediates on L1210 mouse leukemia cells were evaluated by Shioiri et al. (Table 5). Compared with parent compound **1**, analogs **86** and **87**, intermediate tripeptide Boc-Dil-Dap-Doe (**89**), and dipeptide Boc-Dap-Doe (**90**) showed weaker antiproliferative activity, and only intermediate tetrapeptide Boc-Val-Dil-Dap-Doe (**88**) exhibited strong cytotoxicity similar to that of **1**. Therefore, it was speculated that the configuration at C-9 and N,O,O-trimethyl functional groups played a key role in the cytotoxicity of dolastatins [111].

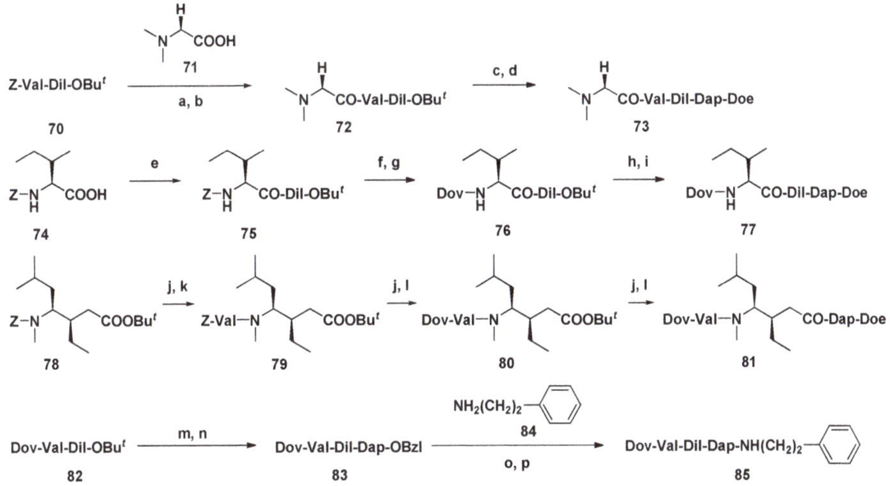

Scheme 6. Synthesis of analogs modified at the Dov, Val, Dil, and Doe units. Reagents and conditions: (a) H_2, Pd-C, *t*-BuOH/H_2O; (b) DEPC, Et_3N, DMF; (c) TFA, CH_2Cl_2; (d) H-Dap-Doe·HCl, DEPC, Et_3N, DMF; (e) H-Dil-OBu^t, DCC, CH_2Cl_2; (f) H_2, Pd-C, *t*-BuOH/H_2O; (g) Dov, DEPC, Et_3N, DMF; (h) TFA, CH_2Cl_2; (i) H-Dap-Doe·HCl, DEPC, Et_3N, DMF; (j) H_2, Pd-C, *t*-BuOH/H_2O; (k) Z-Val-OH, DCC, CH_2Cl_2; (l) Dov, DEPC, Et_3N, DMF; (m) TFA, CH_2Cl_2; (n) H-Dap-OBzl·HCl, DEPC, Et_3N, DMF; (o) H_2, Pd-C, *t*-BuOH/H_2O; (p) DEPC, Et_3N, DMF.

Table 4. Antitumor activity of multiunit modified Dol-10 derivatives. Position: Dov[1]-Val[2]-Dil[3]-Dap[4]-Doe[5].

Compound	Modified Position	ILS$_{max}$ *	Optimal Dose (mg/kg per inj.)
1		50	0.05
73	1	94	0.5
77	2	80	0.5
81	3	74	2.0
85	5	83	0.5

* Maximal increase in life span (please refer to Reference [110]).

Table 5. Chemical structures and cytotoxicity of Dol-10 (1) and its derivatives 86–90.

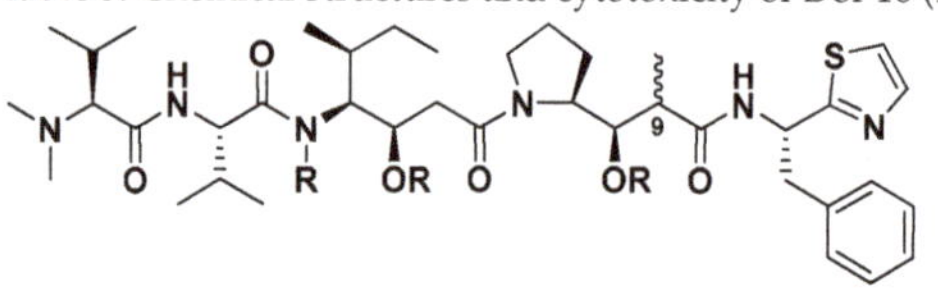

Compound		R	C$_9$-CH$_3$	IC$_{50}$ (µg/mL)
1	Dol-10	CH$_3$	β	2.95×10^{-4}
86	trisnordolastatin 10	H	β	1.0×10^{-1}
87	9-epi-trisnordolastatin 10	H	α	50
88	Boc-Val-Dil-Dap-Doe			4.0×10^{-3}
89	Boc-Dil-Dap-Doe			11
90	Boc-Dap-Doe	CH$_3$	β	>100

3.1.7. Cyclic Analogs

Different from common linear derivatives, the synthesis and activity of cyclic derivatives based on Dol-10 were rarely reported, which had aroused great interest of Poncet et al. Introducing an ester bond between the side chain of Dov residue and thiazole ring of Doe residue of compound **91** (Scheme 7), the modified linear precursor of Dol-10, to achieve the macrocyclic lactonization and obtain the cyclic analog (**92**) of the Dol-10. Compared with the parent compound **1**, the cytotoxicity of **92** against L1210 and HT-29 cell lines significantly decreased. Yet, it still had the submicromolar level inhibitory activity of microtubule polymerization in vitro (IC$_{50}$ = 39 µM). The blocking of Dov residue modified in **91** resulted in a significant decrease in inhibitory activity, which indicated that Dov residue was crucial to the antiproliferative activity of Dol-10 [112].

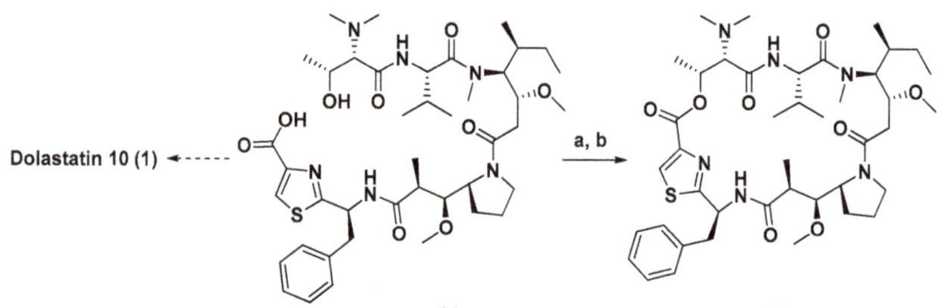

	91	92
HT-29 (IC$_{50}$)	0.06 nM	58.5 nM
L1210 (IC$_{50}$)	0.03 nM	110.8 nM
tubulin polymerization	2.2 µM	39 µM

Scheme 7. Synthesis of the cyclic analog (**92**) of Dol-10. Reagents and conditions: (a) IPCC/DMAP; (b) CH$_2$Cl$_2$, 3 h, r.t., 26%.

3.2. Structure-Activity Relationship

Pentapeptide Dol-10 has nine asymmetric carbon atoms, of which five positions (C-9, 10, 18, 19, and 19a) possess the ability to obtain alternating configurations (Figure 1). The tubulin inhibitory activity of isomers was lost when C-18 and C-19 were modified, and only the reversal of C-19a configuration avoided the decrease of cytotoxicity. Nevertheless, there was no correlation between the effects of these isomers on microtubule assembly and cell growth [34]. Moreover, it was confirmed that both *N*-terminal tripeptide (lacking Dap and Doe), such as tripeptide A (**4**) and the *C*-terminal tetrapeptide (lacking Dov), inhibited tubulin polymerization but did not interrupt tubulin-ligand interaction. Only the antimitotic isomers with reversed configuration on C-6 or C-19a had the same activity as Dol-10. The stable binding (i.e., slow separation) of the peptide to tubulin preceded rapid binding, which significantly inhibited microtubule polymerization and interaction between other ligands and tubulin [33]. In solution, the geometric configurations of the Val-Dil amide bond and the Dil-Dap amide bond were *trans*- and *cis-/trans*-, respectively. According to speculation, the stability and configuration transition of Dil-Dap amide bond might be changed by the polarity of the solvent. However, configurations of the above two amide bonds showed *cis*- and *trans*- in the tubulin co-crystal, respectively (Figure 11). The phenomenon elaborated on the preferential binding mode of Dol-10 had guiding significance for the research of novel analogs with pre-oriented *cis*-Val-Dil amide bond and *trans*-Dil-Dap amide bond [83,85,113].

Some structural modifications are crucial to the antitumor activity of Dol-10 in vivo (Figure 12). For instance, substituting hydrogen for one *N*-methyl group in Dov unit, or *N*-methyl group in Dil unit, or 2-methyl group in Dap unit; replacing methoxy in Dap unit with hydrogen or hydroxyl group, and reversing the configuration of methoxy group in Dil unit failed to bring the significant difference to activity of Dol-10. However, the activity of modified products (such as **85**, Table 4) was significantly enhanced after deleting thiazole group in Doe unit. At the same time, if the thiazole group were deleted and the phenylethylamine moiety was simultaneously replaced by other aralkyl amide moieties, it would lead to the loss of cytotoxicity [84,110].

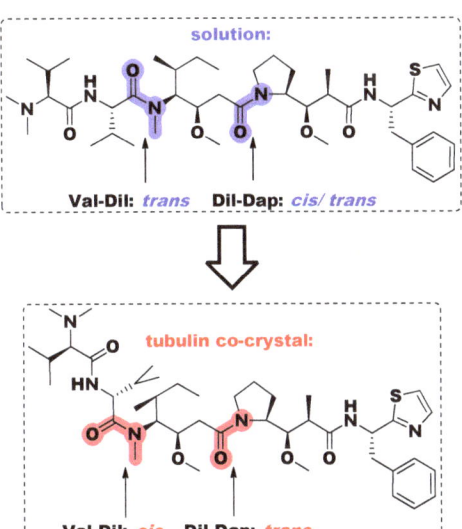

Figure 11. The geometric configurations of the Val-Dil amide bond and Dil-Dap amide bond of Dol-10 under different conditions.

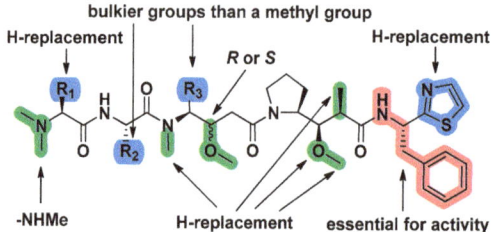

Figure 12. Structure-activity relationship of Dol-10 (**1**). The red marked part was an essential group for antitumor activity, and some modifications (marked with blue) had stronger activity than **1**, while other modifications (marked with green) possessed activity equivalent to **1**.

4. Synthetic Chemistry

The natural sources of the bioactive dolastatins, especially Dol-10, were rather limited (~1.0 mg/100 kg of collected organism from the sea hare *Dolabella Auricularia*, with a yield of 10^{-6}~10^{-7}%). Until the end of the 1980s, based on almost 20,000 times of separation and screening of two tons of raw materials by chromatography and mouse leukemia P388 model, Dol-10 was discovered by Pettit group for the first time [21,30,114]. Therefore, it is necessary to explore a reliable synthetic scheme for large-scale preparation of Dol-10, which will greatly accelerate the synthesis of potentially useful structures, extensive evaluation of biological characteristics and preclinical development. It is worth mentioning that the last three residues of Dol-10, Doe, Dap, and Dil, are particular to *Dolabella auricularia*, and their stereoselective synthesis is the key prerequisite for the total synthesis of the Dol-10 (**1**) and its analogs. In the activity evaluation of P388 lymphoblastic leukemia, the synthetic Dol-10 is equivalent to the corresponding natural product ($ED_{50} = 1\times10^{-4}$ µg/mL) [111]. According to the similarities and differences of synthetic strategies, the repeated or similar synthetic work is summarized (Figure 13), and more synthetic details and the conformational study of Dol-10 are introduced as follows.

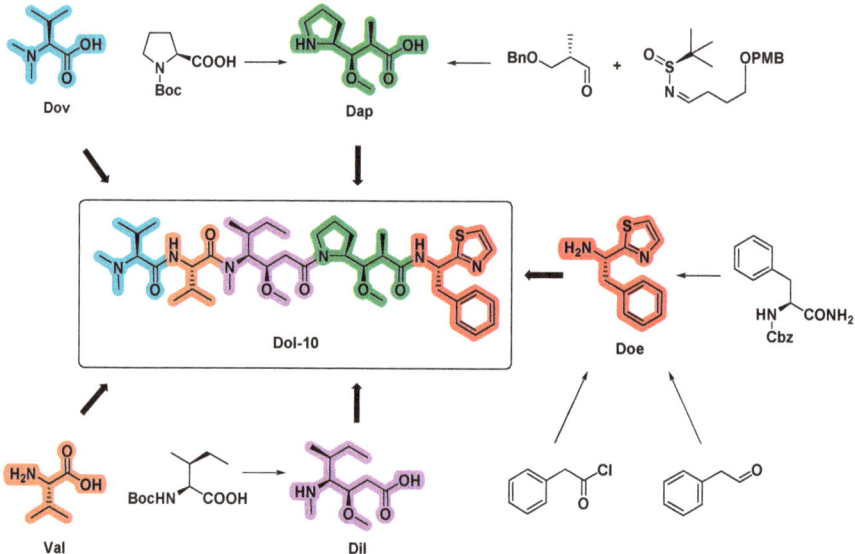

Figure 13. Overview of syntheses of Doe, Dap, Dil, and Dol-10.

4.1. Synthesis of the Doe Unit

A great deal of literatures have reported the synthesis of C-terminal Doe units in detail, which is mostly based on asymmetric addition reaction. compared with the method from Tomioka et al. [115], the asymmetric addition of chiral N-sulfinyl imine 94 (Scheme 8, Panel A) of Zhou et al. [98] was a simpler and more direct scheme to get the protected Doe fragment (95). Utilizing the Z-(S)-Phe-NH$_2$ as raw material and improved Hantzsch method (Scheme 8, Panel B), Z-(S)-Doe (98) was prepared by Shioiri et al. Thioamide converted from Z-(S)-Phe-NH$_2$ reacted with bromoacetaldehyde, and 4-hydroxythiazoline was dehydrated by trifluoroacetic anhydride to obtain the crude product 98. Doe was obtained by repeated recrystallization from hexane-diethyl ether, with a yield of 64% and high optical purity (>97% e.e.) [116]. Later, in the optimization scheme of Burkhart et al., thiazole was synthesized by thio-Ugi reaction, and then Doe was directly synthesized. The improved scheme possessed the numerous advantages, such as simplicity, rapidity, high yield, and almost no racemization [117]. In 1992, Shioiri et al. also developed a brand-new scheme to obtain the key synthesis unit Doe [111], and the advancement of this scheme was verified by Mordant et al. (Scheme 8, Panel C). Phenylacetyl chloride 99 reacted with N-methoxy-N-methylamine hydrochloride to form amide 100, which reacted with thiazolyllithium 101 produced benzyl thiazolyl ketone 102, which was asymmetrically reduced by Brown's reagent (Ipc$_2$BCl) to afford (R)-alcohol 103. With the help of Mitsunobu reaction, optically pure Boc-(S)-dorafenin 105 was finally obtained (44%, two steps) [118].

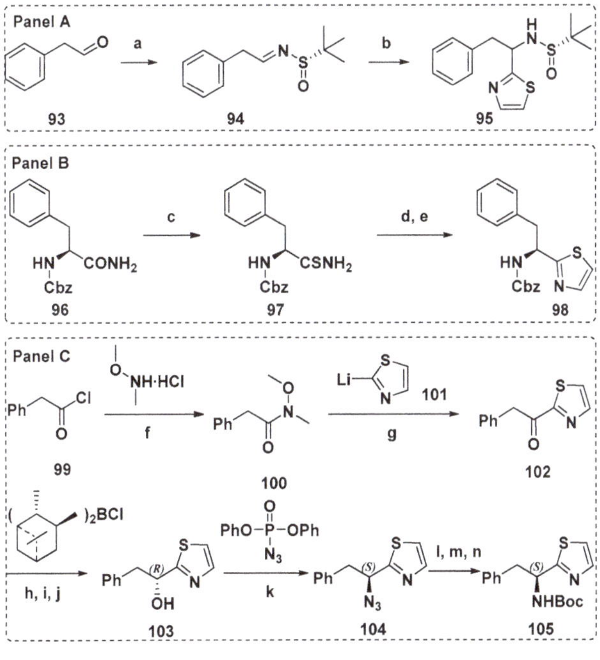

Scheme 8. The preparation of the protected Doe fragments (95, 98, and 105). Reagents and conditions: (a) (S)-tert-Butanesulfinamide, CuSO$_4$, PPTS, DCM, r.t., 36 h, 80%; (b) 2-bromothiazole, n-BuLi, toluene, −78 °C, 3 h, 53% (complete yield 80%); (c) Lawesson's reagent, dioxane, 97%; (d) BrCH$_2$CHO, K$_2$CO$_3$, DMF; (e) (CF$_3$CO)$_2$O, CH$_2$Cl$_2$, 66% in 2 steps; (f) pyridine, CH$_2$Cl$_2$, 0 °C, 2 h; r.t., 12 h, 77%; (g) THF, −78 °C, 30 min; 10 °C, 2 h, 56%; (h) Et$_2$O, −10 °C; (i) NaOH, 0 °C; (j) H$_2$O$_2$, 10 °C to r.t., 81% yield, e.e. 92%, (60% yield, e.e. > 99%, after recrystallization); (k) PPh$_3$, DEAD, THF, 0 °C to r.t., 48 h; (l) PPh$_3$, 50 °C, 2 h; (m) NH$_4$OH; (n) Boc$_2$O, dioxane, 0 °C to r.t., 60 h, 44% (2 steps), e.e. > 99%.

4.2. Synthesis of the Dap Unit

There are many reports about the synthesis of Dap unit, and the typical one is the N-*tert*-butoxy carbonyl derivative **112** of Dap synthesized by Pettit et al. Aldehyde **108** derived from (S)-proline and chiral propionate **109** were assembled through Evans aldol condensation to obtain related diastereomers of Dap. Methyl ether **112** was then produced by hydrogenolysis-based methylation and cleavage of chiral-directed ester groups (Scheme 9) [71,111,116,119]. In addition, there are many other reports on the construction of Dap unit, including crotylation of natural amino acid N-Boc-L-prolinal [97], asymmetric hydrogenation of β-keto esters derived from (S)-Boc-proline under the catalysis of ruthenium-SYNPHOS complex [118], or aldehyde cross-coupling with (S)-N-*tert*-butyrylimine under SmI$_2$ induction (Scheme 9) [98].

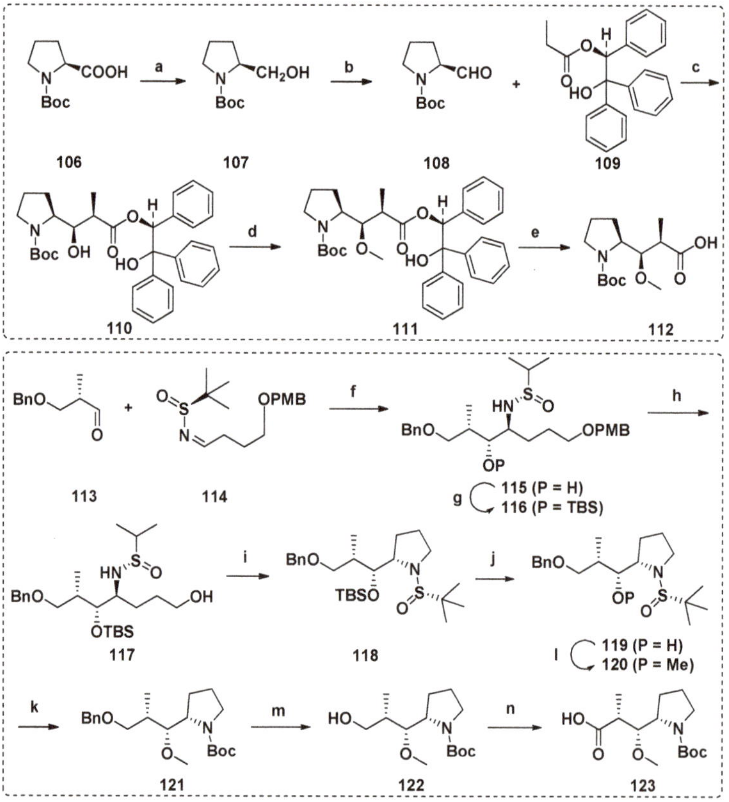

Scheme 9. Synthesis of the Dap units (**112** and **123**). Reagents and conditions: (a) B$_2$H$_6$; (b) SO$_3$·Py, Et$_3$N, DMSO; (c) *i*Pr$_2$NLi, MgBr$_2$, Et$_2$O; (d) (CH$_3$)$_3$OBF$_4$, proton sponge; (e) H$_2$, 10% Pd/C; (f) SmI$_2$, *t*-BuOH, THF, −78 °C, 5 h, 75%; (g) TBSOTf, 2,6-lutidine, DCM, 0 °C to r.t., 4 h, 88%; (h) DDQ, DCM/H$_2$O, 0 °C, 30 min, 68%; (i) (1) MsCl, TEA, DCM, 0 °C, 15 min; (2) *t*-BuOK, THF, 0 °C, 15 min, for two steps 73%; (j) TBAF, THF, 0 °C to r.t., 4 h, 61%; (k) LiHMDS, HMPA, THF, −78 °C, 30 min, and then MeOTf, −15 °C, 15 min, 95%; (l) (1) HCl/dioxane, MeOH, 0 °C, 30 min; (2) Boc$_2$O, TEA, DCM, r.t., 12 h, for two steps 79%; (m) Pd/C, H$_2$, MeOH, 5 h, 72%; (n) (1) DMP, DCM, r.t., 30 min; (2) NaH$_2$PO$_4$·2H$_2$O, NaClO$_2$, 2-methyl-2-butene/*t*-BuOH, r.t., 8 h, for two steps 75%.

4.3. Synthesis of the Dil Unit

The complete preparation scheme of the Dil unit was first developed by the Hamada group [111,116]. With Boc-(S)-isoleucine (**124**) or Boc-(S)-isoleucinal (**126**) as raw materials, the chiral center needed was established in a stereoselective manner, and then the methylation of nitrogen and oxygen realized the efficient synthesis of Dil unit (**129**, Scheme 10). Firstly, **124** was converted into the corresponding imidazoline, which was treated with magnesium enolate of malonate half ester to obtain β-keto ester **125**, subsequently reduced with sodium borohydride to get a mixture of hydroxyl esters **127a** and **127b** with a ratio of 91:9. The reaction of Boc-(S)-isoleucine (**126**) with lithium enol, an ideal alternative method, obtained **127a** and **127b** with a ratio of 38:62. Alkaline hydrolysis of the separated hydroxyl ester **127a** produced carboxylic acid **128**, which was finally treated to yield the target product Dil unit **129**. This synthetic scheme was mature and efficient, and it has been widely used in later related research [97,98,118,119].

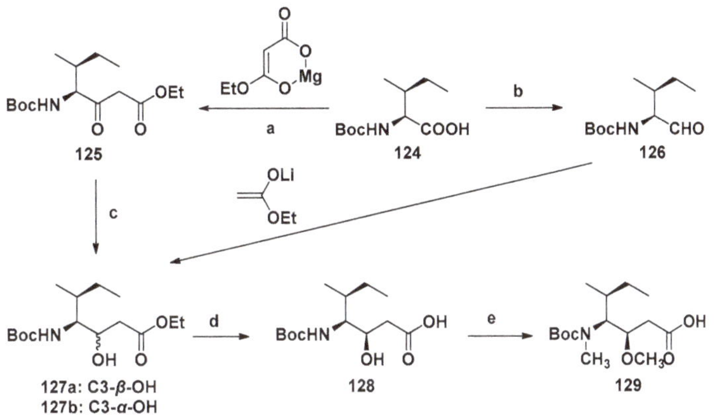

Scheme 10. Synthesis of the Dil unit (**129**). Reagents and conditions: (a) CDI (carbonyl dimidazole), THF; (b) (1) CH$_3$I, KHCO$_3$, (2) LiCl, NaBH$_4$, (3) DMSO, Py·SO$_3$; (c) NaBH$_4$; (d) NaOH; (e) (1) NaH, (2) CH$_3$I.

4.4. Synthesis of Dolastatin 10

According to most reports, two synthetic schemes of Dol-10 based on Evans aldol method are summarized. In the asymmetric synthesis scheme of Pettit and Zhou et al. (Scheme 11) [98,120], the C-terminal subunit (S)-Doe and remaining four amino acid residues were gradually assembled into compound **1** with high stereoselectivity, which were more convenient, effective and acceptable than most linear synthesis patterns starting from C-terminal (Scheme 12) [111,116,118,119].

4.5. Conformational Study

The basic conformational characteristics of Dol-10, the effect of terminal residues on the whole conformation and interaction of peptides were described via nuclear magnetic resonance (NMR), molecular mechanics (MM) and molecular dynamics (MD) calculation techniques [113,121–123].

The ^{1}H NMR spectra and ^{1}H-^{13}C hetero-correlated spectra were analyzed in CD$_2$Cl$_2$ solution, and the conformational energy minimization was systematically studied under limited experimental conditions. According to the NMR data, it was observed that the αCH (25) proton of Dov residue had a huge shielding effect, which indicated that there was an interaction between N-terminal and aromatic C-terminal of the peptide. Therefore, it was speculated that this linear dolastatin molecule might have a ring-like conformation. However, the conformational theory analysis denied the possibility of binding between molecules from head to tail, verified the NMR hypothesis of a folded peptide-like molecule, and speculated a series of possible conformations based on the consistent experimental data (Figure 14) [121]. Molecular mechanics (MM) analysis confirmed that pentapeptide had a comparatively rigid molecular system. Molecular dynamics (MD) simulation of molecular conformation had reached an almost stable state in the gas phase without large degree of conformational freedom. The conformation with the least energy had a pocket-like shape with all groups facing out of the structural framework. In addition, the conformational behavior of Dol-10 mainly depended on the hydrophobicity of its residues. On the C-terminal residue, even slight structural modifications might change the functional position of interaction with biological partners [123]. The model studies indicated that the terminal residues Dov and Doe had certain mobility, while the internal residues Val and Dap had almost no change in cis- and trans- structures. On the contrary, due to the cis-trans isomerization of the C15-C16 amide bond, the central residue Dil changed significantly [113].

To sum up, this work was helpful to understand the structural characteristics of Dol-10 that played a role in microtubule polymerization and mitosis. The folding structure and high flexibility of Dol-10 together realized its excellent biological activity.

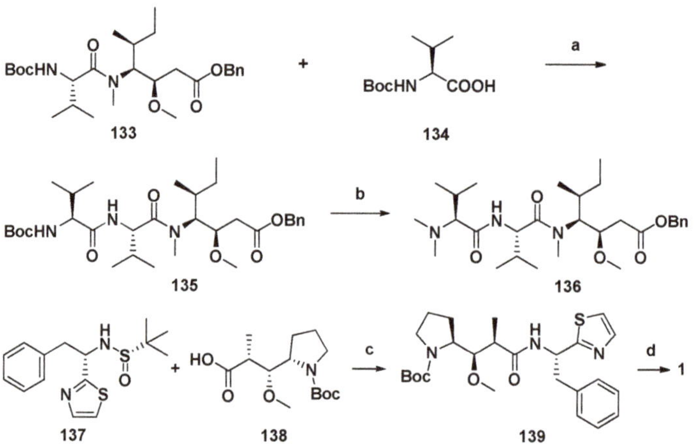

Scheme 11. The asymmetric synthesis of Dol-10 (1). Reagents and conditions: Please refer to Reference [98] for the synthesis of 133. (a) (1) TFA, DCM, 0 °C, 2 h; (2) HATU, HOAt, DIPEA, DCM, r.t., overnight, for two steps 85%; (b) (1) TFA, DCM, r.t., 2 h; (2) 40% HCHO, Na(BH$_3$)CN, CH$_3$CN, r.t., 18 h, for two steps 82%; (c) (1) HCl/dioxane, MeOH, 0 °C, 30 min; (2) HATU, HOAt, DIPEA, DCM, r.t., overnight, for two steps 80%; (d) (1) TFA, DCM, 0 °C, 2 h; (2) 136, Pd/C, H$_2$, MeOH, 2 h; (3) HATU, HOAt, DIPEA, DCM, r.t., 24 h, for three steps 60%.

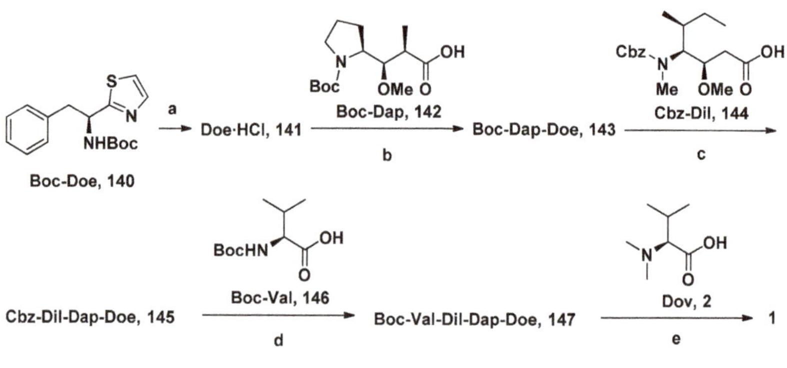

Scheme 12. The linear synthesis pattern of Dol-10 (1) starting from C-terminal. Reagents and conditions: (a) 2.4 N HCl/dioxane, r.t., 80 min, 93%; (b) DEPC, NEt$_3$/DME, 4 °C, 14 h, 78%; (c) 2.4 N HCl/dioxane, r.t., 1 h, DEPC, NEt$_3$/DME, 0 °C, 3 h, 70%; (d) 5% HBr/AcOH, r.t., 2 h, BopCl, NEt$_3$/CH$_2$Cl$_2$, 4 °C, 7 d, 75%; (e) 1.2 N HCl/dioxane, r.t., 1 h, DEPC, NEt$_3$/DME, 4 °C, 12 h, 75%.

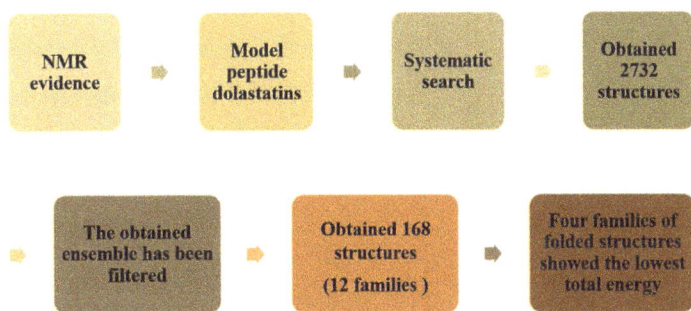

Figure 14. Outline of the procedures for the conformational search performed.

5. Conclusions

Marine bioactive polypeptide Dol-10 has been investigated for more than 30 years, from its first discovery to the approval of the related drug for marketing, which brings a bright prospect for tumor treatment and is still one of the most active antitumor compounds found so far. Dol-10 and its derivatives can effectively inhibit the growth of tumor cells in vitro, but their clinical efficacy as a single drug in phase II clinical trials of solid tumors is frustrating due to adverse effects. For example, the most common peripheral neuropathy had brought a great blow to the clinical research of the marine peptide. Later, chemical researchers coupled monoclonal antibodies with Dol-10 derivatives by ADCs technology, and utilized the specificity of antibodies to transport drug molecules to target tissues for their functions. As a result, the systemic toxic and side effects of drugs were reduced, and the treatment window of drugs was improved. Adcetris®, as a typical representative of listed ADCs, has successfully overcome the obstacles in clinical application of Dol-10 and greatly promoted the research progress of ADCs. Moreover, in the process of systematical antitumor study of Dol-10, it is accidentally found that this antitumor peptide also has potent antifungal [124], antibacterial [86], and anti-*Plasmodium falciparum* [125] biological activities, which points out a new direction for the further development of Dol-10. At present, many excellent studies about Dol-10 have been published, but the related antitumor research based on Dol-10 still faces challenges and opportunities. Reducing the toxicity of Dol-10 in vivo and in clinical research by structural modifications and/or combining with newly emerging medical technology, so that it can be better applied to the treatment of tumors. Considering most reported structural modifications of *N*- and *C*-terminal subunits, it can be predicted that more Dol-10 analogs based on modified central residues Dil, Dap, and Doe will appear soon. And there is no doubt that selecting appropriate monoclonal antibodies to couple with Dol-10 or its derivatives to prepare ADCs into the clinic is still one of the main research directions of Dol-10 in the future.

Funding: This research received no external funding.

Acknowledgments: This paper was financially supported by Public Project of Ningbo (No. 202002N3167), High-level Innovative Project in Shenyang (Young and Middle-aged Technological Innovative Support Plan, RC190483) and Career Development Support Plan in Shenyang Pharmaceutical University. In addition, the work was also sponsored by a K.C. Wong Magna Fund in Ningbo University.

Conflicts of Interest: The authors declare that they have no known competing financial interests or personal relationships that could have appeared to influence the work reported in this paper.

References

1. Blunt, J.W.; Carroll, A.R.; Copp, B.R.; Davis, R.A.; Keyzers, R.A.; Prinsep, M.R. Marine natural products. *Nat. Prod. Rep.* **2018**, *35*, 8–53. [CrossRef]
2. Carroll, A.R.; Copp, B.R.; Davis, R.A.; Keyzers, R.A.; Prinsep, M.R. Marine natural products. *Nat. Prod. Rep.* **2020**, *37*, 175–223. [CrossRef]

3. Faulkner, D.J. Marine natural products. *Nat. Prod. Rep.* **2001**, *19*, 1–48. [CrossRef] [PubMed]
4. Dyshlovoy, S.A.; Honecker, F. Marine Compounds and Cancer: The First Two Decades of XXI Century. *Mar. Drugs* **2019**, *18*, 20. [CrossRef]
5. Stonik, V.A. Marine Natural Products: A Way to New Drugs. *Acta Nat.* **2009**, *1*, 15–25. [CrossRef]
6. Paterson, I.; Anderson, E.A. The Renaissance of Natural Products as Drug Candidates. *Science* **2005**, *310*, 451–453. [CrossRef]
7. Molinski, T.F.; Dalisay, D.S.; Lievens, S.L.; Saludes, J.P. Drug development from marine natural products. *Nat. Rev. Drug Discov.* **2008**, *8*, 69–85. [CrossRef]
8. Jing, Q.; Hu, X.; Ma, Y.; Mu, J.; Liu, W.; Xu, F.; Li, Z.; Bai, J.; Hua, H.; Li, D. Marine-Derived Natural Lead Compound Disulfide-Linked Dimer Psammaplin A: Biological Activity and Structural Modification. *Mar. Drugs* **2019**, *17*, 384. [CrossRef] [PubMed]
9. Chen, J.; Wang, B.; Lu, Y.; Guo, Y.; Sun, J.; Wei, B.; Zhang, H.; Wang, H. Quorum Sensing Inhibitors from Marine Microorganisms and Their Synthetic Derivatives. *Mar. Drugs* **2019**, *17*, 80. [CrossRef] [PubMed]
10. Choudhary, A.; Naughton, L.M.; Montánchez, I.; Dobson, A.D.W.; Rai, D.K. Current Status and Future Prospects of Marine Natural Products (MNPs) as Antimicrobials. *Mar. Drugs* **2017**, *15*, 272. [CrossRef]
11. Pereira, F. Have marine natural product drug discovery efforts been productive and how can we improve their efficiency? *Expert Opin. Drug Discov.* **2019**, *14*, 717–722. [CrossRef]
12. Huang, C.; Zhang, Z.; Cui, W. Marine-Derived Natural Compounds for the Treatment of Parkinson's Disease. *Mar. Drugs* **2019**, *17*, 221. [CrossRef]
13. Wu, Q.; Nay, B.; Yang, M.; Ni, Y.; Wang, H.; Yao, L.; Li, X. Marine sponges of the genus Stelletta as promising drug sources: Chemical and biological aspects. *Acta Pharm. Sin. B* **2019**, *9*, 237–257. [CrossRef] [PubMed]
14. Livingston, D.M.; Kung, A.L. Composition and Method for Imaging Cells. US20090185977A1, 23 July 2009.
15. Nalli, Y.; Gupta, S.; Khajuria, V.; Singh, V.P.; Sajgotra, M.; Ahmed, Z.; Thakur, N.L.; Ali, A. TNF-α and IL-6 inhibitory effects of cyclic dipeptides isolated from marine bacteria *Streptomyces* sp. *Med. Chem. Res.* **2017**, *26*, 93–100. [CrossRef]
16. Zheng, L.; Xu, Y.; Lin, X.; Yuan, Z.; Liu, M.; Cao, S.; Zhang, F.; Linhardt, R.J. Recent Progress of Marine Polypeptides as Anticancer Agents. *Recent Pat. Anti-Cancer Drug Discov.* **2018**, *13*, 445–454. [CrossRef]
17. Sable, R.; Parajuli, P.; Jois, S. Peptides, Peptidomimetics, and Polypeptides from Marine Sources: A Wealth of Natural Sources for Pharmaceutical Applications. *Mar. Drugs* **2017**, *15*, 124. [CrossRef] [PubMed]
18. Hansen, E.; Andersen, J.H. Screening for Marine Natural Products with Potential as Chemotherapeutics for Acute Myeloid Leukemia. *Curr. Pharm. Biotechnol.* **2015**, *17*, 71–77. [CrossRef] [PubMed]
19. Zheng, L.-H.; Wang, Y.-J.; Sheng, J.; Wang, F.; Zheng, Y.; Lin, X.-K.; Sun, M. Antitumor Peptides from Marine Organisms. *Mar. Drugs* **2011**, *9*, 1840–1859. [CrossRef]
20. Daqiao, Y.; Jinxu, W.; Laihao, L.; Xianqing, Y.; Haixia, M. Development of Co-production of Polysaccharides and Polypeptides from Marine Organisms—A Review. *Chin. Fish. Qual. Stand.* **2019**, *9*, 01–08.
21. Cao, W.L.; Song, J.X.R.; Li, F.Q.C. Research advances on marine antitumor peptides dolastatin 10. *J. Med. Postgrad.* **2011**, *24*, 1208–1211.
22. Negi, B.; Kumar, D.; Rawat, D.S. Marine Peptides as Anticancer Agents: A Remedy to Mankind by Nature. *Curr. Protein Pept. Sci.* **2017**, *18*, 885–904. [CrossRef]
23. Cui, Q.; Chen, J.R.; Jiang, X.Y.; Guan, L.L.; Liu, S.M.; Kong, L.C.; Hong-Xia, M.A. Advances in the application of marine bioactive peptide drugs. *Chin. J. Mar. Drugs* **2019**, *38*, 54–60.
24. Ma, W.; Qin, T.; Sun, Y. The classification and advances of bioactive peptides. *Chin. J. Inj. Rep. Wound Heal.* **2019**, *14*, 149–152.
25. Festa, C.; Marino, S.D.; D'Auria, M.; Monti, M.C.; Bucci, M.; Vellecco, V.; Debitus, C.; Zampella, A. Anti-inflammatory cyclopeptides from the marine sponge Theonella swinhoei. *Tetrahedron* **2012**, *68*, 2851–2857. [CrossRef]
26. Donia, M.; Hamann, M.T. Marine natural products and their potential applications as anti-infective agents. *Lancet Infect. Dis.* **2003**, *3*, 338–348. [CrossRef]
27. Ram Singh, M.S.; Joshi, P.; Rawat, D.S. Clinical status of anti-cancer agents derived from marine sources. *Anticancer Agents Med. Chem.* **2008**, *8*, 603–617. [CrossRef]
28. de Castro, R.J.S.; Sato, H.H. Biologically active peptides: Processes for their generation, purification and identification and applications as natural additives in the food and pharmaceutical industries. *Food Res. Int.* **2015**, *74*, 185–198. [CrossRef]
29. Cavé, A.; Cortes, D.; Figadère, B.; Laurens, A.; Pettit, G.R.; Herz, W.; Kirby, G.W.; Moore, R.E.; Steglich, W.; Tamm, C. [Fortschritte der Chemie organischer Naturstoffe/Progress in the Chemistry of Organic Natural Products] Fortschritte der Chemie organischer Naturstoffe Progress in the Chemistry of Organic Natural Products. *Dolastatins* **1997**, *70*, 1–79. [CrossRef]
30. Pettit, G.R.; Kamano, Y.; Herald, C.L.; Tuinman, A.A.; Boettner, F.E.; Kizu, H.; Schmidt, J.M.; Baczynskyj, L.; Tomer, K.B.; Bontems, R.J. The isolation and structure of a remarkable marine animal antineoplastic constituent: Dolastatin 10. *J. Am. Chem. Soc.* **1987**, *109*, 6883–6885. [CrossRef]
31. Pettit, G.R.; Kamano, Y.; Herald, C.L.; Fujii, Y.; Kizu, H.; Boyd, M.R.; Boettner, F.E.; Doubek, D.L.; Schmidt, J.M.; Chapuis, J.-C.; et al. Antineoplastic Agents. Part 247. The Dolastatins. Part 18. Isolation of Dolastatins 10–15 from the Marine Mollusc Dolabella auricularia. *Tetrahedron* **1993**, *49*, 9151–9170. [CrossRef]
32. Kingston, D.G.I. Tubulin-Interactive Natural Products as Anticancer Agents. *J. Nat. Prod.* **2009**, *72*, 507–515. [CrossRef] [PubMed]
33. Bai, R.; Roach, M.C.; Jayaram, S.K.; Barkoczy, J.; Pettit, G.R.; Luduena, R.F.; Hamel, E. Differential effects of active isomers, segments, and analogs of dolastatin 10 on ligand interactions with tubulin. *Biochem. Pharmacol.* **1993**, *45*, 1503–1515. [CrossRef]

34. Bai, R.; Pettit, G.R.; Hamel, E. Structure-activity studies with chiral isomers and with segments of the antimitotic marine peptide dolastatin 10. *Biochem. Pharmacol.* **1990**, *40*, 1859–1864. [CrossRef]
35. Bai, R.; Pettit, G.R.; Hamel, E. Dolastatin 10, a powerful cytostatic peptide derived from a marine animal. Inhibition of tubulin polymerization mediated through the vinca alkaloid binding domain. *Biochem. Pharmacol.* **1990**, *39*, 1941–1949. [CrossRef]
36. Maki, A.; Mohammad, R.; Raza, S.; Saleh, M.; Govindaraju, K.D.; Pettit, G.R.; al-Katib, A. Effect of dolastatin 10 on human non-Hodgkin's lymphoma cell lines. *Anticancer Drugs* **1996**, *7*, 344–350. [CrossRef]
37. Kalemkerian, G.P.; Ou, X.; Adil, M.R.; Rosati, R.; Khoulani, M.M.; Madan, S.K.; Pettit, G.R. Activity of dolastatin 10 against small-cell lung cancer in vitro and in vivo: Induction of apoptosis and bcl-2 modification. *Cancer Chemother. Pharmacol.* **1999**, *43*, 507–515. [CrossRef]
38. Turner, T.; Jackson, W.H.; Pettit, G.R.; Wells, A.; Kraft, A.S. Treatment of human prostate cancer cells with dolastatin 10, a peptide isolated from a marine shell-less mollusc. *Prostate* **1998**, *34*, 175–181. [CrossRef]
39. Pettit, G.R.; Srirangam, J.K.; Williams, M.D.; Durkin, K.P.M.; Barlozzari, T.; Kling, A.; Janssen, B.; Haupt, A. Dolastatin Peptides. US6323315B1, 27 December 2001.
40. Pettit, G.R.; Kamano, Y.; Fujii, Y.; Herald, C.L.; Inoue, M.; Brown, P.; Gust, D.; Kitahara, K.; Schmidt, J.M.; Doubek, D.L.; et al. Marine Animal Biosynthetic Constituents For Cancer Chemotherapy. *J. Nat. Prod.* **1981**, *44*, 482–485. [CrossRef]
41. Butler, M.S. Natural products to drugs: Natural product-derived compounds in clinical trials. *Nat. Prod. Rep.* **2008**, *25*, 475–516. [CrossRef]
42. Pettit, G.R.; Singh, S.B.; Hogan, F.; Lloydwilliams, P.; Herald, D.L.; Burkett, D.D.; Clewlow, P.J. Antineoplastic Agents.189. The Absolute-Configuration and Synthesis of Natural (-)-Dolastatin-10. *J. Am. Chem. Soc.* **1989**, *111*, 5463–5465. [CrossRef]
43. Simmons, T.L.; Andrianasolo, E.; McPhail, K.; Flatt, P.; Gerwick, W.H. Marine natural products as anticancer drugs. *Mol. Cancer Ther.* **2005**, *4*, 333–342.
44. Pitot, H.C.; McElroy, E.A.; Reid, J.M.; Windebank, A.J.; Sloan, J.A.; Erlichman, C.; Bagniewski, P.G.; Walker, D.L.; Rubin, J.; Goldberg, R.M.; et al. Phase I trial of dolastatin-10 (NSC 376128) in patients with advanced solid tumors. *Clin. Cancer Res.* **1999**, *5*, 525–531. [PubMed]
45. Yamamoto, N.; Andoh, M.; Kawahara, M.; Fukuoka, M.; Niitani, H. Phase I study of TZT-1027, a novel synthetic dolastatin 10 derivative and inhibitor of tubulin polymerization, given weekly to advanced solid tumor patients for 3 weeks. *Cancer Sci.* **2009**, *100*, 316–321. [CrossRef] [PubMed]
46. Horti, J.; Juhász, E.; Monostori, Z.; Maeda, K.; Eckhardt, S.; Bodrogi, I. Phase I study of TZT-1027, a novel synthetic dolastatin 10 derivative, for the treatment of patients with non-small cell lung cancer. *Cancer Chemother. Pharmacol.* **2008**, *62*, 173–180. [CrossRef] [PubMed]
47. Senter, P.D.; Sievers, E. The discovery and development of brentuximab vedotin for use in relapsed Hodgkin lymphoma and systemic anaplastic large cell lymphoma. *Nat. Biotechnol.* **2012**, *30*, 631–637. [CrossRef]
48. Hoffman, M.A.; Blessing, J.A.; Lentz, S.S. A phase II trial of dolastatin-10 in recurrent platinum-sensitive ovarian carcinoma: A Gynecologic Oncology Group study. *Gynecol. Oncol.* **2003**, *89*, 95–98. [CrossRef]
49. Verdier-Pinard, P.; Kepler, J.A.; Pettit, G.R.; Hamel, E. Sustained intracellular retention of dolastatin 10 causes its potent antimitotic activity. *Mol. Pharmacol.* **2000**, *57*, 180–187.
50. Beckwith, M.; Urba, W.J.; Longo, D.L. Growth Inhibition of Human Lymphoma Cell Lines by the Marine Products, Dolastatins 10 and 15. *J. Natl. Cancer Inst.* **1993**, *85*, 483–488. [CrossRef]
51. Mohammad, R.M.; Pettit, G.R.; Almatchy, V.P.; Wall, N.; Varterasian, M.; Ai-Katib, A. Synergistic interaction of selected marine animal anticancer drugs against human diffuse large cell lymphoma. *Anti-Cancer Drugs* **1998**, *9*, 149–156. [CrossRef]
52. Vaishampayan, U.; Glode, M.; Du, W.; Kraft, A.; Hudes, G.; Wright, J.; Hussain, M. Phase II study of dolastatin-10 in patients with hormone-refractory metastatic prostate adenocarcinoma. *Clin. Cancer Res.* **2000**, *6*, 4205.
53. Von, M.M.; Balcerzak, S.P.; Kraft, A.S.; Edmonson, J.H.; Okuno, S.H.; Davey, M.; Mclaughlin, S.; Beard, M.T.; Rogatko, A. Phase II Trial of Dolastatin-10, a Novel Anti-Tubulin Agent, in Metastatic Soft Tissue Sarcomas. *Sarcoma* **2004**, *8*, 107–111.
54. Perez, E.A.; Hillman, D.W.; Fishkin, P.A.; Krook, J.E.; Tan, W.W.; Kuriakose, P.A.; Alberts, S.R.; Dakhil, S.R. Phase II trial of dolastatin-10 in patients with advanced breast cancer. *Investig. New Drugs* **2005**, *23*, 257–261. [CrossRef]
55. Kindler, H.L.; Tothy, P.K.; Wolff, R.; McCormack, R.A.; Abbruzzese, J.L.; Mani, S.; Wade-Oliver, K.T.; Vokes, E.E. Phase II trials of dolastatin-10 in advanced pancreaticobiliary cancers. *Investig. New Drugs* **2005**, *23*, 489–493. [CrossRef]
56. Hadfield, J.A.; Ducki, S.; Hirst, N.; McGown, A.T. Tubulin and microtubules as targets for anticancer drugs. *Prog. Cell Cycle Res.* **2003**, *5*, 309–325.
57. Perez, E.A.; Shang, X.; Burlingame, S.M.; Okcu, M.F.; Ge, N.; Russell, H.V.; Egler, R.A.; David, R.D.; Vasudevan, S.A.; Yang, J.; et al. Microtubule inhibitors: Differentiating tubulin-inhibiting agents based on mechanisms of action, clinical activity, and resistance. *Mol. Cancer Ther.* **2009**, *8*, 2086–2095. [CrossRef]
58. Morris, P.G.; Fornier, M.N. Microtubule Active Agents: Beyond the Taxane Frontier. *Clin. Cancer Res.* **2008**, *14*, 7167–7172. [CrossRef]
59. Pasquier, E.; Kavallaris, M. Microtubules: A dynamic target in cancer therapy. *Iubmb Life* **2008**, *60*, 165–170. [CrossRef]
60. Kavallaris, M.; Verrills, N.M.; Hill, B.T. Anticancer therapy with novel tubulin-interacting drugs. *Drug Resist. Updat.* **2001**, *4*, 392–401. [CrossRef] [PubMed]
61. Rai, S.S.; Wolff, J. Localization of the Vinblastine-binding Site on β-Tubulin. *J. Biol. Chem.* **1996**, *271*, 14707–14711. [CrossRef] [PubMed]

62. Li, Y.; Kobayashi, H.; Hashimoto, Y.; Shirai, R.; Hirata, A.; Hayashi, K.; Hamada, Y.; Shioiri, T.; Iwasaki, S. Interaction of marine toxin dolastatin 10 with porcine brain tubulin: Competitive inhibition of rhizoxin and phomopsin A binding. *Chem. Interact.* **1994**, *93*, 175–183. [CrossRef]
63. Luduena, R.F.; Roach, M.C.; Prasad, V.; Pettit, G.R. Interaction of dolastatin 10 with bovine brain tubulin. *Biochem. Pharmacol.* **1992**, *43*, 539–543. [CrossRef]
64. Bai, R.L.; Pettit, G.R.; Hamel, E. Binding of dolastatin 10 to tubulin at a distinct site for peptide antimitotic agents near the exchangeable nucleotide and vinca alkaloid sites. *J. Biol. Chem.* **1990**, *265*, 17141–17149. [CrossRef]
65. Roach, M.C.; Luduena, R.F. Different effects of tubulin ligands on the intrachain cross-linking of beta 1-tubulin. *J. Biol. Chem.* **1984**, *259*, 12063–12071. [CrossRef]
66. Ludueña, R.F.; Roach, M.C. Contrasting effects of maytansine and vinblastine on the alkylation of tubulin sulfhydryls. *Arch. Biochem. Biophys.* **1981**, *210*, 498–504. [CrossRef]
67. Little, M.; Ludueña, R.F. Location of two cysteines in brain beta 1-tubulin that can be cross-linked after removal of exchangeable GTP. *Biochim. Biophys. Acta* **1987**, *912*, 28–33. [CrossRef]
68. Ludueña, R.F.; Roach, M.C.; Prasad, V.; Lacey, E. Effect of phomopsin a on the alkylation of tubulin. *Biochem. Pharmacol.* **1990**, *39*, 1603–1608. [CrossRef]
69. Mitra, A.; Sept, D. Localization of the antimitotic peptide and depsipeptide binding site on beta-tubulin. *Biochemistry* **2004**, *43*, 13955–13962. [CrossRef] [PubMed]
70. Bai, R.; Covell, D.G.; Taylor, G.F.; Kepler, J.A.; Copeland, T.D.; Nguyen, N.Y.; Pettit, G.R.; Hamel, E. Direct photoaffinity labeling by dolastatin 10 of the amino-terminal peptide of beta-tubulin containing cysteine 12. *J. Biol. Chem.* **2004**, *279*, 30731–30740. [CrossRef] [PubMed]
71. Maki, A.; Diwakaran, H.; Redman, B.; Al-Asfar, S.; Pettit, G.R.; Mohammad, R.M.; Al-Katib, A. The bcl-2 and p53 oncoproteins can be modulated by bryostatin 1 and dolastatins in human diffuse large cell lymphoma. *Anti-Cancer Drugs* **1995**, *6*, 392–397. [CrossRef] [PubMed]
72. Haldar, S.; Basu, A.; Croce, C.M. Serine-70 is one of the critical sites for drug-induced Bcl2 phosphorylation in cancer cells. *Cancer Res.* **1998**, *58*, 1609.
73. Pathak, S.; Multani, A.S.; Ozen, M.; Richardson, M.A.; Newman, R.A. Dolastatin-10 induces polyploidy, telomeric associations and apoptosis in a murine melanoma cell line. *Oncol. Rep.* **1998**, *5*, 373–379. [CrossRef]
74. Pathak, S.; Risin, S.; Brown, N.; Berry, K. Telomeric association of chromosomes is an early manifestation of programmed cell death. *Int. J. Oncol.* **1994**, *4*, 323–328. [CrossRef]
75. Pathak, S.; Dave, B.J.; Gagos, S. Chromosome alterations in cancer development and apoptosis. *In Vivo* **1994**, *8*, 843–850.
76. Aherne, G.W.; Hardcastle, A.; Valenti, M.; Bryant, A.; Rogers, P.; Pettit, G.R.; Srirangam, J.K.; Kelland, L.R. Antitumour evaluation of dolastatins 10 and 15 and their measurement in plasma by radioimmunoassay. *Cancer Chemother. Pharmacol.* **1996**, *38*, 225–232. [CrossRef] [PubMed]
77. Garteiz, D.A.; Madden, T.; Beck, D.E.; Huie, W.R.; McManus, K.T.; Abbruzzese, J.L.; Chen, W.; Newman, R.A. Quantitation of dolastatin-10 using HPLC/electrospray ionization mass spectrometry: Application in a phase I clinical trial. *Cancer Chemother. Pharmacol.* **1998**, *41*, 299–306. [CrossRef] [PubMed]
78. Madden, T.; Tran, H.T.; Beck, D.; Huie, R.; Newman, R.A.; Pusztai, L.; Wright, J.J.; Abbruzzese, J.L. Novel marine-derived anticancer agents: A phase I clinical, pharmacological, and pharmacodynamic study of dolastatin 10 (NSC 376128) in patients with advanced solid tumors. *Clin. Cancer Res.* **2000**, *6*, 1293–1301.
79. Mirsalis, J.C.; Schindler-Horvat, J.; Hill, J.R.; Tomaszewski, J.E.; Donohue, S.J.; Tyson, C.A. Toxicity of dolastatin 10 in mice, rats and dogs and its clinical relevance. *Cancer Chemother. Pharmacol.* **1999**, *44*, 395–402. [CrossRef] [PubMed]
80. Thamm, D.H.; MacEwen, G.E.; Phillips, B.S.; Hershey, E.A.; Burgess, K.M.; Pettit, G.R.; Vail, D.M. Preclinical study of dolastatin-10 in dogs with spontaneous neoplasia. *Cancer Chemother. Pharmacol.* **2002**, *49*, 251–255. [CrossRef]
81. Fayette, J.; Coquard, I.R.; Alberti, L.; Boyle, H.; Méeus, P.; Decouvelaere, A.-V.; Thiesse, P.; Sunyach, M.-P.; Ranchère, D.; Blay, J.-Y. ET-743: A novel agent with activity in soft-tissue sarcomas. *Curr. Opin. Oncol.* **2006**, *18*, 347–353. [CrossRef] [PubMed]
82. Toppmeyer, D.L.; Slapak, C.A.; Croop, J.; Kufe, D.W. Role of P-glycoprotein in dolastatin 10 resistance. *Biochem. Pharmacol.* **1994**, *48*, 609–612. [CrossRef]
83. Akaiwa, M.; Martin, T.; Mendelsohn, B.A. Synthesis and Evaluation of Linear and Macrocyclic Dolastatin 10 Analogues Containing Pyrrolidine Ring Modifications. *ACS Omega* **2018**, *3*, 5212–5221. [CrossRef] [PubMed]
84. Dugal-Tessier, J.; Barnscher, S.D.; Kanai, A.; Mendelsohn, B.A. Synthesis and Evaluation of Dolastatin 10 Analogues Containing Heteroatoms on the Amino Acid Side Chains. *J. Nat. Prod.* **2017**, *80*, 2484–2491. [CrossRef] [PubMed]
85. Maderna, A.; Doroski, M.; Subramanyam, C.; Porte, A.; Leverett, C.A.; Vetelino, B.C.; Chen, Z.; Risley, H.; Parris, K.; Pandit, J.; et al. Discovery of Cytotoxic Dolastatin 10 Analogues with N-Terminal Modifications. *J. Med. Chem.* **2014**, *57*, 10527–10543. [CrossRef] [PubMed]
86. Pettit, G.R.; Srirangam, J.K.; Barkoczy, J.; Williams, M.D.; Boyd, M.R.; Hamel, E.; Pettit, R.K.; Hogan, F.; Bai, R.; Chapuis, J.C.; et al. Antineoplastic agents 365. Dolastatin 10 SAR probes. *Anticancer Drug Des.* **1998**, *13*, 243–277. [PubMed]
87. Shnyder, S.D.; Cooper, P.A.; Millington, N.J.; Pettit, G.R.; Bibby, M.C. Auristatin PYE, a novel synthetic derivative of dolastatin 10: Activity and mechanistic studies in a colon adenocarcinoma model. *Cancer Res.* **2005**, *65*, 806–807.

88. Akashi, Y.; Okamoto, I.; Suzuki, M.; Tamura, K.; Iwasa, T.; Hisada, S.; Satoh, T.; Nakagawa, K.; Ono, K.; Fukuoka, M. The novel microtubule-interfering agent TZT-1027 enhances the anticancer effect of radiation in vitro and in vivo. *Br. J. Cancer* **2007**, *96*, 1532–1539. [CrossRef]
89. Watanabe, J.; Minami, M.; Kobayashi, M. Antitumor activity of TZT-1027 (Soblidotin). *Anticancer Res.* **2006**, *26*, 1973–1981.
90. Natsume, T.; Watanabe, J.-I.; Koh, Y.; Fujio, N.; Ohe, Y.; Horiuchi, T.; Saijo, N.; Nishio, K.; Kobayashi, M. Antitumor activity of TZT-1027 (Soblidotin) against vascular endothelial growth factor-secreting human lung cancer in vivo. *Cancer Sci.* **2003**, *94*, 826–833. [CrossRef]
91. Yokosaka, S.; Izawa, A.; Sakai, C.; Sakurada, E.; Morita, Y.; Nishio, Y. Synthesis and evaluation of novel dolastatin 10 derivatives for versatile conjugations. *Bioorganic Med. Chem.* **2018**, *26*, 1643–1652. [CrossRef]
92. Pettit, G.R.; Hogan, F.; Toms, S. Antineoplastic Agents. 592. Highly Effective Cancer Cell Growth Inhibitory Structural Modifications of Dolastatin 10. *J. Nat. Prod.* **2011**, *74*, 962–968. [CrossRef]
93. Pettit, G.R.; Melody, N.; Chapuis, J.-C. Antineoplastic Agents. 607. Emetine Auristatins. *J. Nat. Prod.* **2020**, *83*, 1571–1576. [CrossRef]
94. Pettit, G.R.; Singh, S.B.; Hogan, F.; Burkett, D.D. Chiral modifications of dolastatin 10: The potent cytostatic peptide (19aR)-isodolastatin 10. *J. Med. Chem.* **1990**, *33*, 3132–3133. [CrossRef]
95. Nie, X.-D.; Mao, Z.-Y.; Zhou, W.; Si, C.-M.; Wei, B.-G.; Lin, G.-Q. A diastereoselective approach to amino alcohols and application for divergent synthesis of dolastatin 10. *Org. Chem. Front.* **2020**, *7*, 76–103. [CrossRef]
96. Poncet, J.; Busquet, M.; Roux, F.; Pierre, A.; Atassi, G.; Jouin, P. Synthesis and Biological Activity of Chimeric Structures Derived from the Cytotoxic Natural Compounds Dolastatin 10 and Dolastatin 15. *J. Med. Chem.* **1998**, *41*, 1524–1530. [CrossRef]
97. Wang, X.; Dong, S.; Feng, D.; Chen, Y.; Ma, M.; Hu, W. Synthesis and biological activity evaluation of dolastatin 10 analogues with N-terminal modifications. *Tetrahedron* **2017**, *73*, 2255–2266. [CrossRef]
98. Zhou, W.; Nie, X.-D.; Zhang, Y.; Si, C.-M.; Zhou, Z.; Sun, X.; Wei, B.-G. A practical approach to asymmetric synthesis of dolastatin 10. *Org. Biomol. Chem.* **2017**, *15*, 6119–6131. [CrossRef]
99. Yang, K.; Chen, B.; Gianolio, D.A.; Stefano, J.E.; Busch, M.; Manning, C.; Alving, K.; Gregory, R.C.; Brondyk, W.H.; Miller, R.J.; et al. Convergent synthesis of hydrophilic monomethyl dolastatin 10 based drug linkers for antibody–drug conjugation. *Org. Biomol. Chem.* **2019**, *17*, 8115–8124. [CrossRef] [PubMed]
100. Zhang, S.X.; Chen, M.X.R.; Fang-qiu, L.I. Application of fluorescence imaging in the research of tumor. *J. Med. Postgrad.* **2009**, *22*, 195–197.
101. Lee, J.-W.; Stone, R.L.; Lee, S.J.; Nam, E.J.; Roh, J.-W.; Nick, A.M.; Han, H.-D.; Shahzad, M.M.; Kim, H.-S.; Mangala, L.S.; et al. EphA2 Targeted Chemotherapy Using an Antibody Drug Conjugate in Endometrial Carcinoma. *Clin. Cancer Res.* **2010**, *16*, 2562–2570. [CrossRef]
102. Lee, J.-W.; Han, H.D.; Shahzad, M.M.K.; Kim, S.W.; Mangala, L.S.; Nick, A.M.; Lu, C.; Langley, R.R.; Schmandt, R.; Kim, H.-S.; et al. EphA2 Immunoconjugate as Molecularly Targeted Chemotherapy for Ovarian Carcinoma. *J. Natl. Cancer Inst.* **2009**, *101*, 1193–1205. [CrossRef]
103. Amoroso, L.; Castel, V.; Bisogno, G.; Casanova, M.; Marquez-Vega, C.; Chisholm, J.C.; Doz, F.; Moreno, L.; Ruggiero, A.; Gerber, N.U.; et al. Phase II results from a phase I/II study to assess the safety and efficacy of weekly nab-paclitaxel in paediatric patients with recurrent or refractory solid tumours: A collaboration with the European Innovative Therapies for Children with Cancer Network. *Eur. J. Cancer* **2020**, *135*, 89–97. [CrossRef]
104. Annunziata, C.M.; Kohn, E.C.; Lorusso, P.; Houston, N.D.; Coleman, R.L.; Buzoianu, M.; Robbie, G.; Lechleider, R. Phase 1, open-label study of MEDI-547 in patients with relapsed or refractory solid tumors. *Investig. New Drugs* **2012**, *31*, 77–84. [CrossRef]
105. Bhat, S.A.; Czuczman, M.S. Novel antibodies in the treatment of non-Hodgkin's lymphoma. *Neth. J. Med.* **2009**, *67*, 311.
106. Polson, A.G.; Calemine-Fenaux, J.; Chan, P.; Chang, W.; Christensen, E.; Clark, S.; de Sauvage, F.J.; Eaton, D.; Elkins, K.; Elliott, J.M.; et al. Antibody-drug conjugates for the treatment of non-Hodgkin's lymphoma: Target and linker-drug selection. *Cancer Res.* **2009**, *69*, 2358–2364. [CrossRef]
107. Pettit, G.R.; Melody, N.; Chapuis, J.-C. Antineoplastic Agents. 603. Quinstatins: Exceptional Cancer Cell Growth Inhibitors. *J. Nat. Prod.* **2017**, *80*, 692–698. [CrossRef]
108. Pettit, G.R.; Melody, N.; Chapuis, J.-C. Antineoplastic Agents. 604. The Path of Quinstatin Derivatives to Antibody Drug Conjugates. *J. Nat. Prod.* **2017**, *80*, 2447–2452. [CrossRef]
109. Pettit, G.R.; Melody, N.; Chapuis, J.C. Antineoplastic Agents. 605. Isoquinstatins. *J. Nat. Prod.* **2018**, *81*, 451–457. [CrossRef]
110. Miyazaki, K.; Kobayashi, M.; Natsume, T.; Gondo, M.; Mikami, T.; Sakakibara, K.; Tsukagoshi, S. Synthesis and Antitumor Activity of Novel Dolastatin 10 Analogs. *Chem. Pharm. Bull.* **1995**, *43*, 1706–1718. [CrossRef]
111. Shioiri, T.; Hayashi, K.; Hamada, Y. Stereoselective synthesis of dolastatin 10 and its congeners. *Tetrahedron* **1993**, *49*, 1913–1924. [CrossRef]
112. Poncet, J.; Hortala, L.; Busquet, M.; Guéritte-Voegelein, F.; Thoret, S.; Pierré, A.; Atassi, G.; Jouin, P. Synthesis and antiproliferative activity of a cyclic analog of dolastatin 10. *Bioorg. Med. Chem. Lett.* **1998**, *8*, 2855–2858. [CrossRef]
113. Alattia, T.; Roux, F.; Poncet, J.; Cavé, A.; Jouin, P. Conformational study of dolastatin 10. *Tetrahedron* **1995**, *51*, 2593–2604. [CrossRef]
114. Sone, H.; Kigoshi, H.; Yamada, K. Isolation and stereostructure of dolastatin I, a cytotoxic cyclic hexapeptide from the Japanese sea hare Dolabella auricularia. *Tetrahedron* **1997**, *53*, 8149–8154. [CrossRef]

115. Tomioka, K.; Satoh, M.; Taniyama, D.; Kanai, M.; Iida, A. ChemInform Abstract: Enantioselective Addition of Thiazolyllithium to Aldimines with the Aid of Chiral Ligand. Asymmetric Synthesis of (S)-Doe, a Component of Marine Natural Product, Dolastatin 10. *Cheminform* **1998**, *29*. [CrossRef]
116. Hamada, Y.; Hayashi, K.; Shioiri, T. Efficient stereoselective synthesis of dolastatin 10, an antineoplastic peptide from a sea hare. *Tetrahedron Lett.* **1991**, *32*, 931–934. [CrossRef]
117. Kazmaier, U.; Burkhart, J.L. A Straightforward Approach to Protected (S)-Dolaphenine (Doe), the Unusual Amino Acid Component of Dolastatin 10. *Synthesis* **2011**, *2011*, 4033–4036. [CrossRef]
118. Mordant, C.; Reymond, S.; Tone, H.; Lavergne, D.; Touati, R.; Ben Hassine, B.; Ratovelomanana-Vidal, V.; Genet, J.-P. Total Synthesis of Dolastatin 10 Through Ruthenium-Catalyzed Asymmetric Hydrogenations. *ChemInform* **2007**, *38*, 6115–6123. [CrossRef]
119. Kiyoshi, T.; Motomu, K.; Kenji, K. An expeditious synthesis of dolastatin 10. *Tetrahedron Lett.* **1991**, *32*, 2395–2398.
120. Pettit, G.R.; Singh, S.B.; Hogan, F.; Lloyd-Williams, P.; Herald, D.L.; Burkett, D.D.; Clewlow, P.J. ChemInform Abstract: Antineoplastic Agents. Part 189. The Absolute Configuration and Synthesis of Natural (-)-Dolastatin 10. *ChemInform* **1989**, *20*. [CrossRef]
121. Benedetti, E.; Carlomagno, T.; Fraternali, F.; Hamada, Y.; Hayashi, K.; Paolillo, L.; Shioiri, T. Conformational analysis of dolastatin 10: An nmr and theoretical approach. *Biopolymers* **1995**, *36*, 525–538. [CrossRef]
122. Fantucci, P.; Mattioli, E.; Marino, T.; Russo, N. The Conformational Properties of (-)-Dolastatin 10, a Powerful Antineoplastic Agent. *Mol. Electron.* **1994**, *11*, 205–209. [CrossRef]
123. Fantucci, P.; Marino, T.; Russo, N.; Villa, A.M. Conformational behaviour of the antineoplastic peptide dolastatin-10 and of two mutated derivatives. *J. Comput. Mol. Des.* **1995**, *9*, 425–438. [CrossRef]
124. Pettit, R.K.; Pettit, G.R.; Hazen, K.C. Specific Activities of Dolastatin 10 and Peptide Derivatives against Cryptococcus neoformans. *Antimicrob. Agents Chemother.* **1998**, *42*, 2961–2965. [CrossRef] [PubMed]
125. Fennell, B.J.; Carolan, S.; Pettit, G.R.; Bell, A. Effects of the antimitotic natural product dolastatin 10, and related peptides, on the human malarial parasite Plasmodium falciparum. *J. Antimicrob. Chemother.* **2003**, *51*, 833–841. [CrossRef]

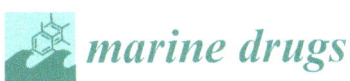

Review

Recent Advances in Small Peptides of Marine Origin in Cancer Therapy

Qi-Ting Zhang [1], Ze-Dong Liu [2], Ze Wang [2], Tao Wang [1], Nan Wang [3], Ning Wang [1,*], Bin Zhang [2,*] and Yu-Fen Zhao [1]

[1] Institute of Drug Discovery Technology, Ningbo University, Ningbo 315211, China; 1811075025@nbu.edu.cn (Q.-T.Z.); 1911074031@nbu.edu.cn (T.W.); zhaoyufen@nbu.edu.cn (Y.-F.Z.)
[2] Li Dak Sum Yip Yio Chin Kenneth Li Marine Biopharmaceutical Research Center, Department of Marine Pharmacy, College of Food and Pharmaceutical Sciences, Ningbo University, Ningbo 315800, China; 1911085033@nbu.edu.cn (Z.-D.L.); 2011085073@nbu.edu.cn (Z.W.)
[3] Quality Assurance Department, Shenzhen Kivita Innovative Drug Discovery Institute, Shenzhen 518057, China; nan.wang@szkivita.com
* Correspondence: wangning2@nbu.edu.cn (N.W.); zhangbin1@nbu.edu.cn (B.Z.)

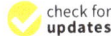

Citation: Zhang, Q.-T.; Liu, Z.-D.; Wang, Z.; Wang, T.; Wang, N.; Wang, N.; Zhang, B.; Zhao, Y.-F. Recent Advances in Small Peptides of Marine Origin in Cancer Therapy. *Mar. Drugs* **2021**, *19*, 115. https://doi.org/10.3390/md19020115

Academic Editor: Tatiana V. Ovchinnikova

Received: 31 December 2020
Accepted: 18 February 2021
Published: 19 February 2021

Publisher's Note: MDPI stays neutral with regard to jurisdictional claims in published maps and institutional affiliations.

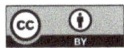

Copyright: © 2021 by the authors. Licensee MDPI, Basel, Switzerland. This article is an open access article distributed under the terms and conditions of the Creative Commons Attribution (CC BY) license (https://creativecommons.org/licenses/by/4.0/).

Abstract: Cancer is one of the leading causes of death in the world, and antineoplastic drug research continues to be a major field in medicine development. The marine milieu has thousands of biological species that are a valuable source of novel functional proteins and peptides, which have been used in the treatment of many diseases, including cancer. In contrast with proteins and polypeptides, small peptides (with a molecular weight of less than 1000 Da) have overwhelming advantages, such as preferential and fast absorption, which can decrease the burden on human gastrointestinal function. Besides, these peptides are only connected by a few peptide bonds, and their small molecular weight makes it easy to modify and synthesize them. Specifically, small peptides can deliver nutrients and drugs to cells and tissues in the body. These characteristics make them stand out in relation to targeted drug therapy. Nowadays, the anticancer mechanisms of the small marine peptides are still largely not well understood; however, several marine peptides have been applied in preclinical treatment. This paper highlights the anticancer linear and cyclic small peptides in marine resources and presents a review of peptides and the derivatives and their mechanisms.

Keywords: marine organism; anticancer medicine; small peptide; liner peptide; cyclic peptide

1. Introduction

Oceans cover about 70% of the earth's surface and 95% of the biosphere. Water was the cradle of the earliest living organisms, containing approximately 75% of all living organisms. The marine environment offers a rich source of natural products with potential therapeutic applications. More than 1 million marine invertebrates and more than 25,000 species of fish have been discovered, and some of these have been shown to contain natural products with potential biological activity [1,2]. In recent years, marine microorganisms, have also been regarded as a valuable source of bioactive compounds, with the advantages of easy cultivation and good compound extraction repeatability [3]. More than 10,000 bioactive molecules that have been isolated from marine organisms, and several have been found to possess anticancer activity [4]. Most of these natural products with anticancer activity originate from microorganisms (bacteria, fungi, protozoa, viruses, and chromista), plantae (flowering plants like mangroves and macroalgae), and animalia (invertebrates such as sponges, tunicates, and vertebrates such as fish and whale), etc.

Cancer is one of the leading causes of death in the world. An estimated 9.6 million people died of cancer in 2018 [5]. Almost 1 in 6 people die of cancer globally. With the application of new theories, modern technologies, and new drugs in basic tumor research and clinical treatment, the rising trend in tumor death in many countries has been effectively controlled [5]. Chemotherapy is part of the major categories of medical oncology. Despite these successes, chemotherapy's lingering toxic side-effects are still a primary cause of morbidity and mortality in cancer survivors [6]. As for traditional chemotherapy drugs, most of these inhibit tumor cell proliferation by acting on the DNA synthesis and the replication of tumor cells, which have been shown to be effective but at the price of high toxicity due to a lack of selectivity. Nowadays, there are novel molecular methods for treatment using cancer drugs, including target therapy by cell surface receptors, immune-directed therapy, therapeutic vaccines, and antibody–drug conjugates (ADCs) [7,8]. According to the 2020 ASCO's Annual Report, a large number of innovative drugs, which can be categorized into targeted drugs and immune drugs, have entered trials and clinical trials [9]. Targeted medicine can restrain tumor cell growth by blocking the signal transduction, but the recurrence rate is extremely high [10]. Antibody–drug conjugates have the potential for increased tumor penetration and drug resistance. It has been demonstrated that a knottin peptide–drug conjugate (KDC) can selectively deliver gemcitabine to malignant cells expressing tumor-associated integrins [11]. In recent years, major pharmaceutical companies and research centers have focused on monoclonal antibody drugs and bi-specific antibody drugs in targeted therapy, as well as CAR-T and immunoassay point inhibitors in immunotherapy [12–14]. Immunotherapy achieves anti-tumor therapy by stimulating the body's immune system. In immunotherapy, mainly immune cell therapy, immune checkpoint inhibitors, tumor vaccines, and immune system regulators, the immune system is used to recognize and regulate the body's attack on abnormal cell functions [14]. Small peptides, such as the thymic peptide, with their unique advantages in immunotherapy, are also very prominent. The thymic peptide used has been a non-specific adjuvant therapy for various tumors, as it can induce T cell differentiation and development, promoting its proliferation and improving T cell response to the antigen at the same time [15]. This kind of drug enhances the patient's immunity, with fewer side effects.

The resistance adaptation ability of small peptides in many drug treatments and their fewer toxic side effects indicate their potential application in further developing novel drugs. Due to these medicines' unique metabolic processes, many new study areas on the pharmaceutical aspects of protein and peptide drugs have recently emerged [16,17]. Many natural and synthetic peptides were characterized in recent decades, and public databases were established, such as APD3 (database of antimicrobial peptides), the Defensins Knowledgebase, the antiviral AVPdb (database of antiviral peptides), the antiparasitic ParaPep, and the CancerPPD (database of anticancer peptides and proteins) [18–22]. Bioactive small peptides are composed of 2–10 amino acids linked by peptide bonds. Studies have found that amino acids such as Trp, Tyr, Met, Gly, Cys, His, and Pro in the peptide chain can significantly improve the bioactivity [23,24]. In other words, compared with traditional chemotherapy drugs, small peptides have several advantages, such as high absorption, small size, well-defined signaling targets, and minimal toxicity. As such, they offer a new promising area of research. Besides, small peptides are just connected by a few peptide linkages, and their small molecular weight makes them easy to be modified and synthesized. Additionally, small peptides can be used as vectors to deliver drugs specifically to every cell and tissue [25]. However, small peptides have some disadvantages, including a short half-life, easy degradation in vivo, poor stability, etc. Many researchers have tried to modify or develop corresponding pseudo-peptide drugs or have combined small peptides with traditional therapy for tumor combination therapy to achieve better results than with a single treatment. The application of several cyclic peptides as noncovalent nuclear targeting molecular transporters of Dox has been reported [26]. Additionally, another work designed new peptides based on the molecular dynamics simulation (MDs) of the matuzumab-EGFR complex in a water environment. These peptides had a higher affinity to the EGFR relative to that previously reported [27]. The peptide modification of anticancer drugs could enhance their activity and selectivity, perhaps even circumventing multi-drug resistance [28].

The marine environment is a crucial biological kingdom with the richest source of novel functional proteins and peptides. Additionally, it is gradually becoming a vital field of drug development [29]. As marine organisms live in a special environment that is hypersaline, high-pressure, hypoxia, and hypothermic, and lacks sunlight, these proteins and peptides have strong bioactivities and a specific structure. There are many effects associated with marine peptides, such as antioxidant, antimicrobial, antitumor, antiviral, cardioprotective, immunomodulatory, and tissue regeneration properties [16,30–32]. Approximately 49 marine-derived active substances or their derivatives have been approved for the market or entered clinical trials globally [33]. Most of these bioactive molecules are extracted from marine sponges, mollusca, and algae. There are 11 kinds of marine drugs approved by European and American drug authorities, of which, four are listed as anticancer drugs: Cytosar-U, Yondelis, Halaven, and Adcetris. In recent years, more and more studies on marine bioactive peptides have appeared. Many bioactive peptides with anticancer potential have been extracted from various marine organisms. Small peptides from marine sources are gradually gaining attention because of their uniqueness. Compared with high-molecular-weight peptides, low-molecular-weight peptides show greater molecular mobility and diffusivity, contributing to their enhanced interaction with cancer cell components and increasing their anticancer activity [34]. Nowadays, several newly discovered anticancer small peptides and their derivatives thereof from marine organisms have been widely applied to clinical research [35–37] (Figure 1). Marine small peptides are molecules that participates in all processes of life activities. They can bear anticancer roles in diversiform aspects in different ways, such as preventing cell migration, induction of apoptosis, disorganization of tubulin structure and inducing cell cycle arrest, and more (Figure 2) [38].

Due to differences in the properties and activities of linear and cyclic peptides, we have generally used these two categories for the review. The first part and the second part of this article introduce the research progress of marine-derived antitumor linear peptides and cyclic peptides, respectively. Finally, we systematically summarized the small peptides and their derivatives that have entered the stage of clinical research.

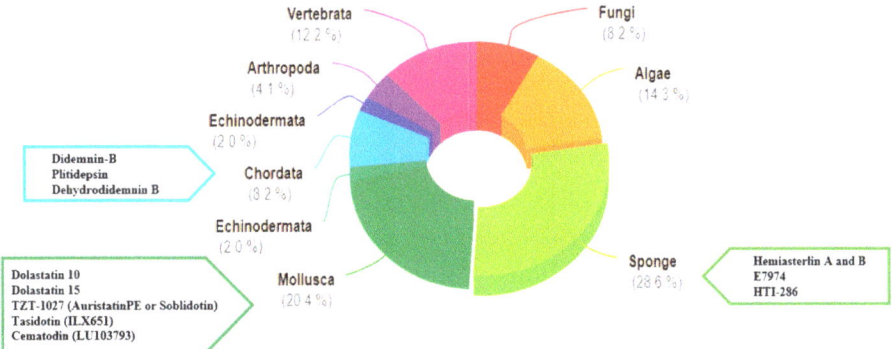

Figure 1. Sources of marine natural products or derivatives that have been approved or entered clinical trials, as well as anticancer small peptides and their derivatives which have entered clinical studies.

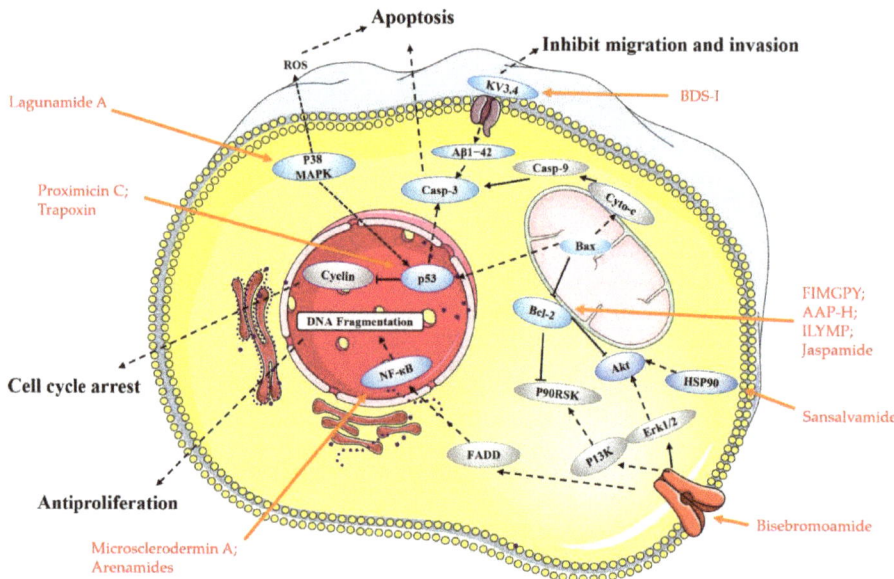

Figure 2. Main molecular mechanism of actions deployed by the anticancer peptides presented in this review. Blue represents the targets mentioned in the paper, and gray represents the proteins involved in the signaling pathway that are not present in this paper, the anticancer peptides mentioned in the article are highlighted in red.

2. Linear Peptides and Derivatives

2.1. Animals

In recent years, some anticancer peptides have been discovered from proteolytic products and secondary metabolites of marine animals, and these purified anticancer peptides have cytotoxic, anti-proliferative and protease inhibition effects [39].

The early discovery of the anti-tumor effect of small marine peptides was mostly based on cytotoxicity assessment, and the subsequent mechanism is not clear. Ding Guo-Fang et al. discovered a tripeptide QPK (Table 1) with anticancer activity shows that it inhibited the growth of DU-145 cells (human prostate cancer cells) in a dose-dependent manner, the IC_{50} (half-maximal inhibitory concentration) fell from 9.50 mg/mL at 24 h to 1.00 mg/mL at 48 h [40]. Three novel cytotoxic peptides, AGAPGG, AERQ, and RDTQ (Table 1), were successfully purified and identified from the papain hydrolysate of *Sarcophyton glaucum*. They displayed relatively high cytotoxicity on HeLa cells (human cervical cancer cells), which was 3.3-, 5.8-, and 5.1-fold stronger than that of the anticancer drug 5-FU, respectively. Additionally, their IC_{50} values to inhibit the growth of Hela cells were 8.6, 4.9, and 5.6 mmol/L, respectively [41].

Marine natural products are an important source of topological enzyme inhibitors and DNA damaging agents. Virenamides A–C (Table 1 and Figure 3) have been isolated from extracts of the Didemnid ascidian *Diplosoma virens*. It is reported that Virenamide A exhibited topoisomerase II inhibitory activity and had modest cytotoxicity toward a panel of cultured cells: gave an IC_{50} of 2.5 µg/mL against P388 (mouse leukemia cells), and 10 µg/mL against A549 (human non-small cells lung cancer cells), HT-29 (human colon cancer cells), and CV1 (kidney cells) cells. Additionally, Virenamides B and C both had an IC_{50} of 5 µg/mL against P388, A549, HT-29, and CV1 cells [42]. SCAP1 (Table 1) is an anticancer and antioxidative peptide that was shown to initiate cancer cell death by inhibiting cancer cell growth and increasing DNA damage and apoptosis in HT-29 with IC_{50} values of 90.31 to 60.21 µg/mL [43,44].

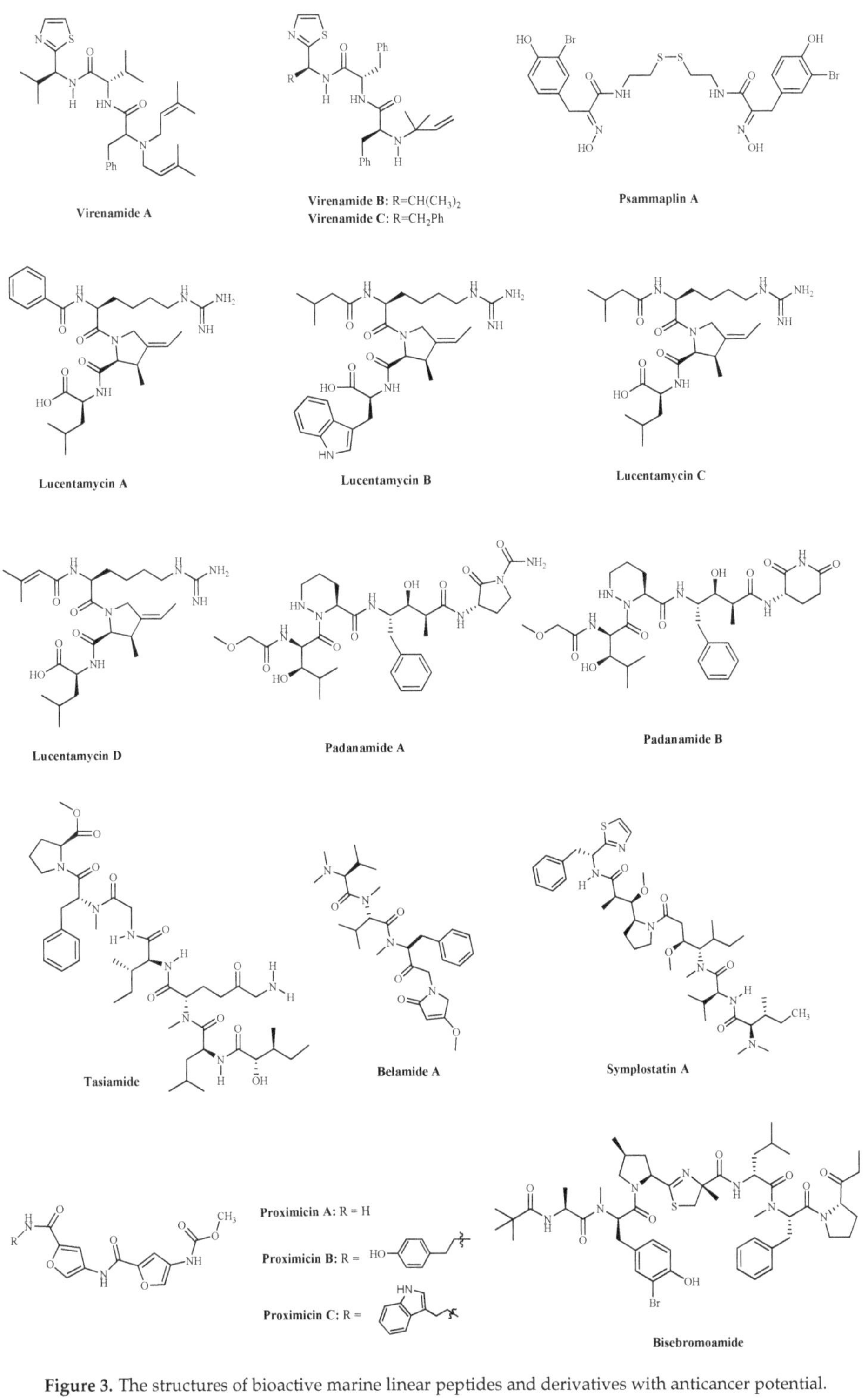

Figure 3. The structures of bioactive marine linear peptides and derivatives with anticancer potential.

With the deepening of understanding, researchers have discovered that a variety of marine small peptides can induce tumor cell apoptosis to exert anti-tumor effects. The peptide sequence was identified as YALPAH (Table 1), isolated from half-fin *Setipinna taty* anchovy, it has been found to induce PC-3 cells (human prostate cancer cells) apoptosis and inhibit cells proliferation, with an IC_{50} value of 8.1 mg/mL [45]. Additionally, three modified peptides were synthesized ulteriorly. It was revealed that the guanidine portion of arginine (R) forms hydrogen bonds with phosphates, sulfates, and carboxylate salts, which affect the proliferative activity [46]. A tripeptide, BCP-A (Table 1), was isolated from the protein hydrolysate of blood clam (*Tegillarca granosa*) muscle, showing a strong cytotoxicity toward PC-3, DU-145, H-1299 (human lung cancer cells), and HeLa cells with an IC_{50} of 1.99, 2.80, 3.3 and 2.54 mg/mL, respectively. Additionally, it was also displaying a high anti-proliferation activity on the PC-3 cells by inducing apoptosis. In addition, BCP-A has a significant anti-lipid peroxidation effect, which is not conducive to tumor formation [47]. A novel peptide obtained from the sea anemone toxin, BDS-I (Table 1), had been successfully identified as a new inhibitor of the KV3.4 channel subunits. In particular, it had been reported that KV3.4 channels play a crucial role in cancer cell migration [48]. BDS-I blocking KV3.4 currents prevented (the neurotoxic β-amyloid peptide1–42) Aβ1–42-induced caspase-3 activation and apoptotic processes [49,50].

Moreover, several small peptides are closely associated with the mitochondrial-mediated apoptosis pathway. The hexapeptide FIMGPY (Table 1), from the skate (*Raja porosa*) cartilage protein hydrolysate, displayed high anti-proliferation activities in HeLa cells with an IC_{50} of 4.81 mg/mL. It also could induce apoptosis by upregulating the Bax/Bcl-2 ratio and caspase-3 activation [51]. The anticancer peptide AAP-H (Table 1) is a pentapeptide from the sea anemone *Anthopleura anjunae* with an amino acid sequence Tyr-Val-Pro-Gly-Pro. It has been shown that AAP-H induces apoptosis by decreasing the mitochondrial membrane potential and increasing Bax/Bcl-2 ratio, cytochrome-C, caspase-3, and caspase-9 [52]. An antiproliferative pentapeptide ILYMP (Table 1), was isolated from the protein hydrolysate of *Cyclina sinensis*. It has been demonstrated that *ILYMP* enhances Bax and cleaved caspase-3/9 expression and the suppression of Bcl-2 expression in DU-145 cells [53].

Apoptosis is closely related to cell cycle arrest. At present, some small peptides discovered cannot only induce cancer cells apoptosis, but also cause cell cycle arrest and ultimately lead to cell death. The sequences of SCH-P9 and SCH-P10 (Table 1), identified as Leu-Pro-Gly-Pro and Asp-Tyr-Val-Pro, were obtained from *Sinonovacula constricta* hydrolysates. The researches illustrated that SCH-P9 and SCH-P10 inhibited the growth of DU-145 cells and PC-3 cells by reducing the number of cells in the G0/G1 phase, thus increasing the number in the sub G1 phase and inducing apoptosis [54]. SIO (Table 1) is another tripeptide found in *sepia* ink. The research found that it significantly inhibited the proliferation of DU-145, PC-3, LNCaP (human prostate cancer cells), A549 and H-1299 cells, in a time and dose-dependent manner by inducing apoptosis and arresting cell at S or G2/M phase [55,56]. The anticancer mechanism is similar to another decapeptide SHP, which is accompanied by the activation of cellular tumor antigen p53 and caspase-3, the upregulation of pro-apoptosis regulator Bax, and the downregulation of anti-apoptosis regulator Bcl-2 [57]. Psammaplin A (PsA) (Table 1 and Figure 3) is a natural product that has been isolated from sponges and has been suggested to be a promising novel HDAC (histone deacetylase) inhibitor. Some researchers found that PsA exhibited antiproliferative effects on cancer cells by the induction of cell cycle arrest and apoptosis. However, the psammaplin class has the disadvantage of physiologic instability [58,59]. Latest research reports that the indole derivatives of Psammaplin are more potent modulators of epigenetic enzymes than the original natural product. Additionally, positional isomers at the bromoindole ring also showed cell cycle block and apoptosis induction [59]. NVP-LAQ824 (Table 1) is a more stable indolic cinnamyl hydroxamate analogue of Psammaplin A, has entered phase I clinical trials in patients with solid tumors or leukemia [60]. A toxicity evaluation in rats identified the hematopoietic and lymphatic systems as the primary target organs, with a reversible dose-dependent reduction in RBC (red blood cell) and WBC (white blood cell) counts and lymphoid atrophy [60].

2.2. Fungi and Bacteria

Hundreds of secondary metabolites obtained from marine fungal strains revealed potent pharmacological and biological activities [61]. Lucentamycins A–D (Table 1 and Figure 3), have been isolated from the fermentation broth of a marine-derived actinomycete identified by phylogenetic methods as *Nocardiopsis lucentensis*. Lucentamycins A and B showed significant in vitro cytotoxicity against HCT-116 cells (human colon cancer cells) with IC_{50} values of 0.20 and 11 μM [62]. Two highly modified linear tetrapeptides, Padanamides A and B (Table 1 and Figure 3), were obtained from sediment in the culture of *Streptomyces* sp. It demonstrated that Padanamide B is cytotoxic to Jurkat cells (human leukemia cells) with an IC_{50} value of 30.9 μM [63]. Tasiamide (Table 1 and Figure 3) was predicted to be the best active cyanobacterial compound derived from *Symploca* sp. It has been shown that it was cytotoxic against KB (human nasopharyngeal cancer cells) and LoVo (human colon cancer cells) cells, with IC_{50} values of 0.48 and 3.47 μg/mL, respectively [64]. Cathepsin D (Cath D) has been considered a potential target to treat cancer [65]. Tasiamide's C-terminal modified derivatives have inhibitory activity against Cath D/Cath E/BACE1, potentially making them highly potent and selective Cath D inhibitors [66]. Belamide A (Table 1 and Figure 3) is a highly methylated linear tetrapeptide, with a structural analogy to the important linear peptides, Dolastatins 10 and 15. It has a moderate intensity of cytotoxicity to HCT-116 cells (IC_{50}: 0.74 μM). At a concentration of 20 μM, it destroyed the micro-tubule network in rat aortic smooth muscle A-10 cells and showed the classic tubulin destabilizing mitotic characteristics [67]. Symplostatin *A* (Table 1 and Figure 3), a Dolastatin 10 analogue from the cyanobacterium *Symploca hydnoides*, can cause a loss of interphase micro-tubules, G2/M arrest, and active caspase 3 and initiate the phosphorylation of Bcl-2 [68]. Proximicins A, B, and C (Table 1 and Figure 3) are a family of three novel aminofuran antibiotics isolated from actinomycetes of the genus *Verrucosispora*. It was illustrated that Proximicins could activate cell-cycle regulatory proteins involved in the transition of cells from G1 to S phase and induce apoptotic cell death in L1236 (Hodgkin's Lymphoma cells) Jurkat 16 (T-cell leukemia cells) cells. Moreover, Proximicin C can induce up-regulation of p53 and p21 in gastric adenocarcinoma cells, and inhibit the U-87 MG (human glioblastoma cells) and MDA-MB-231 (human breast cancer cells) cells proliferation, with IC_{50} values of 12.7 and 11.4 μg/mL, respectively [69]. Bisebromoamide (Table 1 and Figure 3), a cyanobacterial metabolite from a cyanobacterium of the genus, *Lyngbya* sp., was shown to have an antiproliferative activity at nanomolar levels of 40 nM that average a 50% growth inhibition (GI_{50}) value across all of the cell lines (a panel of 39 human cancer cell lines (termed JFCR39)) [70]. Additionally, it can also inhibit the Raf/MEK/ERK and PI3K/Akt/mTOR pathways, showing a potent protein kinase inhibitor effect [71].

2.3. Other Small Peptides

Currently, the number of small linear anti-cancer peptides derived from marine plants is relatively small. The peptide, HVLSRAPR (Table 1), exhibited strong inhibitory activity on HT-29 cells, with an IC_{50} value of 99.88 μg/mL, while it had little inhibitory activity on LO2 cells (normal liver cells) (5.37% at 500 μg/mL). It was also shown to be selectively active on cancer cells, including Hep G2 (human liver cancer cells), MCF-7 (human breast cancer cells), SGC-7901 (human gastric cancer cells), and A549 cells [72].

Most of the small peptides are still in the stage of structural optimization and in vitro activity verification. The lack of progress in subsequent research on their mechanisms prevents them from entering clinical development. Additionally, these small peptides merit further investigation as a potential therapeutic agent.

Table 1. Marine sources of bioactive linear peptides with anticancer potential.

Compound	Source	Mechanism	Cell Lines	IC$_{50}$/(GI$_{50}$) [b]	Reference
QPK	Sepia ink	Cytotoxicity [a]	DU-145	9.50 mg/mL (24 h); 1.00 mg/mL (48 h)	[40]
AGAPGG; AERQ; RDTQ	Sarcophyton glaucum	Cytotoxicity [a]	HeLa	8.6 mmol/L; 4.9 mmol/L; 5.6 mmol/L	[41]
Virenamides A;	The Didemnid ascidian Diplosoma virens	Inhibiting the Topoisomerase II	P388; A549; HT-29; CV1	2.5 µg/mL; 10 µg/mL; 10 µg/mL; 10 µg/mL	[42]
Virenamides B	The Didemnid ascidian Diplosoma virens	Inhibiting the Topoisomerase II	P388; A549; HT-29; CV1	5 µg/mL; 5 µg/mL; 5 µg/mL; 5 µg/mL	[42]
Virenamides C	The Didemnid ascidian Diplosoma virens	Inhibiting the Topoisomerase II	P388; A549; HT-29; CV1	5 µg/mL; 5 µg/mL; 5 µg/mL; 5 µg/mL	[42]
SCAP1; (Leu-Ala-Asn-Ala-Lys)	Oyster (Saccostrea cucullata)	Enhancing oxidative DNA damage; Inducing apoptosis	HT-29	90.31 mg/mL (24 h); 70.87 mg/mL (48 h); 60.21 mg/mL (72 h)	[43,44]
YALPAH	Half-fin anchovy (Setipinna taty)	Inducing apoptosis	PC-3	8.1 mg/mL	[45,46]
BCP-A (Trp-Pro-Pro)	Blood clam (Tegillarca granosa) muscle	Inducing apoptosis and inhibiting lipid peroxidation	PC-3; DU-145; H-1299; HeLa	1.99 mg/mL; 2.80 mg/mL; 3.3 mg/mL; 2.54 mg/mL	[47]
BDS-I; (Ala-Ala-Pro-Ala-Phe-Ala-Ser-Gly)	The sea anemone toxin	Blocking KV3.4 currents prevented (the neurotoxic β-amyloid peptide1-42) Aβ1–42-induced caspase-3 activation and apoptotic processes	PC-12	75 nM	[49,50]
FIMGPY	The skate (R. porosa) cartilage protein hydrolysate	Inducing apoptosis by upregulating the Bax/Bcl-2 ratio and caspase-3 activation	HeLa	4.81 mg/mL	[51]
AAP-H; (Tyr-Val-Pro-Gly-Pro)	The sea anemone Anthopleura anjunae	Inducing apoptosis, decreasing the mitochondrial membrane potential, and increasing Bax/Bcl-2 ratio, cytochrome-C, caspase-3, and caspase-9	DU-145	9.605 mM (24 h); 7.910 mM (48 h); 2.298 mM (72 h)	[52]
ILYMP	Cyclina sinensis	Enhancing expression of Bax, cleaved caspase-3/9 as well as suppression of Bcl-2 expression	DU-145	11.25 mM	[53]

Table 1. Cont.

Compound	Source	Mechanism	Cell Lines	IC$_{50}$/(GI$_{50}$) [b]	Reference
SCH-P9 (Leu-Pro-Gly-Pro)	Sinonovacula constricta hydrolysates	Inducing apoptosis and sub-G1 phase cell cycle arrest	DU-145;	1.21 mg/mL (24 h);	[54]
			PC-3	1.09 mg/mL (24 h)	
SCH-P10 (Asp-Tyr-Val-Pro)			DU-145;	1.41 mg/mL (24 h);	
			PC-3	0.91 mg/mL (24 h)	
SIO	Sepia ink	Inducing apoptosis, and S and G2/M phase cell cycle arrest	DU-145;	<5 mg/mL	[55,56]
			PC-3;	<5 mg/mL	
			LNCaP	<10 mg/mL	
Psammaplin A (PsA)	The two Sponges, Jaspis sp. and Poecillastra wondoensis.	Inducing S or S-G2/M phase cell cycle arrest; Inhibting HDAC	P388; HCT-116; A549	(40 nM)	[58,59]
NVP-LAQ824	Psammaplysilla sp.	Inducing S or S-G2/M phase cell cycle arrest; Inhibting HDAC	H-1299	150 nM	[60]
			HCT-116	10 nM	
Lucentamycins A;	The fermentation broth of a marine-derived actinomycete	Cytotoxicity [a]	HCT-116	0.20 µM;	[62]
Lucentamycins B				11 µM	
Padanamides A and B	Sediment in the culture of Streptomyces sp.	Cytotoxicity [a]	Jurkat	30.9 µM	[63]
Tasiamide	Cyanobacterial compound derived from Symploca sp.	Inhibiting the expression of Cath D	KB;	0.48 µg/mL;	[64,66]
			LoVo	3.47 µg/mL	
Belamide A	Cyanobacterium	Tubulin polymerization inhibition	HCT-116;	0.74 µM;	[67]
			A-10	20 µM	
Symplostatin A	Cyanobacterium	Microtubule assembly Inhibiting cell cycle arrest	MDA-MB-435	0.15 µM	[68]
			SK-OV-3;	0.09 µM	
			NCI/ADR;	2.90 µM	
			NCI/ADR with Verapamil;	0.09 µM	
			A-10;	1.8 µM	
			HUVEC	0.16 µM	
Proximicins C	Actinomycetes of the genus Verrucosispora,	Inducing Cell cycle G1 to S phase arrest and inducing apoptotic cell death	U-87 MG;	12.7 µg/mL	[69]
			MDA-MD-231	11.4 µg/mL	
Bisebromoamide	Cyanobacterium of the genus Lyngbya sp.	Inhibiting both the Raf/MEK/ERK and PI3K/Akt/mTOR pathways	JFCR39	(40 nM)	[70,71]
HVLSRAPR	Spirulina platensis	Cytotoxicity [a]	HT-29;	99.88 µg/mL	[72]

Notes: [a] Mechanism is yet to be investigated; [b] If there are parentheses around the value, it means the GI$_{50}$ value is displayed.

3. Cyclic Peptides and Derivatives

Cyclic peptides combine several favorable properties, such as a good binding affinity, target selectivity, and low toxicity, which make them attractive in anticancer drug researches [73]. Besides, most of the small peptides are concentrated in marine animals, and they are found to be secondary metabolites from sponges, sea squirts, cnidaria, and mollusks.

3.1. Animals

3.1.1. Metabolites of Ascidians

A significant number of compounds with unusual structures and bioactivities have been isolated from various ascidians. The cyclic hexapeptides, Mollamides B and C (Table 2 and Figure 4), were isolated from an Indonesian tunicate *Didemnum mole* in 1994, along with the known peptide, Keenamide A (Table 2 and Figure 4) [74]. Keenamide A and Mollamides B show antiproliferation activity against several cancer cell lines [74]. Keenamide A show cytotoxicity against a range of cell lines, with IC_{50} values of 2.5 μg/mL toward P388, A549 and MEL-20, and 5.0 μg/mL against HT-29 cells [75]. Mollamides B inhibited the proliferation of H460 (human non-small cell lung cancer cells) and MCF-7 and SF-268 cells, but the GI_{50} values are all greater than 100 μM [74]. Subsequently, the cyclic depsipeptides Trunkamide A (Table 2 and Figure 4) was isolated from the colonial ascidian *Lissoclinum* sp., which was collected by Bowden and co-workers in 1996, and its structure was similar to Didemnin B. It has been found to have a cytotoxic effect on several human cancer cell lines, such as HeLa, AGS (human gastric cancer adenocytes cells), and DLD-1 (human colonic adenocarcinoma cells) cells [76]. Tamandarins A and B (Table 2 and Figure 4), were isolated from the unidentified species of didemnid ascidian in 2000 and determined to be cyclic depsipeptides closely related to Didemnins. They were found to possess a very similar structure and biological activity to that of the Didemnin B. They were evaluated against various human cancer cell lines and slightly more potent than Didemnin B [77]. Cycloxazoline (Table 2 and Figure 4) is an asymmetrical cyclic hexapeptide isolated from species of didemnid ascidians in 1992. It can delay S-phase cells entering the G2/M phase and induce apoptosis in HL-60 human leukemia cells [78]. These peptides are structurally similar to Didemnin B, but it's unclear whether they have a better effect or mechanism on tumor cells.

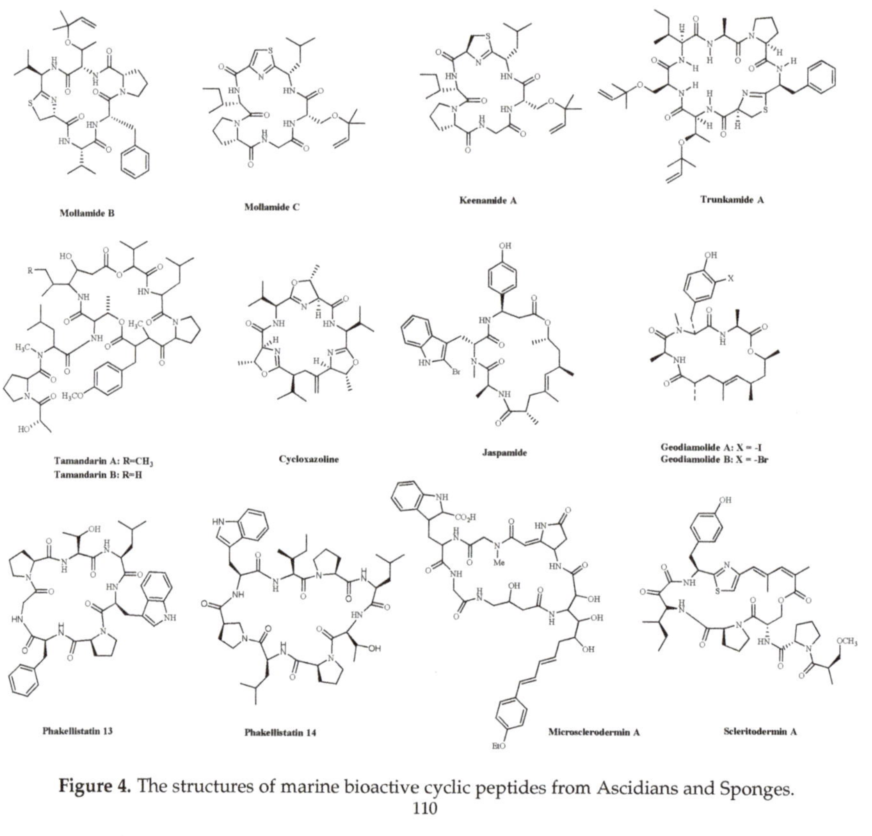

Figure 4. The structures of marine bioactive cyclic peptides from Ascidians and Sponges.

3.1.2. Metabolites of Sponges

Sponges are an excellent source of bioactive metabolites with novel chemical architectures. They produce a diverse array of highly modified peptides, especially cyclic peptides with nonproteinogenic amino acids and polyketide-derived moieties. The depsipeptides isolated from sponges or associated organisms are usually described as cytotoxic substances, such as Jaspamide (Jasplakinolide) [79], Geodiamolides [80], Phakellistatin [81], Microsclerodermin A [82] and Scleritodermin A [83]. However, some of those researched have an anticancer mechanism for a specific cancer cell. Jaspamide (jasplakinolide, NSC-613009, Table 2 and Figure 4), isolated from the sponge, *Jaspis Johnstoni* in 1986, has been considered a classical actin stabilizer [84]. Jaspamide-induced apoptosis is associated with caspase-3 activation, and increased Bax level, and decreased Bcl-2 protein expression. It exhibits antitumor activity in multiple in vitro tumor models for prostate and breast carcinomas and acute myeloid leukemia [85,86]. Geodiamolides A, B (Table 2 and Figure 4) were isolated from the sponge *Geodia* sp. in 1987 [87,88]. In a way similar to other depsipeptides (Jaspamide and Dolastatins), it keeps the normal microtubule organization and regulates actin cytoskeleton, migration, and invasion of breast cancer cells [89,90]. Phakellistatins, a class of cycloheptapeptides, isolated from *Phalkellia* sp., are potent anti-proliferative agents against the leukemia cell line. Phakellistatin 14 (Table 2 and Figure 4) showed cancer cell growth inhibitory activity (GI_{50}: 5 µg/mL) against P388 cells, and Phakellistatins 13 is reported to be cytotoxic at an effective dose of 10 ng/mL (GI_{50}) against BEL-7404 (human liver cancer cells) cells [91,92]. Due to its good antitumor activity in vitro and in vivo, many researchers have modified this structure in the hope of synthesizing potential Marine drugs with a better anti-cancer effect [93]. The Microsclerodermins are cyclic hexapeptides isolated from a deep-water sponge of the genus *Microscleroderma* in 1994. Microsclerodermin A (Table 2 and Figure 4) has been demonstrated to inhibit NF-κB and induce apoptosis in the AsPC-1, BxPC-3, and PANC-1 pancreatic cancer cell lines, its IC_{50} values were 2.3, 0.8, 4.3, and 4.0 µM against the four cells, respectively [82]. Additionally, recent research has discovered the congeners of the Microsclerodermins, Microsclerodermins N and O. They exhibit cytotoxic activity against HeLa cells with IC_{50} values of 0.77 mM and 0.81 mM, respectively [94]. Scleritodermin A (Table 2 and Figure 4) was isolated from the lithistid sponge *Scleritoderma nodosum* in 2004. Scleritodermin A has significant in vitro cytotoxicity against a panel of human tumor cell lines and acts through tubulin polymerization inhibition and the resulting disruption of microtubules [83]. Subsequent studies have led to discovering several novel cyclopeptides, but their antitumor activity is relatively weak, and the mechanism of action is unclear [95]. These peptides have unique structures as compared with those from other sources. This attribute makes sponge- and tunicate-derived peptides highly attractive as potential drug and molecular probes.

Table 2. Marine bioactive cyclic peptides from Ascidians and Sponges.

Compound	Source	Mechanism	Cell Lines	IC$_{50}$/(GI$_{50}$) [b]	Reference
Mollamide B	Tunicate Didemnum	Cytotoxicity [a]	H460; MCF-7; SF-268	(>100 µM)	[74]
Keenamide A	Tunicate Didemnum.	Cytotoxicity [a]	P-388; A-549; MEL-20; HT-29	2.5 µg/mL; 2.5 µg/mL; 2.5 µg/mL; 5.0 µg/mL	[75]
Trunkamide A	Didemnid ascidians	Cytotoxicity [a]	DU-145; IGROV; SK-BR-3; Hela	7.08 nM; 7.31 nM; 5.44 nM; 3.90 nM	[76]
Tamandarin A	Didemnid ascidians	Cytotoxicity [a]	NCI-60	1.4 µM (2.3 µM)	[77]
Tamandarin B			NCI-60	1.4 µM (2.3 µM)	
Cycloxazoline	Didemnid ascidians	Cell cycle G2/M arrest, Induction of apoptosis	MRC5CV1; T24	0.5 µg/mL	[77]
Jaspamide (Jasplakinolide, NSC-613009)	Sponge *Jaspis johnstoni*	Induced apoptosis is associated with caspase-3 activation, increased Bax level, and decreased Bcl-2 protein expression	T24; MCF-7; 15NCI/ADR; A-10	60 to 150 µg/mL	[85,86]
Geodiamolide A	Sponge *Geodia corticostylifera*	Induction of apoptosis; Tubulin polymerization inhibition	T47D; MCF7	18.82 nM; 17.83 nM;	[89]
Geodiamolides B			T47D; MCF7	113.90 nM; 9.82 nM;	
Phakellistatin 13	Sponge *Phakellia* sp.	Induction of both intrinsic and extrinsic apoptosis	BEL-7404	(10 ng/mL)	[91,92]
Phakellistatin 14			P388	(5 µg/mL)	
Microsclerodermin A	Sponge of the genus *Amphibleptula*	Inhibit NFκB, Induction of apoptosis;	AsPC-1; BxPC-3; MIA PaCa-2; PANC-1;	2.3 µM; 0.8 µM; 4.3 µM; 4.0 µM	[82]
Scleritodermin A	Sponge *Scleritoderma nodosum*	Tubulin polymerization inhibition	HCT-116; A2780; SKBR3	1.9 µM; 0.940 µM; 0.670 µM	[83]

Notes: [a] Mechanism is yet to be investigated; [b] If there are parentheses around the value, it means the GI$_{50}$ value is displayed.

3.2. Fungi

Zygosporamide (Table 3 and Figure 5), a new cyclic pentadepsipeptide, was isolated from the seawater-based fermentation broth of a fungus identified as *Zygosporium masonii*. Zygosporamide showed a significant cytotoxicity in the NCI's 60 cell line panel (GI$_{50}$ = 9.1 µM), with a highly enhanced selectivity against the central nervous system cancer cells SF-268 (GI$_{50}$ = 6.5 nM), and the renal cancer cells RXF 393 (GI$_{50}$ = 5.0 nM) [96].

Three new cycloheptapeptides, Cordyheptapeptides C–E (Table 3 and Figure 5), were isolated from the fungus fermentation extract, *Acremonium persicinum* SCSIO 115. The compounds displayed cytotoxicity against SF-268 (Human neuro cancer cell), MCF-7, and NCI-H460 tumor cell lines, with IC_{50} values ranging from 2.5 to 12.1 µM [97]. A new cytotoxic and antiviral cyclic tetrapeptide, Asperterrestide A (Table 3 and Figure 5), showed cytotoxicity against U937 and MOLT4 (human acute T lymphoblastic leukaemia cells) cells and inhibitory effects on influenza virus strains H1N1 and H3N2 [98]. Unfortunately, although these compounds have good anti-cancer activity in vitro, their specific anti-cancer mechanism is not clear.

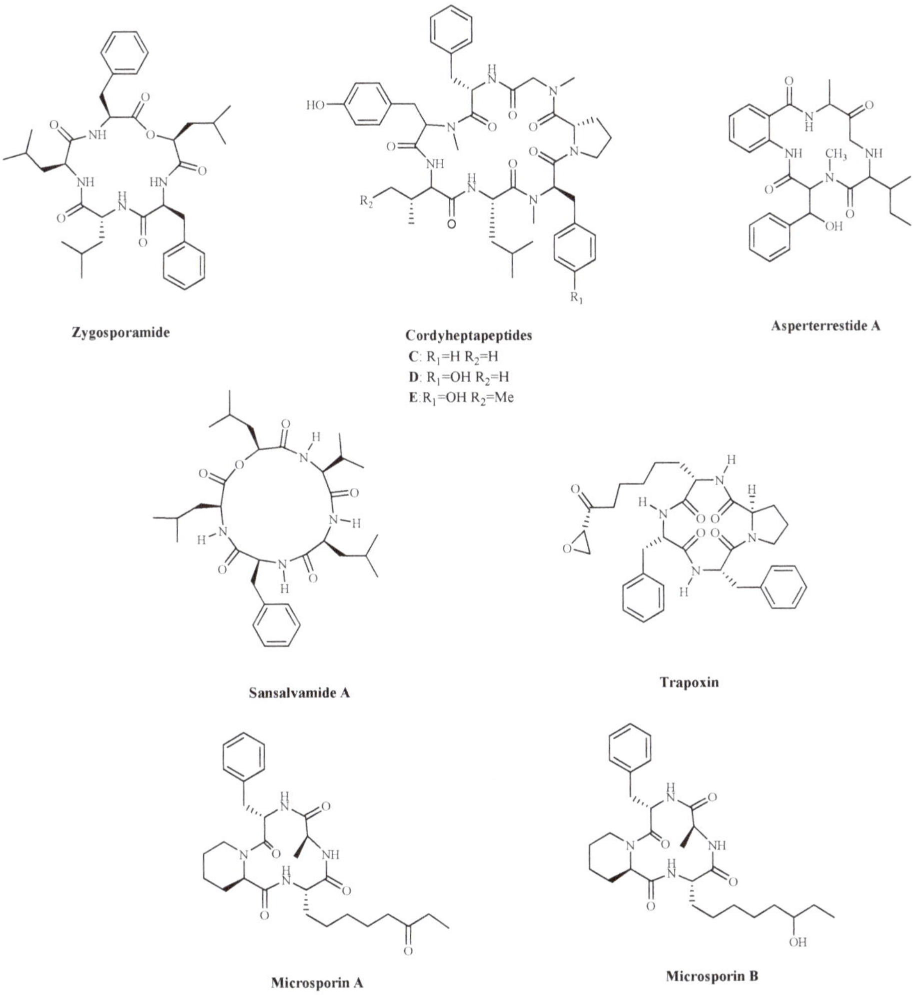

Figure 5. The structures of marine bioactive cyclic peptides from Fungi.

Sansalvamide A (Table 3 and Figure 5) is a cyclic depsipeptide produced by the fungi *Microsporum* cf. *gypseum*. Since ring-opening enzymes easily inactivate natural products, many analogues have been synthesized and modified to provide better stability, and 86 analogues have been reported synthesized [99]. Recently researchers have shown that Sansalvamide A and Sansalvamide analogues inhibit cell growth and proliferation, and induce cell apoptosis by regulating the expression of HSP90 [99,100]. New research has shown that HSP90A strengthens AKT activation through TCL1A-stabilization, promoting multi-aggressive properties in tumor cells [101].

Trapoxin (Table 3 and Figure 5), is a known potent irreversible inhibitor of histone deacetylase. The report indicated that the inhibitory warhead is the α, β-epoxyketone side-chain of (2S,9S)-2-amino-8-oxo-9,10-epoxydecanoic acid (L-Aoe) [102,103]. Some finding displayed that the primary target molecule of the agent in vivo is the histone deacetylase itself, and it also induced growth inhibition in several cell lines regardless of their p53 status [104,105]. Other cyclic peptides, Microsporins A and B (Table 3 and Figure 5) were isolated from culture extracts of the fungus, *Microsporum* cf. *gypseum*. Microsporins A and B are potent inhibitors of histone deacetylase, with IC_{50} values equal to 0.6 mg/mL and 8.5 mg/mL against HCT-116 cells. The results of the HDAC enzyme activity inhibition experiment showed that Microsporins A had a greater inhibitory effect against $HDAC_5$ and HDAC8 than SAHA, with IC_{50} values of 0.14 and 0.55 μM, respectively [106].

Table 3. Marine bioactive cyclic peptides from fungi.

Compound	Source	Mechanism	Cell Lines	$IC_{50}/(GI_{50})$ [b]	Reference
Zygosporamide	*Zygosporium masonii*	Cytotoxicity [a]	SF-268;	(6.5 nM)	[96]
			RXF 393	(5.0 nM)	
Cordyheptapeptide C	*Acremonium persicinum*	Cytotoxicity [a]	SF-268;	3.7 μM;	
			MCF-7;	3.0 μM;	
			NCI-H460	11.6 μM	
Cordyheptapeptide D	*Acremonium persicinum*	Cytotoxicity [a]	SF-268;	45.6 μM;	[97]
			MCF-7;	82.7 μM;	
			NCI-H460	>100 μM	
Cordyheptapeptide E	*Acremonium persicinum*	Cytotoxicity [a]	SF-268;	3.2 μM;	
			MCF-7;	2.7 μM;	
			NCI-H460	4.5 μM	
Asperterrestide A	*Aspergillus terreus*	Cytotoxicity [a]	U937;	6.4 μM;	[98]
			MOLT4	6.2 μM	
Sansalvamide A	*Microsporum* cf. *gypseum*	Inhibiting cell growth, and proliferation, and inducing cell apoptosis by regulating the expression of HSP90	HCT-116;	1.5 μM;	[99,100]
			HCT-15	1 μM	
Trapoxin	Fungal product the culture broth of *Helicoma ambiens* RF-1023	Inhibiting HDAC	NIH3T3	200 ng/mL	[104,105]
Microsporin A	*Microsporum* cf. *gypseum*	Inhibiting HDAC	HCT-116	0.6 mg/mL;	[106]
Microsporin B			HCT-116	8.5 mg/mL	

Notes: [a] Mechanism is yet to be investigated; [b] If there are parentheses around the value, it means the GI_{50} value is displayed.

3.3. Bacteria

Bacterial proteins and peptides are a class of promising bioactive compounds and potential anticancer drugs [107]. Mixirins are cyclic acyl-peptides derived from the bacterium *Bacillus* species. Mixirins A, B and C (Table 4 and Figure 6) blocked the growth of the HCT-116 with an IC_{50} value at the level of 0.65, 1.6, and 1.26 μM, respectively [108]. A new cytotoxic substance named Mechercharmycin A (Table 4 and Figure 6) was isolated from *Thermoactinomyces* sp. YM3-251 showed relatively strong antitumor activity against A549 and Jurkat cells with an IC$_{50}$ value of 40 nM and 46 nM, respectively [109]. Urukthapelstatin A (Table 4 and Figure 6), a novel cyclic peptide, was isolated from the cultured mycelia of Thermoactinomycetaceae bacterium *Mechercharimyces asporophorigenens* YM11-542. Research showed that Urukthapelstatin A inhibited human growth lung cancer A549 cells with an IC$_{50}$ value of 12 nM. Recently analogues of Urukthapelstatin A were synthesized. Cytotoxicity data showed the phenyl ring attached to the eastern oxazole and the rigid, lipophilic tripeptide section are critical structural features of the bio-activity [110]. Three new cyclohexadepsipeptides, Arenamides A–C (Table 3 and Figure 6), were isolated from the fermentation broth of a bacterial strain, identified as *Salinispora arenicola*. Arenamide A and B's effect on NF-κB activity was studied with stably transfected 293/NF-κB-Luc human embryonic kidney cells, induced by treatment with tumor necrosis factor (TNF). Arenamides A and B blocked TNF-induced activation in a dose- and time-dependent manner with IC$_{50}$ values of 3.7 and 1.7 µM, respectively [111].

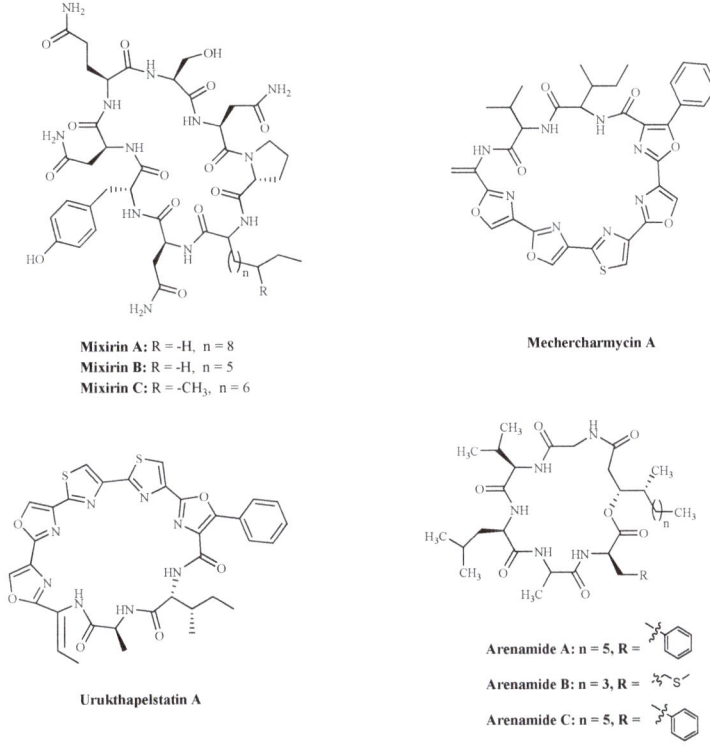

Figure 6. The structures of marine bioactive cyclic peptides from Bacteria.

Table 4. Marine bioactive cyclic peptides from Bacteria.

Compound	Source	Mechanism	Cell Lines	IC$_{50}$	Reference
Mixirin A	Bacillus species.	Cytotoxicity [a]	HCT-116	0.65 µM;	[108]
Mixirin B			HCT-116	1.6 µM;	
Mixirin C			HCT-116	1.26 µM;	
Mechercharmycin A	Thermoactinomyces sp. YM3-251	Cytotoxicity [a]	A549;	40 nM;	[109]
			Jurkat	46 nM;	
Urukthapelstatin A	Thermoactinomycetaceae bacterium Mechercharimyces asporophigenens YM11-542	Cytotoxicity [a]	A549	12 nM;	[110]
Arenamide A	Salinispora Arenicola.	Inhibiting NF kappa B	293/NF-κB-Luc	3.7 µM;	[111]
Arenamide B			293/NF-κB-Luc	1.7 µM	

Notes: [a] Mechanism is yet to be investigated.

Cyanobacterial Metabolites

The potential of marine cyanobacteria, as anticancer agents, displays selective cytotoxicity in tumor cell lines. The mechanism of action of these compounds is not the same, including induction of apoptosis, inhibition of protease, inhibition of HDAC and other mechanisms.

Coibamide A (Table 5 and Figure 7) is a new, potent anti-proliferative depsipeptide, which was isolated from the *Leptolyngbya* cyanobacterium. It displayed a potent cytotoxicity against NCI-H460 lung cancer cells and mouse neuro-2a cells (IC$_{50}$ < 23 nM) [112]. Samoamide A (Table 5 and Figure 7) is a cyclic peptide extracted from *Symploca* sp., collected in American Samoan. It has shown a good cytotoxicity in vitro activity tests, with an IC$_{50}$ value of < 10 µM against colorectal cancer cells and between 1.1 and 4.5 µM against non-small lung cancer cells, breast cancer cells, and others [113,114]. Lagunamide A (Table 5 and Figure 7), a cytotoxic cyclodepsipeptide isolated from cyanobacterium, *Lyngbya majuscule*, has been found to induce caspase-mediated mitochondrial apoptosis, accompanied by the dissipation of mitochondrial membrane potential (Δφm) and the overproduction of reactive oxygen species (ROS) [115]. Furthermore, Lagunamide D (Table 5 and Figure 7) displayed potent activity in triggering apoptosis in a dose- and time-dependent manner [116]. Its structure is closely related to a series of marine-originated compounds from cyanobacteria, including Aurilides [117], Odoamide [118], Palau'amide [119]. The cyanobacterial metabolite Apratoxins (Table 5 and Figure 7) are a family of potent anticancer and antiangiogenic agents. Apratoxins A (Table 5 and Figure 7) down-regulated receptors and growth factor ligands for cancer cells that rely on autocrine loops [120]. Recently, a novel Apratoxin analogue, Apratoxin S10 (Apra S10), has been reported. It inhibited pancreatic cancer cell secretion and reduced the factors secreted by other cell types active within the tumor microenvironment [121]. Lyngyabellins A and B (Table 5 and Figure 7) display anti-proliferative activities in various cell types. Lyngbyabellin A has been demonstrated to have potent cytotoxic activities against human cancer cell lines. It induces apoptosis through the disruption of cellular microfilament network cytokinesis [122].

Cyanobacterial serine protease inhibitors are the most predominant secondary metabolites isolated from cyanobacteria. Some new protease inhibitor compounds were found in cyanobacteria, such as Symplocamide A (Table 5 and Figure 7) [123]. The presence of several unusual structural features in Symplocamide A provides new insights into the pharmacophore model for protease selectivity in this drug class. It has been found that it inhibits serine proteases, with a 200-fold greater inhibition of chymotrypsin over trypsin, which may underlie the potent cytotoxicity to H-460 lung cancer cells (IC$_{50}$ = 40 nM), as well as neuro-2a neuroblastoma cells (IC$_{50}$ = 29 nM) [123].

Largazole (Table 5 and Figure 7), isolated from a cyanobacterium of the *Symploca* genus, was shown to be effective in inhibiting tumor growth and induced apoptosis in a tumor. This selectivity is attributed to its very potent class I HDAC inhibitory activity. As it has various biological activities, most Largazole analogues have been synthesized to improve its activity [124,125].

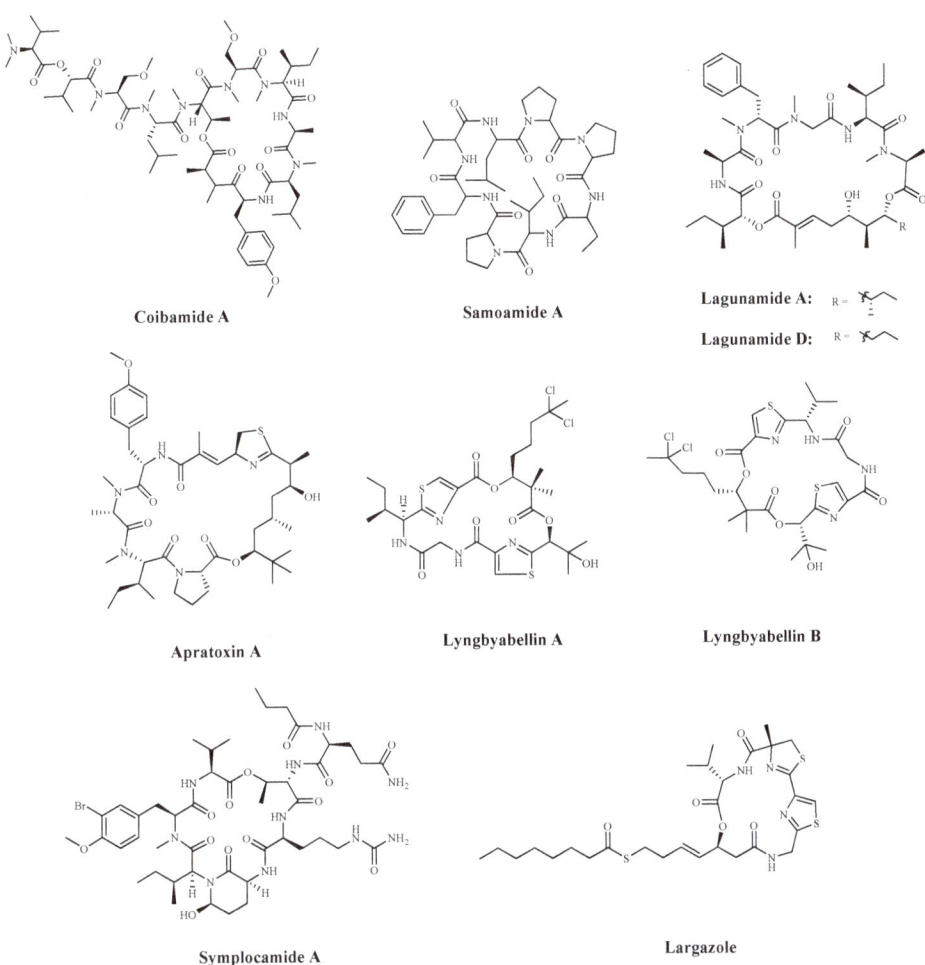

Figure 7. The structures of marine bioactive cyclic peptides from cyanobacteria.

Table 5. Marine bioactive cyclic peptides from Cyanobacterial metabolites.

Compound	Source	Mechanism	Cell Lines/Target protein	IC$_{50}$	Reference
Coibamide A	*Leptolyngbya* cyanobacterium	Cytotoxicity [a]	NCI-H460	<23 nM	[112]
Samoamide A	*Symploca* sp.	Cytotoxicity [a]	H460; H116	1.1 µM; 4.5 µM	[113,114]
Lagunamide A	cyanobacterium, *Lyngbya majuscule,*	Cytotoxicity; Caspase-mediated mitochondrial apoptosis	A549	7.1 nM;	[116]
Lagunamide D			A549	6.7 nM	
Apratoxin A	Cyanobacterial metabolite	Down-regulating receptors and growth factor ligands for cancer cells that rely on autocrine loop	HCT-116	5.97 nM	[120]
Lyngyabellin A	cyanobacterium *Lyngbya majuscula*	Antiproliferation; Disruption of cellular microfilament network cytokinesis	KB; LoVo	0.03 µg/mL; 0.50 µg/mL	[122]
Symplocamide A	Cyanobacteria *Symploca* sp.	Inhibiting Protease	Chymotrypsin H-460; Neuro-2a neuroblastoma	0.234 µM 40 nM 29 nM	[123]
Largazole	cyanobacteria *Symploca* sp.	Inhibiting HDAC	HCT-116 Inhibit HDAC1	44 nM 25 nM	[124,125]

Notes: [a] Mechanism is yet to be investigated.

4. Marine-Derived Small Peptides in Clinical Trials

Some marine small peptides have entered the clinical stage. However, due to their shortcomings such as low activity and large side effects, some have been terminated. What is gratifying is that a large number of researchers have synthesized a series of derivatives by optimizing their structures, and some of them are currently in the clinical stage. In this review, we collected the current clinical information and the latest clinical progress of anti-tumor small peptides through clinicaltrials.gov, PubMed, and Scopus, etc.

4.1. Linear Peptides

The Hemiasterlins (Figure 8) are a family of potent cytotoxic peptides isolated from sponges [126]. Like other peptide molecules with a diversity of structure, Hemiasterlins bind to the "Vinca-peptide site" in tubulin, disrupts the normal microtubule dynamics, and, at stoichiometric amounts, depolymerizes microtubules [127,128]. They progressed into Phase II, but the trials were discontinued due to significant bone marrow toxicity and neuropathy. The structural motif of the Hemiasterlins would appear to be readily amenable to the rapid generation of analogues by combinatorial chemistry. Two novel synthetic analogues of Hemiasterlin are known as HTI-286 (Taltobulin, Table S1 and Figure 8) and E7974 (Table S1 and Figure 8). They have been reported to have potent activity against tumor cells with a potentially high therapeutic index [129–136]. A synthetic analogue of Hemiasterlin, HTI-286, has significantly improved the drug resistance [130]. Some researchers found the N-isopropyl-D-pipecolic acid derivative E7974, which retains the potent in vitro antitumor activity of Hemiasterlin and induces a long-lasting mitotic blockade that ultimately triggers apoptosis [129]. The development of Hemiasterlin derivatives *BF65* synergized with a colchicine site microtubule inhibitor stilbene 5c both in vitro and in vivo, which may provide a potential drug combination in future clinical application [132]. It was reported that the stereospecific diastereomer (R)(S)(S)-BF65 (Figure 8) could synergize with an allosteric Akt inhibitor MK-2206 to suppress the growth of SKOV3 ovarian cancer cells [130].

Hemiasterlin derivatives HTI-286 and E7974 are poor substrates for P-glycoprotein and can circumvent drug resistance. All of them have entered the clinical stage (clinical information is shown in Table S1). However, it remains to be determined whether Hemiasterlins and derivatives have a better therapeutic profile for clinical development.

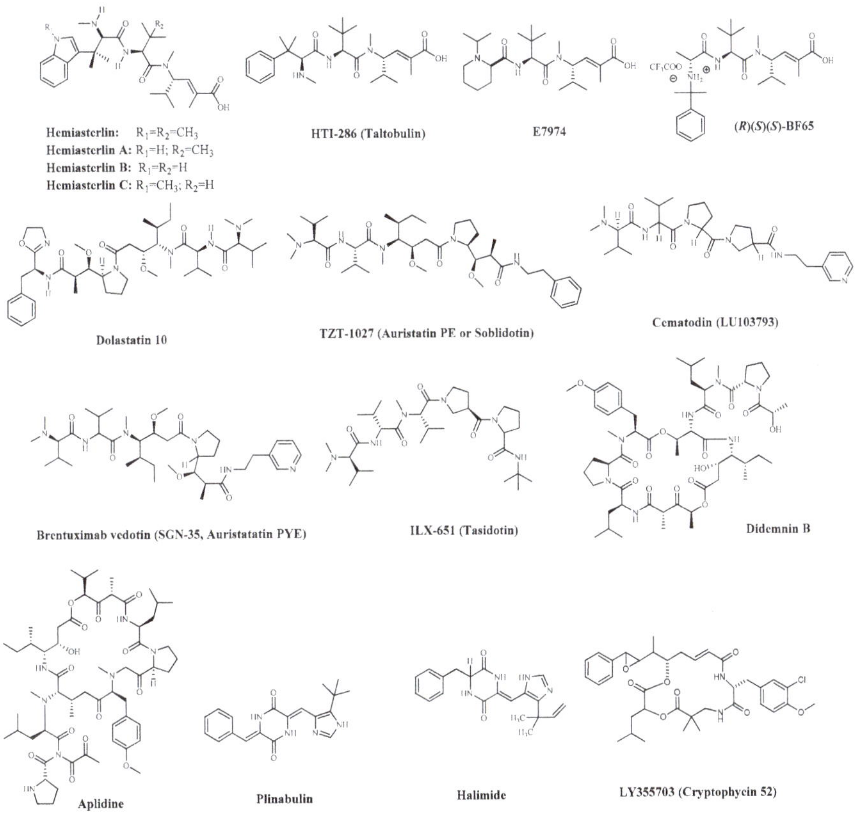

Figure 8. Marine-derived clinical small peptides and some of their derivatives.

Dolastatins are a series of cytotoxic peptides that were originally isolated from the sea hare *Dolabella Auricularia* as early as 1972 and recently obtained from a cyanobacterium. However, the most potent constituent Dolastatin 10 (Table S1 and Figure 8) was not until 1987 that it was isolated and characterized. Dolastatin 10 was a linear pentapeptide with four distinctive amino acids and exhibited potent inhibitory activity against a battery of human cancer cell lines [133]. It has been shown that Dolastatin 10 inhibits the binding of vincristine alkaloids to tubulin in a competitive inhibitory manner and binds adjacent to the exchangeable GTP site on the β-tubulin [134,135]. Dolastatin 10 progressed through to Phase II trials as a single agent. However, it did not demonstrate significant antitumor activity in a Phase II trial, together with problems of complex chemical synthesis with low yields and poor water solubility. Therefore, a large number of derivatives have been synthesized to optimize the structure and enhance the antitumor activity. Specific clinical information is shown in Table S1. Due to various harmful side effects with these series of cytotoxic peptides, they have been synthesized and modified largely, some of the derivatives are already in clinical trials, such as TZT-1027 (Auristatin PE or Soblidotin, Table S1 and Figure 8) [136–139]. Cematodin (LU103793, Figure 8) [140] and Glembatumumab vedotin (CDX-011, Table S1) [141]. Their clinical information is shown in Table S1. TZT-1027 is an anti-microtubule agent, which has been demonstrated to have a potent anti-vascular effect in the advanced stage of vascular-rich SBC-3/VEGF tumors and is currently in Phase II clinical trials [138]. However, significant side effects were observed in clinical trials at dose levels that were insufficient to attain clinical efficacy [142]. Auristatin PYE (SGN 35, Table S1 and Figure 8) is a novel synthetic derivative of Dolastatin 10 with a structural modification of phenol to a pyridine from Auristatin PE. It was reported that Auristatin PYE was less potent in vitro than Dolastatin 10, but it was significantly more effective ($p < 0.01$) in vivo against both human colon adenocarcinoma cell lines [143]. Owing to the drug resistance of tumor cells, Auristatin PYE could be exploited in combination therapy to improve the efficacy of the standard agent [144].

Similar to the drug Dolastatin 10, Dolastatin 15 is an anti-neoplastic pseudopeptide that represses tubulin-dependent GTP hydrolysis to tubulin. The derivative of Dolastatin 15 is known as Cematodin or LU-103793 (Figure 8). It has been illustrated that Cemadotin inhibits cell proliferation by blocking mitosis at the G2/M phase in lymphoma cell lines and was entered into Phase I clinical trials for treatment of breast cancer. It progressed into Phase II, but trials appear to have been discontinued to strong side-effects [140]. A new generation of Dolastatins represented by Tasidotin (ILX-651, Table S1 and Figure 8) and its major metabolite Tasidotin C-carboxylate, restrain dynamic instability at the plus ends of purified microtubules in vitro at concentrations that are 10 to 20 times lower than those which inhibit microtubule polymerization, and the metabolite is considerably more potent than that of the parent compound [145]. In Phase I clinical trials, Tasidotin was found to have several advantages over other Dolastatins for treating patients with advanced solid tumors, including reduced toxicity and the absence of long-term accumulation [146–148].

While it was designed as a single-agent drug from a Dolastatin analogue, ADCs selectively transport drugs to target sites, increasing drug activity while reducing side effects through selectivity. Monomethyl auristatin E (MMAE), as an ADC, has been utilized to increase antitumor activity. For example, Glembatumumab vedotin (CDX-011; formerly CR011-vcMMAE, Table S1) is an antibody–drug conjugate consisting of CR011, a fully human IgG2monoclonal antibody against gpNMB, conjugated via a valine-citrulline link to the potent microtubule inhibitor, MMAE [149]. Therefore, the FDA granted Fast Track designation to CDX-011 for the treatment of advanced, refractory, or resistant GPNMB-expressing breast cancer and was entered into phase II study to evaluate the overall response rate and safety of GV, glycoprotein NMB (GPNMB) expression, and survival in patients with metastatic uveal melanoma [141,150]. Similarly, Brentuximab vedotin (SGN-35, Table S1 and Figure 8) is an ADC comprising an anti-CD30 antibody conjugated by a protease-cleavable linker to the potent anti-microtubule agent, MMAE [149,151]. It gained the United States Food and Drug Administration (FDA) approval in 2011 for the treatment of Hodgkin lymphoma and systemic anapla sms known to stic large cell lymphoma [36].

4.2. Cyclic Peptides

The peptide metabolite Didemnin B (Table S1 and Figure 8) is a classic type of anticancer cyclic peptides that was the first marine natural product to enter phase I and II clinical trials. It has a number of non-proteinogenic amino acids and contains l-2-hydroxyisovalerylproprionic acid and l-isostatin within its ring structure. It was shown to induce the death of various transformed cells with apoptotic morphology and DNA fragmentation within the cytosol and the generation of DNA ladders. It also behaved as a potent inhibitor of protein synthesis. However, NCI trials were terminated in 1990 due to toxicity issues [152,153]. Aplidine (Plitidepsin and Dehydrodidemnin B, Table S1 and Figure 8) is a new marine anticancer depsipeptide with a chemical structure very similar to that of Didemnin B, has an oxidized pyruvate instead of lactate [154,155]. It has nearly entered a phase II clinical trial with metastatic, relapsed/refractory Dedifferentiated Liposarcoma, but it also can cause common adverse events like nausea, vomiting, and transient transaminitis [156]. It was recently used to evaluate the safety profile of Aplidine in Patients With COVID-19 (APLICOV-PC) [157] (shown in Table S1). Plinabulin (NPI-2358,

Table S1 and Figure 8), a potent microtubule-targeting agent derived from the natural diketopiperazine, 'phenylahistin' with a colchicine-like tubulin depolymerization activity, is an anticancer agent undergoing Phase II clinical trials in four countries, including the United States [158,159]. Another cyclic dipeptide, Halimide (Table S1 and Figure 8), can inhibit spindle formation in cells, thus reducing or inhibiting the ability of the cells to proceed through mitosis, arresting the cells in a premeiotic stage, and inhibiting tubulin polymerization [160]. Cryptophycin (Crp) is a cyanobacterial depsipeptide, which is a new potent cytotoxic anti-microtubule agent. The treatment of cells with Cryptophycin can rapidly cause morphological changes and DNA strand breakage [161,162]. LY355703 (Cryptophytic 52) (Table S1 and Figure 8) is a synthetic derivative of the cryptophycins, it is a cytotoxic agent that induce mitotic arrest by binding at the microtubule vinca binding domain. At present, it has entered phase I clinical treatment [163].

5. Conclusions

Due to its nonspecific selectivity and multidrug resistance (MDR), chemotherapy still has numerous cancer treatment challenges [164]. Nowadays, many scientists focused on using delivery systems with nanoscale therapeutics to improve the accuracy and precision of drugs [165]. The chemical diversity and structural complexity of marine natural products show that they may be an unexploited source of structures for use as biological probes or in drug discovery and development. It is reported that some anticancer peptides have high efficacy and selectivity in cancer treatment [166]. Additionally, they are expected to become the ideal drug carriers due to due to their superior targeting ability and low immunogenicity [167]. Among anticancer peptides, cyclic peptides have significant structural advantages. They display a large surface area, which provides a high affinity and selectivity for protein targets. Furthermore, cyclic peptides have little to no toxicity due to their benign amino acid make-up. Thus, they are simple to modify, handle, and characterize, which are all essential properties for therapeutics [168].

Personalized cancer vaccines targeting patient-specific neoantigens constitute a novel model of cancer treatment [169]. However, the neoantigen physicochemical variability is a primary problem associated with the optimal format for combatting cancer by manufacturing personalized cancer vaccines [170]. Anticancer peptide-conjugate vaccine modalities constitute a new potential cancer treatment [171].

Marine small peptides have the unique advantage of less adverse effects than other anti-cancer drugs, and are considered to have better therapeutic effects. At present, a variety of small peptide drugs have entered clinical research (Table S1). Understanding the molecular mechanisms of action about some new bioactive small peptides obtained from natural sources on specific cellular targets contributes to the development of peptides as promising lead drug candidates. This article reviewed small peptides of marine origin with antitumor activity and their action mechanism in recent years. Hopefully, it will serve as a reference for the development of novel marine antitumor agents.

Supplementary Materials: The following are available online at https://www.mdpi.com/1660-3397/19/2/115/s1, Table S1: Clinical information on Marine small peptide drugs.

Author Contributions: Conceptualization, B.Z. and N.W. (Ning Wang); literature review and analysis, Q.-T.Z., Z.-D.L., Z.W., T.W. and N.W. (Nan Wang); writing—original draft preparation, Q.-T.Z. and Z.-D.L.; review and editing, B.Z., N.W. (Ning Wang) and Y.-F.Z. All authors have read and agreed to the published version of the manuscript.

Funding: This work was funded by the National Natural Science Foundation of China (91856126), the Natural Science Foundation of Ningbo City (2018A610410), Foundation of Ningbo University for Grant (XYL20023), the National 111 Project of China (D16013), the Li Dak Sum Yip Yio Chin Kenneth Li Marine Biopharmaceutical Development Fund, and the K.C. Wong Magna Fund in Ningbo University.

Institutional Review Board Statement: Not applicable. The animal studies and clinical trials discussed in this review article were not conducted by the authors of the manuscript.

Informed Consent Statement: Not applicable.

Data Availability Statement: Not applicable.

Conflicts of Interest: The authors declare no conflict of interest.

Abbreviations

ADCs	Antibody–drug conjugates
A549	Human non-small cell lung cancer cells
AGS	Human gastric cancer adenocytes cells
APD3	Database of antimicrobial peptides
A-10	Rat aortic smooth muscle cells
AsPC-1	Human metastatic pancreatic cancer cells
AVPdb	Database of antiviral peptides
BACE1	Beta-secretase 1
BEL-7404	Human liver cancer cells
BxPC-3	Human in situ adenocarcinoma cells
CAR-T	Chimeric Antigen Receptor T-Cell Immunotherapy
CancerPPD	Database of anticancer peptides and proteins
Cath D	Cathepsin D
Cath E	Cathepsin E
CDX-011	Glembatumumab vedotin
CV1	African green monkey kidney cells
DLD-1	Human colonic adenocarcinoma cells
DU-145	Human prostate cancer cells
FDA	United States Food and Drug Administration
5-FU	5-Fluorouracil
GI_{50}	Half-maximal growth inhibitory concentration
GPNMB	Glycoprotein NMB
HCT 8	Human cecal adenocarcinoma cell
HCT-116	Human colon cancer cells
HDAC	Histone Deacetylase
HeLa	Human cervical cancer cells
Hep G2	Human liver cancer cells
H460	Human non-small cell lung cancer cells
H-1299	Human non-small cell lung cancer cells
HSP90A	Heat Shock Protein 90 Alpha Family Class A
HT-29	Human colon cancer cells
IC_{50}	Half-maximal inhibitory concentration
Jurkat 16	T-cell leukemia cells
JFCR39	A panel of 39 human cancer cell lines
KB	Human nasopharyngeal cancer cells
KDC	Knottin peptide–drug conjugate
LNCaP	Human prostate cancer cells
LO2	Normal liver cells
L1236	Hodgkin's Lymphoma cells
LoVo	Human colon cancer cells
MCF-7	Human breast cancer cells
MDA-MB-231	Human breast cancer cells
MDR	Multidrug resistance
MDs	Molecular dynamics simulation
MMAE	Monomethyl auristatin E
MOLT4	Human acute T lymphoblastic leukaemia cells
NF-κB	Nuclear factor kappa B
PANC-1	Human pancreatic cancer cells
PC-3	Human prostate cancer cells
P388	Mouse leukemia cells
PsA	Psammaplin A

RBC	Red blood cell
ROS	Overproduction of reactive oxygen species
RXF 393	Human kidney cancer cells
SGC-7901	Human gastric cancer cells
SK-OV3	Human ovarian cancer cell
SF-268	Human neurocancer cells
TNF	Tumor necrosis factor
293/NFκB-	Stably transfected NFκB human embryonic kidney cells
U-87 MG	Human glioblastoma cells
U937	Human histiocytic lymphoma cells
WBC	White blood cell

References

1. Molinski, T. Marine natural products. *Clin. Adv. Hematol. Oncol.* **2009**, *7*, 383–385.
2. de Vries, D.J.; Beart, P.M. Fishing for drugs from the sea: Status and strategies. *Trends Pharmacol. Sci.* **1995**, *16*, 275–279. [CrossRef]
3. Blunt, J.W.; Copp, B.R.; Keyzers, R.A.; Munro, M.H.; Prinsep, M.R. Marine natural products. *Nat. Prod. Rep.* **2015**, *32*, 116–211. [CrossRef]
4. Dyshlovoy, S.A.; Honecker, F. Marine compounds and cancer: 2017 updates. *Mar. Drugs* **2018**, *16*, 41. [CrossRef] [PubMed]
5. Siegel, R.L.; Miller, K.D.; Jemal, A. Cancer statistics, 2020. *CA Cancer J. Clin.* **2020**, *70*, 7–30. [CrossRef] [PubMed]
6. Nazish, S.; Mohamed, A. Personalized medicine in cardio-oncology: The role of induced pluripotent stem cell. *Cardiovasc. Res.* **2019**, *115*, 949–959. [CrossRef]
7. Vora, C.; Gupta, S. Targeted therapy in cervical cancer. *ESMO Open* **2019**, *3*, e000462. [CrossRef] [PubMed]
8. Turner, K.A.; Kalafatis, M. The case back on the TRAIL: Death receptors as markers for rhTRAIL sensitivity. *J. Appl. Lab. Med.* **2017**, *2*, 176–185. [CrossRef] [PubMed]
9. Salazar, R.; Cortés-Funes, H.; Casado, E.; Pardo, B.; López-Martín, A.; Cuadra, C.; Tabernero, J.; Coronado, C.; García, M.; Soto Matos-Pita, A.; et al. Phase I study of weekly kahalalide F as prolonged infusion in patients with advanced solid tumors. *Cancer Chemother. Pharmacol.* **2013**, *72*, 75–83. [CrossRef]
10. Jiao, S.; Wang, H.; Shi, Z.; Dong, A.; Zhang, W.; Song, X.; He, F.; Wang, Y.; Zhang, Z.; Wang, W.; et al. A peptide mimicking VGLL4 function acts as a YAP antagonist therapy against gastric cancer. *Cancer Cell* **2014**, *25*, 166–180. [CrossRef]
11. Cox, N.; Kintzing, J.R.; Smith, M.; Grant, G.A.; Cochran, J.R. Integrin-targeting knottin peptide-drug conjugates are potent inhibitors of tumor cell proliferation. *Angew. Chem. Int. Ed. Engl.* **2016**, *55*, 9894–9897. [CrossRef] [PubMed]
12. Bjork, R.L. Bi-Specific Monoclonal Antibody (Specific for Both CD3 and CD11b) Therapeutic Drug. U.S. Patent WO2007US14524, 22 June 2007.
13. Isazadeh, A.; Hajazimian, S.; Garshasbi, H.; Shadman, B.; Baradaran, B. Resistance mechanisms to immune checkpoints blockade by monoclonal antibody drugs in cancer immunotherapy: Focus on myeloma. *J. Cell. Physiol.* **2020**, *236*, 791–805. [CrossRef] [PubMed]
14. Shahidian, A.; Ghassemi, M.; Mohammadi, J.; Hashemi, M. Immunotherapy. In *Bio-Engineering Approaches to Cancer Diagnosis and Treatment*; Academic Press: Cambridge, MA, USA, 2020; pp. 69–114.
15. Lian, Q.; Cheng, Y.; Zhong, C.; Wang, F. Inhibition of the IgE-mediated activation of RBL-2H3 cells by TIPP, a novel thymic immunosuppressive pentapeptide. *Int. J. Mol. Sci.* **2015**, *16*, 2252–2268. [CrossRef] [PubMed]
16. Patil, S.; Vhora, I.; Amrutiya, J.; Lalani, R.; Misra, A. Role of nanotechnology in delivery of protein and peptide drugs. *Curr. Pharm. Des.* **2015**, *21*, 4155–4173. [CrossRef]
17. Tatiana, R.; Andreas, B.; Yves, S.; Christopher, K.; Alison, B.; Fabien, F.; Luca, M.; Ismael, Z.; Andrea, M. Software-aided approach to investigate peptide structure and metabolic susceptibility of amide bonds in peptide drugs based on high resolution mass spectrometry. *PLoS ONE* **2017**, *12*, e0186461. [CrossRef]
18. Wang, G.; Li, X.; Wang, Z. APD3: The antimicrobial peptide database as a tool for research and education. *Nucleic Acids Res.* **2016**, *44*, D1087–D1093. [CrossRef]
19. Seebah, S.; Suresh, A.; Zhuo, S.; Choong, Y.H.; Chua, H.; Chuon, D.; Beuerman, R.; Verma, C. Defensins knowledgebase: A manually curated database and information source focused on the defensins family of antimicrobial peptides. *Nucleic Acids Res.* **2007**, *35*, D265–D268. [CrossRef]
20. Qureshi, A.; Thakur, N.; Tandon, H.; Kumar, M. AVPdb: A database of experimentally validated antiviral peptides targeting medically important viruses. *Nucleic Acids Res.* **2014**, *42*, D1147–D1153. [CrossRef]
21. Divya, M.; Priya, A.; Vineet, K.; Anshika, J.; Deepika, M.; Sandeep, S.; Abhishek, T.; Kumardeep, C.; Gautam, S.K.; Ankur, G. ParaPep: A web resource for experimentally validated antiparasitic peptide sequences and their structures. *Database (Oxf.)* **2014**. [CrossRef]
22. Atul, T.; Abhishek, T.; Priya, A.; Sudheer, G.; Minakshi, S.; Deepika, M.; Anshika, J.; Sandeep, S.; Ankur, G.; Raghava, G.P.S. CancerPPD: A database of anticancer peptides and proteins. *Nucleic Acids Res.* **2015**, *43*, 837–843. [CrossRef]
23. Zhang, W.J.; Wang, S.; Kang, C.Z.; Lv, C.G.; Zhou, L.; Huang, L.Q.; Guo, L.P. Pharmacodynamic material basis of traditional chinese medicine based on biomacromolecules: A review. *Plant Methods* **2020**, *16*, 26. [CrossRef]

24. Chalamaiah, M.; Yu, W.; Wu, J. Immunomodulatory and anticancer protein hydrolysates (peptides) from food proteins: A review. *Food Chem.* **2018**, *245*, 205–222. [CrossRef] [PubMed]
25. Blanco-Míguez, A.; Gutiérrez-Jácome, A.; Pérez-Pérez, M.; Pérez-Rodríguez, G.; Catalán-García, S.; Fdez-Riverola, F.; Lourenço, A.; Sánchez, B. From amino acid sequence to bioactivity: The biomedical potential of antitumor peptides. *Protein Sci.* **2016**, *25*, 1084–1095. [CrossRef]
26. Nasrolahi Shirazi, A.; Tiwari, R.; Chhikara, B.S.; Mandal, D.; Parang, K. Design and biological evaluation of cell-penetrating peptide-doxorubicin conjugates as prodrugs. *Mol. Pharm.* **2013**, *10*, 488–499. [CrossRef]
27. Ebrahimi, M.; Mani-Varnosfaderani, A.; Khayamian, T.; Gharaghani, S. An in silico approach to design peptide mimetics based on docking and molecular dynamics simulation of EGFR-matuzumab complex. *J. Iran Chem. Soc.* **2016**, *13*, 1805–1817. [CrossRef]
28. Gellerman, G.; Baskin, S.; Galia, L.; Gilad, Y.; Firer, M.A. Drug resistance to chlorambucil in murine B-cell leukemic cells is overcome by its conjugation to a targeting peptide. *Anticancer Drugs* **2013**, *24*, 112–119. [CrossRef] [PubMed]
29. Khalifa, S.A.M.; Elias, N.; Farag, M.A.; Chen, L.; Saeed, A.; Hegazy, M.F.; Moustafa, M.S.; Abd El-Wahed, A.; Al-Mousawi, S.M.; Musharraf, S.G.; et al. Marine natural products: A source of novel anticancer drugs. *Mar. Drugs* **2019**, *17*, 491. [CrossRef] [PubMed]
30. Ganesan, A.R.; Mohanram, M.S.G.; Balasubramanian, B.; Kim, I.H.; Seedevi, P.; Mohan, K.; Kanagasabai, S.; Arasu, M.V.; Al-Dhabi, N.A.; Ignacimuthu, S. Marine invertebrates' proteins: A recent update on functional property. *J. King Saud Univ. Sci.* **2020**, *32*, 1496–1502. [CrossRef]
31. Cheung, R.C.; Ng, T.B.; Wong, J.H. Marine peptides: Bioactivities and applications. *Mar. Drugs* **2015**, *13*, 4006–4043. [CrossRef] [PubMed]
32. Narayanasamy, A.; Balde, A.; Raghavender, P.; Shashanth, D.; Abraham, J.; Joshi, I.; Nazeer, R.A. Isolation of marine crab (Charybdis natator) leg muscle peptide and its anti-inflammatory effects on macrophage cells. *Biocatal. Agric. Biotechnol.* **2020**, *25*, 101577. [CrossRef]
33. Wang, C.; Zhang, G.J.; Liu, W.D.; Yang, X.Y.; Zhu, N.; Shen, J.M.; Wang, Z.C.; Liu, Y.; Cheng, S.; Yu, G.L.; et al. Recent progress in research and development of marine drugs. *Chin. J. Mar. Drugs* **2019**, *38*, 35–69.
34. Kim, S.M. Antioxidant and anticancer activities of enzymatic hydrolysates of solitary tunicate (Styela clava). *Food Sci. Biotechnol.* **2011**, *20*, 1075–1085. [CrossRef]
35. Shakeel, E.; Arora, D.; Jamal, Q.M.S.; Akhtar, S.; Khan, M.K.A.; Kamal, M.A.; Siddiqui, M.H.; Lohani, M.; Arif, J.M. Marine drugs: A hidden wealth and a new epoch for cancer management. *Curr. Drug Metab.* **2018**, *19*, 523–543. [CrossRef]
36. Dyshlovoy, S.; Honecker, F. Marine compounds and cancer: Updates 2020. *Mar. Drugs* **2020**, *18*, 643. [CrossRef] [PubMed]
37. Dyshlovoy, S.; Honecker, F. Marine compounds and cancer: The first two decades of XXI century. *Mar. Drugs* **2019**, *18*, 20. [CrossRef]
38. Srinivasan, N.; Dhanalakshmi, S.; Pandian, P. Encouraging leads from marine sources for cancer therapy—A review approach. *Pharmacogn. J.* **2020**, *12*, 1475–1481. [CrossRef]
39. Ming-Jia, Z.; Dong-Mei, Z.; Jun-Hui, C. Research advances of antitumor peptides. *Chin. J. Biochem. Pharm.* **2007**, *28*, 139–141. [CrossRef]
40. Ding, G.-F.; Huang, F.-F.; Yang, Z.-S.; Yu, D.; Yang, Y.-F. Anticancer activity of an oligopeptide isolated from hydrolysates of Sepia Ink. *Chin. J. Nat. Med.* **2011**, *9*, 151–155. [CrossRef]
41. Quah, Y. Purification and identification of novel cytotoxic oligopeptides from soft coral Sarcophyton glaucum. *J. Zhejiang Univ. Sci. B Biomed. Biotechnol.* **2019**, *20*, 59–70. [CrossRef]
42. Gan, H. Concise and efficient total syntheses of virenamides A and D. *J. Adv. Chem.* **2008**, *4*, 488–493. [CrossRef]
43. Umayaparvathi, S.; Arumugam, M.; Meenakshi, S.; Dräger, G.; Kirschning, A.; Balasubramanian, T. Purification and characterization of antioxidant peptides from oyster (Saccostrea cucullata) hydrolysate and the anticancer activity of hydrolysate on human colon cancer cell lines. *Int. J. Pept. Res. Ther.* **2014**, *20*, 231–243. [CrossRef]
44. Umayaparvathi, S.; Meenakshi, S.; Vimalraj, V.; Arumugam, M.; Sivagami, G.; Balasubramanian, T. Antioxidant activity and anticancer effect of bioactive peptide from enzymatic hydrolysate of oyster (Saccostrea cucullata). *Biomed. Prev. Nutr.* **2014**, *4*, 343–353. [CrossRef]
45. Song, R.; Wei, R.B.; Luo, H.Y.; Yang, Z.S. Isolation and identification of an antiproliferative peptide derived from heated products of peptic hydrolysates of half-fin anchovy (Setipinna taty). *J. Funct. Foods* **2014**, *10*, 104–111. [CrossRef]
46. Ratih, P.; Se-Kwon, K. Bioactive peptide of marine origin for the prevention and treatment of non-communicable diseases. *Mar. Drugs* **2017**, *15*, 67. [CrossRef]
47. Chi, C.-F.; Hu, F.-Y.; Wang, B.; Li, T.; Ding, G.-F. Antioxidant and anticancer peptides from the protein hydrolysate of blood clam (Tegillarca granosa) muscle. *J. Funct. Foods* **2015**, *15*, 301–313. [CrossRef]
48. Aissaoui, D.; Mlayah Bellalouna, S.; Jebali, J.; Abdelkafi Koubaa, Z.; Souid, S.; Moslah, W.; Othman, H.; Luis, J.; Elayeb, M.; Marrakchi, N. Functional role of Kv1.1 and Kv1.3 channels in the neoplastic progression steps of three cancer cell lines, elucidated by scorpion peptides. *Int. J. Biol. Macromol.* **2018**, *111*, 1146–1155. [CrossRef]
49. Ciccone, R.; Piccialli, I.; Grieco, P.; Merlino, F.; Annunziato, L.; Pannaccione, A. Synthesis and pharmacological evaluation of a novel peptide based on anemonia sulcata BDS-I toxin as a new KV3.4 inhibitor exerting a neuroprotective effect against amyloid-β peptide. *Front. Chem.* **2019**, *9*, 497. [CrossRef]

50. Min, S.; Su, P.; Jeong, P.; Jin, B.; Hee, J.; Seung, S.; Pan, R.; So, L. Kv3.1 and Kv3.4, are involved in cancer cell migration and invasion. *Int. J. Mol. Sci.* **2018**, *19*, 1061. [CrossRef]
51. Pan, X.; Zhao, Y.Q.; Hu, F.Y.; Chi, C.F.; Wang, B. Anticancer activity of a hexapeptide from skate (*Raja porosa*) cartilage protein hydrolysate in HeLa cells. *Mar. Drugs* **2016**, *14*, 153. [CrossRef]
52. Wu, Z.Z.; Ding, G.F.; Huang, F.F.; Yang, Z.S.; Yu, F.M.; Tang, Y.P.; Jia, Y.L.; Zheng, Y.Y.; Chen, R. Anticancer activity of anthopleura anjunae oligopeptides in prostate cancer DU-145 cells. *Mar. Drugs* **2018**, *16*, 125. [CrossRef]
53. Fangmiao, Y.; Yaru, Z.; Lei, Y.; Yunping, T.; Guofang, D.; Xiaojun, Z.; Zuisu, Y. A novel antiproliferative pentapeptide (ILYMP) isolated from cyclinasinensis protein hydrolysate induces apoptosis of DU145 prostate cancer cells. *Mol. Med. Rep.* **2018**, *18*, 771–778. [CrossRef]
54. Huang, F.; Ding, G.; Yang, Z.; Yu, F. Two novel peptides derived from *Sinonovacula constricta* inhibit the proliferation and induce apoptosis of human prostate cancer cells. *Mol. Med. Rep.* **2017**, *16*, 6697–6707. [CrossRef]
55. Zhang, Z.; Sun, L.; Zhou, G.; Xie, P.; Ye, J. Sepia ink oligopeptide induces apoptosis and growth inhibition in human lung cancer cells. *Oncotarget* **2017**, *8*, 23202–23212. [CrossRef] [PubMed]
56. Huang, F.; Yang, Z.; Yu, D.; Wang, J.; Li, R.; Ding, G. Sepia ink oligopeptide induces apoptosis in prostate cancer cell lines via caspase-3 activation and elevation of Bax/Bcl-2 ratio. *Mar Drugs* **2012**, *10*, 2153–2165. [CrossRef]
57. Huang, F.; Jing, Y.; Ding, G.; Yang, Z. Isolation and purification of novel peptides derived from *Sepia* ink: Effects on apoptosis of prostate cancer cell PC-3. *Mol. Med. Rep.* **2017**, *16*, 4222–4228. [CrossRef] [PubMed]
58. Baud, M.G.J.; Leiser, T.; Haus, P.; Samlal, S.; Wong, A.C.; Wood, R.J.; Petrucci, V.; Gunaratnam, M.; Hughes, S.M.; Buluwela, L. Defining the mechanism of action and enzymatic selectivity of Psammaplin A against its epigenetic targets. *J. Med. Chem.* **2012**, *55*, 1731–1750. [CrossRef] [PubMed]
59. Kumar M, S.L.; Ali, K.; Chaturvedi, P.; Meena, S.; Datta, D.; Panda, G. Design, synthesis and biological evaluation of oxime lacking Psammaplin inspired chemical libraries as anti-cancer agents. *J. Mol. Struct.* **2021**, *1225*. [CrossRef]
60. Simmons, T.L.; Andrianasolo, E.; McPhail, K.; Flatt, P.; Gerwick, W.H. Marine natural products as anticancer drugs. *Mol. Cancer Ther.* **2005**, *4*, 333–342. [PubMed]
61. Youssef, F.S.; Ashour, M.L.; Singab, A.N.B.; Wink, M. A Comprehensive review of bioactive peptides from marine fungi and their biological significance. *Mar. Drugs* **2019**, *17*, 559. [CrossRef]
62. Cho, J.Y.; Williams, P.G.; Kwon, H.C.; Jensen, P.R.; Fenical, W. Lucentamycins A–D, cytotoxic peptides from the marine-derived actinomycete nocardiopsis lucentensis. *J. Nat. Prod.* **2007**, *70*, 1321–1328. [CrossRef]
63. Williams, D.E.; Dalisay, D.S.; Patrick, B.O.; Matainaho, T.; Andrusiak, K.; Deshpande, R.; Myers, C.L.; Piotrowski, J.S.; Boone, C.; Yoshida, M.; et al. Padanamides A and B, highly modified linear tetrapeptides produced in culture by a *Streptomyces* sp. isolated from a marine sediment. *Org. Lett.* **2011**, *13*, 3936–3939. [CrossRef] [PubMed]
64. Williams, P.G.; Yoshida, W.Y.; Moore, R.E.; Paul, V.J. Tasiamide, a cytotoxic peptide from the marine cyanobacterium *Symploca* sp. *J. Nat. Prod.* **2002**, *65*, 1336. [CrossRef]
65. Pranjol, M.Z.I.; Gutowski, N.J.; Hannemann, M.; Whatmore, J.L. Cathepsin D non-proteolytically induces proliferation and migration in human omental microvascular endothelial cells via activation of the ERK1/2 and PI3K/AKT pathways. *Biochim. Biophys. Acta. Mol. Cell. Res.* **2018**, *1865*, 25–33. [CrossRef]
66. Li, Z.; Bao, K.; Xu, H.; Wu, P.; Li, W.; Liu, J.; Zhang, W. Design, synthesis, and bioactivities of tasiamide B derivatives as cathepsin D inhibitors. *J. Pept. Sci.* **2019**, *25*, e3154. [CrossRef]
67. Simmons, T.L.; Mcphail, K.L.; Ortega-Barría, E.; Mooberry, S.L.; Gerwick, W.H. Belamide A, a new antimitotic tetrapeptide from a Panamanian marine cyanobacterium. *Tetrahedron Lett.* **2006**, *37*, 3387–3390. [CrossRef]
68. Corbett, T.H. The molecular pharmacology of symplostatin 1: A new antimitotic dolastatin 10 analog. *Int. J. Oncol.* **2010**, *104*, 512–521. [CrossRef]
69. Brucoli, F.; Natoli, A.; Marimuthu, P.; Borrello, M.T.; Stapleton, P.; Gibbons, S.; Schätzlein, A. Efficient synthesis and biological evaluation of proximicins A, B and C. *Bioorg. Med. Chem.* **2012**, *20*, 2019–2024. [CrossRef]
70. Teruya, T.; Sasaki, H.; Fukazawa, H.; Suenaga, K. Bisebromoamide, a potent cytotoxic peptide from the marine cyanobacterium *Lyngbya* sp.: Isolation, stereostructure, and biological activity. *Org. Lett.* **2010**, *41*, 5062–5065. [CrossRef]
71. Suzuki, K.; Mizuno, R.; Suenaga, K.; Teruya, T.; Tanaka, N.; Kosaka, T.; Oya, M. Bisebromoamide, an extract from *Lyngbya* species, induces apoptosis through ERK and mTOR inhibitions in renal cancer cells. *Cancer Med.* **2013**, *2*, 32–39. [CrossRef] [PubMed]
72. Wang, Z.; Zhang, X. Isolation and identification of anti-proliferative peptides from *Spirulina platensis* using three-step hydrolysis. *J. Sci. Food Agric.* **2017**, *97*, 918–922. [CrossRef] [PubMed]
73. Choi, J.S.; Joo, S.H. Recent trends in cyclic peptides as therapeutic agents and biochemical tools. *Biomol. Ther.* **2020**, *28*, 18–24. [CrossRef]
74. Donia, M.S.; Wang, B.; Dunbar, D.C.; Desai, P.V.; Hamann, M.T. Mollamides B and C, cyclic hexapeptides from the indonesian tunicate Didemnum molle. *Planta Med.* **2008**, *71*, 941–945. [CrossRef]
75. Wesson, K.J.; Hamann, M.T. Keenamide A, a bioactive cyclic peptide from the marine mollusk *Pleurobranchus forskalii*. *J. Nat. Prod.* **1996**, *59*, 629–631. [CrossRef] [PubMed]
76. Mckeever, B.; Pattenden, G. Total synthesis of trunkamide A, a novel thiazoline-based prenylated cyclopeptide metabolite from *Lissoclinum* sp. *Tetrahedron* **2003**, *59*, 2713–2727. [CrossRef]

77. Liang, B.; Richard, D.J.; Portonovo, P.S.; Joullié, M.M. Total syntheses and biological investigations of tamandarins A and B and tamandarin A analogs. *J. Am. Chem. Soc.* **2001**, *123*, 4469–4474. [CrossRef]
78. Watters, D.J.; Beamish, H.J. Accumulation of HL-60 leukemia cells in G2/M and inhibition of cytokinesis caused by two marine compounds, bistratene A and cycloxazoline. *Cancer Chemoth. Pharm.* **1994**, *33*, 399–409. [CrossRef]
79. Robinson, S.J.; Morinaka, B.I.; Amagata, T.; Tenney, K.; Crews, P. New structures and bioactivity properties of jasplakinolide (jaspamide) analogues from marine sponges. *J. Med. Chem.* **2010**, *53*, 1651–1661. [CrossRef] [PubMed]
80. Rangel, M.; Ionta, M.; Pfister, C.S.; Ferreira, A.S.A.R.; Machado-Santelli, M.G. Marine sponge depsipeptide increases gap junction length in HTC cells transfected with Cx43–GFP. *Cell Biol. Int. Rep.* **2013**, *17*, 13–18. [CrossRef] [PubMed]
81. Pettit, G.R.; Cichacz, Z.; Barkoczy, J.; Dorsaz, A.C.; Herald, D.L.; Williams, M.D.; Doubek, D.L.; Schmidt, J.M.; Tackett, L.P.; Brune, D.C. Isolation and structure of the marine sponge cell growth inhibitory cyclic peptide phakellistatin 1. *J. Nat. Prod.* **1993**, *56*, 260–267. [CrossRef]
82. Guzmán, E.A.; Maers, K.; Roberts, J.; Kemami-Wangun, H.V.; Harmody, D.; Wright, A.E. The marine natural product microsclerodermin A is a novel inhibitor of the nuclear factor kappa B and induces apoptosis in pancreatic cancer cells. *Investig. New Drugs.* **2015**, *33*, 86. [CrossRef]
83. Schmidt, E.W.; Raventos Suarez, C.; Bifano, M.; Menendez, A.T.; Fairchild, C.R.; Faulkner, D.J. Scleritodermin A, a cytotoxic cyclic peptide from the lithistid sponge scleritoderma nodosum. *J. Nat. Prod.* **2004**, *67*, 475–478. [CrossRef]
84. Wang, S.; Crevenna, A.H.; Ugur, I.; Marion, A.; Antes, I.; Kazmaier, U.; Hoyer, M.; Lamb, D.C.; Gegenfurtner, F.; Kliesmete, Z.; et al. Actin stabilizing compounds show specific biological effects due to their binding mode. *Sci. Rep.* **2019**, *9*, 9731. [CrossRef] [PubMed]
85. Schweikart, K.; Guo, L.; Shuler, Z.; Abrams, R.; Chiao, E.T.; Kolaja, K.L.; Davis, M. The effects of jaspamide on human cardiomyocyte function and cardiac ion channel activity. *Toxicol. In Vitro* **2013**, *27*, 745–751. [CrossRef]
86. Cioca, D.P.; Kitano, K. Induction of apoptosis and CD10/neutral endopeptidase expression by jaspamide in HL-60 line cells. *Cell Mol. Life Sci.* **2002**, *59*, 1377–1387. [CrossRef] [PubMed]
87. Chan, W.R.; Tinto, W.F.; Manchand, P.S.; Todaro, L.J. Stereostructures of Geodiamolides A and B, novel cyclodepsipeptides from the marine sponge *Geodia* sp. *J. Org. Chem.* **1987**, *52*, 3091–3093. [CrossRef]
88. Tinto, W.F.; Lough, A.J.; McLean, S.; Reynolds, W.F.; Yu, M.; Chan, W.R. Geodiamolides H and I, further cyclodepsipeptides from the marine sponge *Geodia* sp. *Tetrahedron* **1998**, *54*, 4451–4458. [CrossRef]
89. Rangel, M.; Prado, M.P.; Konno, K.; Naoki, H.; Freitas, J.C.; Machado-Santelli, G.M. Cytoskeleton alterations induced by *Geodia corticostylifera* depsipeptides in breast cancer cells. *Peptides* **2006**, *27*, 2047–2057. [CrossRef]
90. Freitas, V.M.; Rangel, M.; Bisson, L.F.; Jaeger, R.G.; Machado-Santelli, G.M. The geodiamolide H, derived from Brazilian sponge *Geodia corticostylifera*, regulates actin cytoskeleton, migration and invasion of breast cancer cells cultured in three-dimensional environment. *J. Cell. Physiol.* **2008**, *216*, 583–594. [CrossRef]
91. Meli, A.; Tedesco, C.; Della Sala, G.D.; Schettini, R.; Albericio, F.; De Riccardis, F.; Izzo, I. Phakellistatins: An underwater unsolved puzzle. *Mar. Drugs* **2017**, *15*, 78. [CrossRef]
92. Pettit, G.R.; Tan, R. Isolation and structure of phakellistatin 14 from the western pacific marine sponge *Phakellia* sp. *J. Nat. Prod.* **2005**, *68*, 60–63. [CrossRef]
93. Bao, Y.; Jiang, S.; Zhao, L.; Jin, Y.; Yan, R.; Wang, Z. Photoinduced synthesis and antitumor activity of a phakellistatin 18 analog with an isoindolinone fragment. *New J. Chem.* **2020**, *44*, 19174–19178. [CrossRef]
94. Tian, T.; Takada, K.; Ise, Y.; Ohtsuka, S.; Okada, S.; Matsunaga, S. Microsclerodermins N and O, cytotoxic cyclic peptides containing a p-ethoxyphenyl moiety from a deep-sea marine sponge *Pachastrella* sp. *Tetrahedron* **2020**, *76*, 130997. [CrossRef]
95. Vinothkumar, S.; Parameswaran, P.S. Recent advances in marine drug research. *Biotechnol. Adv.* **2013**, *31*, 1826–1845. [CrossRef]
96. Oh, D.C.; Jensen, P.R.; Fenical, W. Zygosporamide, a cytotoxic cyclic depsipeptide from the marine-derived fungus *Zygosporium masonii*. *Tetrahedron Lett.* **2006**, *47*, 8625–8628. [CrossRef]
97. Chen, Z.; Song, Y.; Chen, Y.; Huang, H.; Zhang, W.; Ju, J. Cyclic heptapeptides, cordyheptapeptides C–E, from the marine-derived fungus *Acremonium persicinum* SCSIO 115 and their cytotoxic activities. *J. Nat. Prod.* **2012**, *75*, 1215–1219. [CrossRef]
98. He, F.; Bao, J.; Zhang, X.Y.; Tu, Z.C.; Shi, Y.M.; Qi, S.H. Asperterrestide A, a cytotoxic cyclic tetrapeptide from the marine-derived fungus *Aspergillus terreus* SCSGAF0162. *J. Nat. Prod.* **2013**, *76*, 1182–1186. [CrossRef]
99. Ujiki, M.B.; Milam, B.; Ding, X.Z.; Roginsky, A.B.; Salabat, M.R.; Talamonti, M.S.; Bell, R.H.; Gu, W.; Silverman, R.B.; Adrian, T.E. A novel peptide sansalvamide analogue inhibits pancreatic cancer cell growth through G0/G1 cell-cycle arrest. *Biochem. Biophys. Res. Commun.* **2006**, *340*, 1224–1228. [CrossRef] [PubMed]
100. Wang, X.; Zhang, J.; Wu, H.; Li, Y.; Conti, P.S.; Chen, K. PET imaging of Hsp90 expression in pancreatic cancer using a new 64 Cu-labeled dimeric Sansalvamide A decapeptide. *Amino Acids* **2018**, *50*, 897–907. [CrossRef]
101. Song, K.H.; Oh, S.J.; Kim, S.; Cho, H.; Lee, H.J.; Song, J.S.; Chung, J.Y.; Cho, E.; Lee, J.; Jeon, S.; et al. HSP90A inhibition promotes anti-tumor immunity by reversing multi-modal resistance and stem-like property of immune-refractory tumors. *Nat. Commun.* **2020**, *11*, 562. [CrossRef]
102. Porter, N.J.; Christianson, D.W. Binding of the microbial cyclic tetrapeptide Trapoxin A to the class i histone deacetylase HDAC8. *ACS Chem. Biol.* **2017**, *12*, 2281–2286. [CrossRef] [PubMed]

103. Itazaki, H.; Nagashima, K.; Sugita, K.; Yoshida, H.; Kawamura, Y.; Yasuda, Y.; Matsumoto, K.; Ishii, K.; Uotani, N.; Nakai, H.; et al. Isolation and structural elucidation of new cyclotetrapeptides, trapoxins A and B, having detransformation activities as antitumor agents. *J. Antibiot. (Tokyo)* **1990**, *43*, 1524–1532. [CrossRef] [PubMed]
104. Kijima, M.; Yoshida, M.; Sugita, K.; Horinouchi, S.; Beppu, T. Trapoxin, an antitumor cyclic tetrapeptide, is an irreversible inhibitor of mammalian histone deacetylase. *J. Biol. Chem.* **1993**, *268*, 22429–22435. [CrossRef]
105. Jung, M.; Hoffmann, K.; Brosch, G.; Loidl, P. Analogues of trichostatin A and trapoxin B as histone deacetylase inhibitors. *Bioorg. Med. Chem. Lett.* **1997**, *7*, 1655–1658. [CrossRef]
106. Gu, W.; Cueto, M.; Jensen, P.R.; Fenical, W.; Silverman, R.B. Microsporins A and B: New histone deacetylase inhibitors from the marine-derived fungus *Microsporum* cf. *gypseum* and the solid-phase synthesis of microsporin A. *Tetrahedron* **2007**, *63*, 6535–6541. [CrossRef]
107. Karpiński, T.; Adamczak, A. Anticancer activity of bacterial proteins and peptides. *Pharmaceutics* **2018**, *10*, 54. [CrossRef]
108. Zhang, H.L.; Hua, H.M.; Pei, Y.H.; Yao, X.S. Three new cytotoxic cyclic acylpeptides from marine *Bacillus* sp. *Chem. Pharm. Bull. (Tokyo)* **2004**, *52*, 1029–1030. [CrossRef] [PubMed]
109. Kanoh, K.; Matsuo, Y.; Adachi, K.; Imagawa, H.; Nishizawa, M.; Shizuri, Y. Mechercharmycins A and B, cytotoxic substances from marine-derived *Thermoactinomyces* sp. YM3-251. *J. Antibiot. (Tokyo)* **2005**, *58*, 289–292. [CrossRef] [PubMed]
110. Oberheide, A.; Schwenk, S.; Ronco, C.; Semmrau, L.M.; Gorls, H.; Arndt, H.D. Synthesis, structure, and cytotoxicity of urukthapelstatin A polyazole cyclopeptide analogs. *Eur. J. Org. Chem.* **2019**, *2019*, 4320–4326. [CrossRef]
111. Asolkar, R.N.; Freel, K.C.; Jensen, P.R.; Fenical, W.; Pezzuto, J.M. Arenamides A–C, cytotoxic NFkappaB inhibitors from the marine actinomycete *Salinispora arenicola*. *J. Nat. Prod.* **2009**, *72*, 396–402. [CrossRef]
112. Medina, R.A.; Goeger, D.E.; Hills, P.; Mooberry, S.L.; Huang, N.; Romero, L.I.; Ortega-BarriA, E.; Gerwick, W.H.; Mcphail, K.L. Coibamide A, a potent antiproliferative cyclic depsipeptide from the Panamanian marine cyanobacterium *Leptolyngbya* sp. *J. Am. Chem. Soc.* **2008**, *130*, 6324–6325. [CrossRef] [PubMed]
113. Ge, F.; Zhang, C.; Zhu, L.; Li, W.; Song, P.; Tao, Y.; Du, G. Synthesis and antitumor activity of cyclic octapeptide, samoamide A, and its derivatives. *Med. Chem. Res.* **2019**, *28*, 768–777. [CrossRef]
114. Naman, C.B.; Rattan, R.; Nikoulina, S.E.; Lee, J.; Miller, B.W.; Moss, N.A.; Armstrong, L.; Boudreau, P.D.; Debonsi, H.M.; Valeriote, F.A.; et al. Integrating molecular networking and biological assays to target the isolation of a cytotoxic cyclic octapeptide, Samoamide A, from an American samoan marine cyanobacterium. *J. Nat. Prod.* **2017**, *80*, 625–633. [CrossRef]
115. Huang, W.; Ren, R.-G.; Dong, H.-Q.; Wei, B.-G.; Lin, G.-Q. Diverse synthesis of marine cyclic depsipeptide Lagunamide A and its analogues. *J. Org. Chem.* **2014**, *45*, 10747–10762. [CrossRef]
116. Luo, D.; Putra, M.Y.; Ye, T.; Paul, V.J.; Luesch, H. Isolation, structure elucidation and biological evaluation of lagunamide D: A new cytotoxic macrocyclic depsipeptide from marine cyanobacteria. *Mar. Drugs* **2019**, *17*, 83. [CrossRef] [PubMed]
117. Han, B.; Gross, H.; Goeger, D.E.; Mooberry, S.L.; Gerwick, W.H. Aurilides B and C, cancer cell toxins from a papua new guinea collection of the marine cyanobacterium *Lyngbya majuscula*. *J. Nat. Prod.* **2006**, *69*, 572–575. [CrossRef] [PubMed]
118. Kaneda, M.; Sueyoshi, K.; Teruya, T.; Ohno, H.; Fujii, N.; Oishi, S. Total synthesis of odoamide, a novel cyclic depsipeptide, from an okinawan marine cyanobacterium. *Org. Biomol. Chem.* **2016**, *14*, 9093–9104. [CrossRef] [PubMed]
119. Williams, P.G.; Yoshida, W.Y.; Quon, M.K.; Moore, R.E.; Paul, V.J. The structure of Palau'amide, a potent cytotoxin from a species of the marine cyanobacterium *Lyngbya*. *J. Nat. Prod.* **2003**, *66*, 1545–1549. [CrossRef]
120. Chen, Q.Y.; Liu, Y.; Luesch, H. Systematic chemical mutagenesis identifies a potent novel Apratoxin A/E hybrid with improved in vivo antitumor activity. *ACS Med. Chem. Lett.* **2011**, *2*, 861–865. [CrossRef]
121. Cai, W.; Ratnayake, R.; Gerber, M.H.; Chen, Q.Y.; Yu, Y.; Derendorf, H.; Trevino, J.G.; Luesch, H. Development of apratoxin S10 (Apra S10) as an anti-pancreatic cancer agent and its preliminary evaluation in an orthotopic patient-derived xenograft (PDX) model. *Investig. New Drugs* **2019**, *37*, 364–374. [CrossRef]
122. Luesch, H.; Yoshida, W.Y.; Moore, R.E.; Paul, V.J.; Mooberry, S.L. Isolation, structure determination, and biological activity of Lyngbyabellin A from the marine cyanobacterium *Lyngbya majuscula*. *J. Nat. Prod.* **2000**, *63*, 611–615. [CrossRef]
123. Linington, R.G.; Edwards, D.J.; Shuman, C.F.; Mcphail, K.L.; Matainaho, T.; Gerwick, W.H. Symplocamide A, a potent cytotoxin and chymotrypsin inhibitor from the marine *Cyanobacterium symploca* sp. *J. Nat. Prod.* **2008**, *71*, 22–27. [CrossRef]
124. Ying, Y.; Taori, K.; Kim, H.; Hong, J.; Luesch, H. Total synthesis and molecular target of largazole, a histone deacetylase inhibitor. *J. Am. Chem. Soc.* **2008**, *130*, 8455–8459. [CrossRef] [PubMed]
125. Kim, B.; Park, H.; Salvador, L.A.; Serrano, P.E.; Kwan, J.C.; Zeller, S.L.; Chen, Q.Y.; Ryu, S.; Liu, Y.; Byeon, S.; et al. Evaluation of class I HDAC isoform selectivity of largazole analogues. *Bioorg. Med. Chem. Lett.* **2014**, *24*, 3728–3731. [CrossRef] [PubMed]
126. Anderson, H.J.; Coleman, J.E.; Andersen, R.J.; Roberge, M. Cytotoxic peptides hemiasterlin, hemiasterlin A and hemiasterlin B induce mitotic arrest and abnormal spindle formation. *Cancer Chemother. Pharmacol.* **1996**, *39*, 223–226. [CrossRef] [PubMed]
127. Frank LoVecchio, D.O.; Jane Klemens, R.N.; Ba, B.A.R.; Annie Klemens, B.A. HTI-286, a synthetic analogue of the tripeptide hemiasterlin, is a potent antimicrotubule agent that circumvents P-glycoprotein-mediated resistance in vitro and in vivo. *Cancer Res.* **2003**, *63*, 1838–1845. [CrossRef]
128. Bai, R.; Durso, N.A.; Sackett, D.L.; Hamel, E. Interactions of the sponge-derived antimitotic tripeptide hemiasterlin with tubulin: Comparison with dolastatin 10 and cryptophycin 1. *Biochemistry* **1999**, *38*, 14302. [CrossRef]

129. Kuznetsov, G.; TenDyke, K.; Towle, M.J.; Cheng, H.; Liu, J.; Marsh, J.P.; Schiller, S.E.R.; Spyvee, M.R.; Yang, H.; Seletsky, B.M.; et al. Tubulin-based antimitotic mechanism of E7974, a novel analogue of the marine sponge natural product hemiasterlin. *Mol. Cancer Ther.* **2009**, *8*, 2852–2860. [CrossRef] [PubMed]

130. Poruchynsky, M.S.; Kim, J.H.; Nogales, E.; Annable, T.; Loganzo, F.; Greenberger, L.M.; Sackett, D.L.; Fojo, T. Tumor cells resistant to a microtubule-depolymerizing hemiasterlin analogue, HTI-286, have mutations in alpha- or beta-tubulin and increased microtubule stability. *Biochemistry* **2004**, *43*, 13944–13954. [CrossRef]

131. Lai, W.T.; Cheng, K.L.; Baruchello, R.; Rondanin, R.; Marchetti, P.; Simoni, D.; Lee, R.M.; Guh, J.H.; Hsu, L.C. Hemiasterlin derivative (R)(S)(S)-BF65 and Akt inhibitor MK-2206 synergistically inhibit SKOV3 ovarian cancer cell growth. *Biochem. Pharmacol.* **2016**, *113*, 12–23. [CrossRef]

132. Hsu, L.C.; Durrant, D.E.; Huang, C.C.; Chi, N.W.; Baruchello, R.; Rondanin, R.; Rullo, C.; Marchetti, P.; Grisolia, G.; Simoni, D.; et al. Development of hemiasterlin derivatives as potential anticancer agents that inhibit tubulin polymerization and synergize with a stilbene tubulin inhibitor. *Investig. New Drugs* **2012**, *30*, 1379–1388. [CrossRef]

133. Pettit, G.; Kamano, Y.; Herald, C.; Tuinman, A.; Boettner, F.; Kizu, H.; Schmidt, J.; Baczynskyj, L.; Tomer, K.; Bontems, R. The isolation and structure of a remarkable marine animal antineoplastic constituent: Dolastatin 10. *J. Am. Chem. Soc.* **1986**, *109*, 6883–6885. [CrossRef]

134. Hamel, E. Interactions of antimitotic peptides and depsipeptides with tubulin. *Biopolymers* **2002**, *66*, 142–160. [CrossRef] [PubMed]

135. Bai, R.L.; Pettit, G.R.; Hamel, E. Binding of dolastatin 10 to tubulin at a distinct site for peptide antimitotic agents near the exchangeable nucleotide and vinca alkaloid sites. *J. Biol. Chem.* **1990**, *265*, 17141–17149. [CrossRef]

136. Ebbinghaus, S.; Hersh, E.; Cunningham, C.C.; O'Day, S.; Mcdermott, D.; Stephenson, J.; Richards, D.A.; Eckardt, J.; Haider, O.L.; Hammond, L.A. Phase II study of synthadotin (SYN-D; ILX651) administered daily for 5 consecutive days once every 3 weeks (qdx5q3w) in patients (Pts) with inoperable locally advanced or metastatic melanoma. *J. Clin. Oncol.* **2004**, *22*, 7530. [CrossRef]

137. Mross, K.; Herbst, K.; Berdel, W.E.; Korfel, A.; von Broen, I.M.; Bankmann, Y.; Hossfeld, D.K. Phase I clinical and pharmacokinetic study of LU103793 (Cemadotin Hydrochloride) as an intravenous bolus injection in patients with metastatic solid tumors. *Onkologie* **1996**, *19*, 490–495. [CrossRef]

138. Natsume, T.; Watanabe, J.I.; Koh, Y.; Fujio, N.; Kobayashi, M. Antitumor activity of TZT-1027 (Soblidotin) against vascular endothelial growth factor-secreting human lung cancer in vivo. *Cancer Sci.* **2010**, *94*, 826–833. [CrossRef]

139. Newman, D.; Cragg, G. Natural products from marine invertebrates and microbes as modulators of antitumor targets. *Curr. Drug Targets* **2006**, *7*, 279–304. [CrossRef]

140. Beckwith, M.; Urba, W.J.; Longo, D.L. Growth inhibition of human lymphoma cell lines by the marine products, Dolastatins 10 and 15. *J. Natl. Cancer Inst.* **1993**, *85*, 483–488. [CrossRef]

141. Keir, C.H.; Vahdat, L.T. The use of an antibody drug conjugate, glembatumumab vedotin (CDX-011), for the treatment of breast cancer. *Expert. Opin. Biol. Ther.* **2012**, *12*, 259–263. [CrossRef]

142. Yamamoto, N.; Andoh, M.; Kawahara, M.; Fukuoka, M.; Niitani, H. Phase I study of TZT-1027, a novel synthetic dolastatin 10 derivative and inhibitor of tubulin polymerization, given weekly to advanced solid tumor patients for 3 weeks. *Cancer Sci.* **2009**, *100*, 316–321. [CrossRef]

143. Shnyder, S.D.; Cooper, P.A.; Millington, N.J.; Pettit, G.R.; Bibby, M.C. Auristatin PYE, a novel synthetic derivative of dolastatin 10, is highly effective in human colon tumour models. *Int. J. Oncol.* **2007**, *31*, 353. [CrossRef]

144. Prokopiou, E.M.; Cooper, P.A.; Pettit, G.R.; Bibby, M.C.; Shnyder, S.D. Potentiation of the activity of cisplatin in a human colon tumour xenograft model by auristatin PYE, a structural modification of dolastatin 10. *Mol. Med. Rep.* **2010**, *3*, 309–313. [CrossRef] [PubMed]

145. Ray, A.; Okouneva, T.; Manna, T.; Miller, H.P.; Schmid, S.; Arthaud, L.; Luduena, R.; Jordan, M.A.; Wilson, L. Mechanism of action of the microtubule-targeted antimitotic depsipeptide tasidotin (formerly ILX651) and its major metabolite tasidotin C-carboxylate. *Cancer Res.* **2007**, *67*, 3767–3776. [CrossRef]

146. Cunningham, C.; Appleman, L.J.; Kirvan-Visovatti, M.; Ryan, D.P.; Regan, E.; Vukelja, S.; Bonate, P.L.; Ruvuna, F.; Fram, R.J.; Jekunen, A.; et al. Phase I and pharmacokinetic study of the dolastatin-15 analogue tasidotin (ILX651) administered intravenously on days 1, 3, and 5 every 3 weeks in patients with advanced solid tumors. *Clin. Cancer Res.* **2005**, *11*, 7825–7833. [CrossRef] [PubMed]

147. Ebbinghaus, S.; Rubin, E.; Hersh, E.; Cranmer, L.D.; Bonate, P.L.; Fram, R.J.; Jekunen, A.; Weitman, S.; Hammond, L.A. A phase I study of the dolastatin-15 analogue tasidotin (ILX651) administered intravenously daily for 5 consecutive days every 3 weeks in patients with advanced solid tumors. *Clin. Cancer Res.* **2005**, *11*, 7807–7816. [CrossRef] [PubMed]

148. Mita, A.C.; Hammond, L.A.; Bonate, P.L.; Weiss, G.; McCreery, H.; Syed, S.; Garrison, M.; Chu, Q.S.C.; DeBono, J.S.; Jones, C.B.; et al. Phase I and pharmacokinetic study of tasidotin hydrochloride (ILX651), a third-generation dolastatin-15 analogue, administered weekly for 3 weeks every 28 days in patients with advanced solid tumors. *Clin. Cancer Res.* **2006**, *12*, 5207–5215. [CrossRef]

149. Naumovski, L.; Junutula, J.R. Glembatumumab vedotin, a conjugate of an anti-glycoprotein non-metastatic melanoma protein B mAb and monomethyl auristatin E for the treatment of melanoma and breast cancer. *Curr. Opin. Mol. Ther.* **2010**, *12*, 248–257. [CrossRef] [PubMed]

150. Hasanov, M.; Rioth, M.J.; Kendra, K.; Hernandez-Aya, L.; Joseph, R.W.; Williamson, S.; Chandra, S.; Shirai, K.; Turner, C.D.; Lewis, K.; et al. A phase ii study of glembatumumab vedotin for metastatic uveal melanoma. *Cancers* **2020**, *12*, 2270. [CrossRef] [PubMed]
151. Horwitz, S.M.; Advani, R.H.; Bartlett, N.L.; Jacobsen, E.D.; Sharman, J.P.; O'Connor, O.A.; Siddiqi, T.; Kennedy, D.A. Objective responses in relapsed T-cell lymphomas with single-agent brentuximab vedotin. *Blood* **2014**, *123*, 3095–3100. [CrossRef]
152. Rinehart, K.L.J.; Gloer, J.B.; Cook, J.C.J. Structures of the didemnins, antiviral and cytotoxic depsipeptides from a Caribbean tunicate. *J. Am. Chem. Soc.* **1981**, *12*, 1857–1859. [CrossRef]
153. Urdiales, J.; Morata, P.; Castro, I.N.D.; Sánchez-Jiménez, F. Antiproliferative effect of dehydrodidemnin B (DDB), a depsipeptide isolated from Mediterranean tunicates. *Cancer Lett.* **1996**, *102*, 31–37. [CrossRef]
154. Singh, R.; Sharma, M.; Joshi, P.; Rawat, D.S. Clinical status of anti-cancer agents derived from marine sources. *Anticancer Agents Med. Chem.* **2008**, *8*, 603–617. [CrossRef]
155. Maroun, J.A.; Belanger, K.; Seymour, L.; Matthews, S.; Roach, J.; Dionne, J.; Soulieres, D.; Stewart, D.; Goel, R.; Charpentier, D. Phase I study of Aplidine in a daily×5 one-hour infusion every 3 weeks in patients with solid tumors refractory to standard therapy. *Ann. Oncol.* **2006**, *17*, 1371–1378. [CrossRef] [PubMed]
156. Toulmonde, M.; Le Cesne, A.; Piperno-Neumann, S.; Penel, N.; Chevreau, C.; Duffaud, F.; Bellera, C.; Italiano, A. Aplidin in patients with advanced dedifferentiated liposarcomas: A french sarcoma group single-arm phase II study. *Ann. Oncol.* **2015**, *26*, 1465–1470. [CrossRef]
157. White, K.M.; Rosales, R.; Yildiz, S.; Kehrer, T.; Miorin, L.; Moreno, E.; Jangra, S.; Uccellini, M.B.; Rathnasinghe, R.; Coughlan, L.; et al. Plitidepsin has potent preclinical efficacy against SARS-CoV-2 by targeting the host protein eEF1A. *Science* **2021**, *10*, 1126. [CrossRef]
158. Yamazaki, Y.; Sumikura, M.; Hidaka, K.; Yasui, H.; Kiso, Y.; Yakushiji, F.; Hayashi, Y. Anti-microtubule 'plinabulin' chemical probe KPU-244-B3 labeled both α- and β-tubulin. *Bioorg. Med. Chem.* **2010**, *18*, 3169–3174. [CrossRef] [PubMed]
159. Millward, M.; Mainwaring, P.; Mita, A.; Federico, P.; Lloyd, G.K.; Reddinger, N.; Nawrocki, S.; Mita, M.; Spear, M.A. Phase 1 study of the novel vascular disrupting agent plinabulin (NPI-2358) and docetaxel. *Investig. New Drugs* **2012**, *30*, 1065–1073. [CrossRef]
160. Fenical, W.; Jensen, P.R.; Cheng, X.C. Halimide, a Cytotoxic Marine Natural Product, and Derivatives Thereof. U.S. Patent No. 6,069,146, 30 May 2000.
161. Mooberry, S.L.; Busquets, L.; Tien, G. Induction of apoptosis by cryptophycin 1, a new antimicrotubule agent. *Int. J. Cancer* **1997**, *73*, 440–448. [CrossRef]
162. Ding, Y.; Rath, C.M.; Bolduc, K.L.; Hakansson, K.; Sherman, D.H. Chemoenzymatic synthesis of cryptophycin anticancer agents by an ester bond-forming non-ribosomal peptide synthetase module. *J. Am. Chem. Soc.* **2011**, *133*, 14492–14495. [CrossRef]
163. Sessa, C.; Weigang-Köhler, K.; Pagani, O.; Greim, G.; Mora, O.; De Pas, T.; Burgess, M.; Weimer, I.; Johnson, R. Phase I and pharmacological studies of the cryptophycin analogue LY355703 administered on a single intermittent or weekly schedule. *Eur. J. Cancer* **2002**, *38*, 2388–2396. [CrossRef]
164. Liu, L.; Bao, Y.; Zhang, Y.; Xiao, C.; Chen, L. Acid-responsive dextran-based therapeutic nanoplatforms for photodynamic-chemotherapy against multidrug resistance. *Int. J. Biol. Macromol.* **2020**, *155*, 233–240. [CrossRef]
165. Pei, X.; Zhu, Z.; Gan, Z.; Chen, J.; Zhang, X.; Cheng, X.; Wan, Q.; Wang, J. PEGylated nano-graphene oxide as a nanocarrier for delivering mixed anticancer drugs to improve anticancer activity. *Sci. Rep.* **2020**, *10*, 2717. [CrossRef] [PubMed]
166. Conibear, A.C.; Schmid, A.; Kamalov, M.; Becker, C.F.W.; Bello, C. Recent advances in peptide-based approaches for cancer treatment. *Curr. Med. Chem.* **2020**, *27*, 1174–1205. [CrossRef]
167. Zhao, Y.; Cai, C.; Liu, M.; Zhao, Y.; Wu, Y.; Fan, Z.; Ding, Z.; Zhang, H.; Wang, Z.; Han, J. Drug-binding albumins forming stabilized nanoparticles for co-delivery of paclitaxel and resveratrol: In vitro/in vivo evaluation and binding properties investigation. *Int. J. Biol. Macromol.* **2020**, *153*, 873–882. [CrossRef] [PubMed]
168. Zorzi, A.; Deyle, K.; Heinis, C. Cyclic peptide therapeutics: Past, present and future. *Curr. Opin. Chem. Biol.* **2017**, *38*, 24–29. [CrossRef] [PubMed]
169. Hogervorst, T.P.; Li, R.J.E.; Marino, L.; Bruijns, S.C.M.; Meeuwenoord, N.J.; Filippov, D.V.; Overkleeft, H.S.; van der Marel, G.A.; van Vliet, S.J.; van Kooyk, Y.; et al. C-Mannosyl lysine for solid phase assembly of mannosylated peptide conjugate cancer vaccines. *ACS Chem. Biol.* **2020**, *15*, 728–739. [CrossRef] [PubMed]
170. Lynn, G.M.; Sedlik, C.; Baharom, F.; Zhu, Y.; Ramirez-Valdez, R.A.; Coble, V.L.; Tobin, K.; Nichols, S.R.; Itzkowitz, Y.; Zaidi, N.; et al. Peptide-TLR-7/8a conjugate vaccines chemically programmed for nanoparticle self-assembly enhance CD8 T-cell immunity to tumor antigens. *Nat. Biotechnol.* **2020**, *38*, 320–332. [CrossRef]
171. Habault, J.; Kaci, A.; Pasquereau-Kotula, E.; Fraser, C.; Chomienne, C.; Dombret, H.; Braun, T.; Pla, M.; Poyet, J.L. Prophylactic and therapeutic antileukemic effects induced by the AAC-11-derived Peptide RT53. *Oncoimmunology* **2020**, *9*, 1728871. [CrossRef] [PubMed]

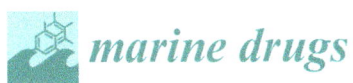

Article

Structure Elucidation and Functional Studies of a Novel β-hairpin Antimicrobial Peptide from the Marine Polychaeta *Capitella teleta*

Pavel V. Panteleev [1], Andrey V. Tsarev [1], Victoria N. Safronova [1], Olesia V. Reznikova [1], Ilia A. Bolosov [1], Sergei V. Sychev [1], Zakhar O. Shenkarev [1] and Tatiana V. Ovchinnikova [1,2,*]

1. M.M. Shemyakin & Yu.A. Ovchinnikov Institute of Bioorganic Chemistry, the Russian Academy of Sciences, Miklukho-Maklaya str., 16/10, 117997 Moscow, Russia; ibch@inbox.ru (P.V.P.); tsarev@nmr.ru (A.V.T.); victoria.saf@ibch.ru (V.N.S.); olesya-r@nmr.ru (O.V.R.); bolosov@ibch.ru (I.A.B.); svs@ibch.ru (S.V.S.); zakhar.shenkarev@nmr.ru (Z.O.S.)
2. Department of Biotechnology, I.M. Sechenov First Moscow State Medical University, Trubetskaya str., 8–2, 119991 Moscow, Russia
* Correspondence: ovch@ibch.ru; Tel.: +7-495-336-44-44

Received: 21 October 2020; Accepted: 2 December 2020; Published: 4 December 2020

Abstract: Endogenous antimicrobial peptides (AMPs) are evolutionary ancient molecular factors of innate immunity that play a key role in host defense. Among the most active and stable under physiological conditions AMPs are the peptides of animal origin that adopt a β-hairpin conformation stabilized by disulfide bridges. In this study, a novel BRICHOS-domain related AMP from the marine polychaeta *Capitella teleta*, named capitellacin, was produced as the recombinant analogue and investigated. The mature capitellacin exhibits high homology with the known β-hairpin AMP family—tachyplesins and polyphemusins from the horseshoe crabs. The β-hairpin structure of the recombinant capitellacin was proved by CD and NMR spectroscopy. In aqueous solution the peptide exists as monomeric right-handed twisted β-hairpin and its structure does not reveal significant amphipathicity. Moreover, the peptide retains this conformation in membrane environment and incorporates into lipid bilayer. Capitellacin exhibits a strong antimicrobial activity in vitro against a wide panel of bacteria including extensively drug-resistant strains. In contrast to other known β-hairpin AMPs, this peptide acts apparently via non-lytic mechanism at concentrations inhibiting bacterial growth. The molecular mechanism of the peptide antimicrobial action does not seem to be related to the inhibition of bacterial translation therefore other molecular targets may be assumed. The reduced cytotoxicity against human cells and high antibacterial cell selectivity as compared to tachyplesin-1 make it an attractive candidate compound for an anti-infective drug design.

Keywords: antimicrobial peptide; polychaeta; innate immunity; BRICHOS domain; recombinant peptide; β-hairpin structure; nuclear magnetic resonance (NMR)

1. Introduction

The spike in antimicrobial resistance along with challenges of conventional antibiotics discovery point out the urgent need for development of new approaches to control infections. Among them, implementation of AMPs which are important components of the innate host defense in many organisms including humans [1]. Invertebrates lack acquired immunity and rely on their innate immunity on pathogens invasion, and AMPs play a key role in such a rapid immune response. In contrast to other marine invertebrate animals, polychaeta is a relatively underexplored class in terms of discovery of new host-defense peptides. AMPs have been identified in several species of polychaetes: 21-residue β-hairpin arenicins from *Arenicola marina* [2], 22-residue β-hairpin alvinellacin from *Alvinella pompejana* [3], 33-residue nicomicins from *Nicomache minor*, combining an amphipathic *N*-terminal α-helix and *C*-terminal extended part with a six-residue loop stabilized by a disulfide bridge [4], 51-residue perinerin from *Perinereis aibuhitensis*, 22-residue α-helical hedistin containing bromo-tryptophans from *Nereis diversicolor* [5], and theromacin from *Perinereis linea*—a first representative of the cysteine-rich macin family among polychaeta species [6].

Here we described a novel β-hairpin antimicrobial peptide, named capitellacin, that was earlier predicted based on the genome data of the polychaeta *Capitella teleta* [3]. *C. teleta* is a small segmented worm found in the sediment of organically enriched areas such as sewage treatment plants, and is well known as a bioindicator of disturbed habitats [7]. This worm is also used as a model organism in tissue regeneration studies [8]. Capitellacin exhibits the highest homology with tachyplesins and polyphemusins—known β-hairpin AMP families, both originating from the horseshoe crabs [9]. At the same time, like arenicins, alvinellacin, and nicomicins, capitellacin is synthesized as the C-terminal part of corresponding precursor protein containing the BRICHOS domain [4]. Therefore, all the above-mentioned peptides could be designated as BRICHOS domain-related antimicrobial peptides. The precursor proteins that contain the BRICHOS domain are characterized by low sequence identities but highly conserved overall domain architecture [10]. BRICHOS domain presumably functions as intramolecular chaperone guiding the aggregation-prone region, in particular a hydrophobic AMP part, into the correct conformation during biosynthesis.

In this study, the most probable variant of the natural mature capitellacin processed by furin protease was expressed as the recombinant peptide in *Escherichia coli*. The peptide structure in aqueous solution and membrane environment was investigated by NMR, CD, FTIR, and fluorescent spectroscopy. A comparative analysis of biological activity of capitellacin and tachyplesin-1 was performed. In particular, antibacterial activity against a wide panel of ESKAPE pathogens as well as cytotoxic properties of capitellacin were analyzed. We also compared the ability of the peptides to compromise the integrity of bacterial membranes using both living cells and proteoliposome model. The effect of capitellacin on bacterial translation was accessed using the cell-free enhanced green fluorescent protein (EGFP) expression system.

2. Results and Discussion

2.1. Recombinant Production of the Capitellacin

Earlier the nucleotide sequence encoding capitellacin was identified by blasting the preproalvinellacin in the *C. teleta* whole genome shotgun (WGS) database [3]. Expression of the preprocapitellacin gene was verified by analysis of *C. teleta* transcripts (NCBI sequence read archives SRX2653646-SRX2653653) deposited in GenBank with the use of nucleotide BLAST instruments. The nucleotide sequence of procapitellacin corresponded to data obtained by genome sequencing (GenBank: AMQN01012506.1, Figure 1A). The sequence analysis with the use of SignalP 5.0 pointed to the Thr22-Thr23 bond as the most probable cleavage site for eukaryotic signal peptidase. In its turn, procapitellacin could be processed by furin protease that frequently cleaves the peptide bond after the dibasic Lys-Arg site. Thus, the 20-residue C-terminal fragment of procapitellacin was chosen for further investigations as the most probable variant of the natural mature peptide. Bioinformatic analysis revealed that the mature capitellacin does not bear similarity higher than ~52% with any known AMPs listed in different AMP databases. The peptide exhibits the highest homology with tachyplesin-1 from the horseshoe crab *Tachypleus tridentatus* (Figure 1B).

Like other known polychaeta β-hairpin AMPs, in particular arenicin-3 and alvinellacin, the peptide is stabilized by two disulfide bonds [11]. In this study, we used bacterial heterologous expression of target peptides fused with modified thioredoxin A–a highly soluble carrier protein that was successfully used for recombinant production of other β-hairpin AMPs [12]. The fusion proteins were expressed in *E. coli* BL21 (DE3) cells, and the obtained total cell lysates were fractionated by affinity chromatography. After purification and cleavage of the fusion proteins, reverse-phase high performance liquid chromatography (RP-HPLC) was used to obtain target AMPs. MALDI mass spectrometry analysis of the main fractions showed that the measured monoisotopic m/z matched well with the calculated molecular masses of protonated ions [M + H]⁺ of corresponding peptides indicating formation of two disulfide bonds and the absence of any other modifications (Table 1, Figure S1). The final yield of the capitellacin was of 6.1 mg per 1 L of the culture that is comparable to that of tachyplesin-1.

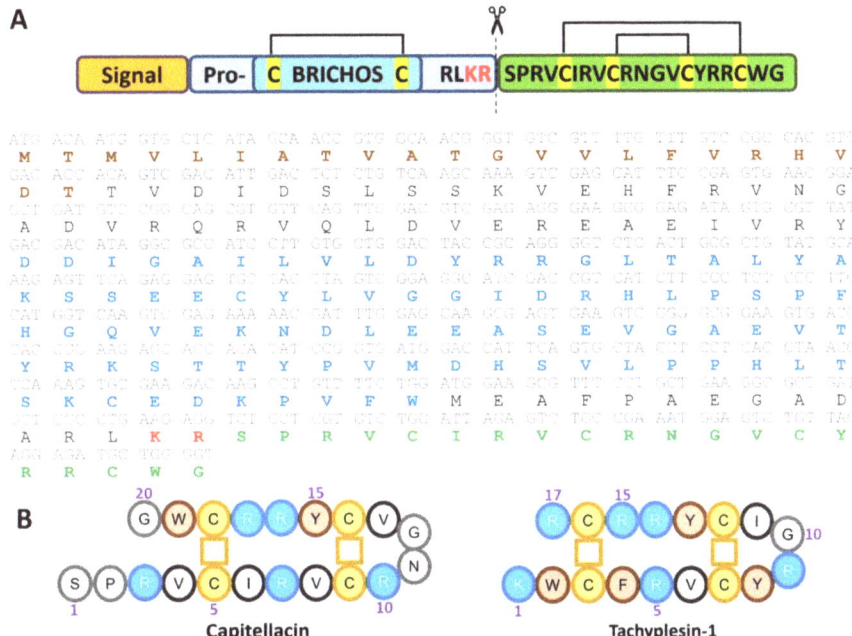

Figure 1. (**A**) Capitellacin precursor protein organization and amino acid sequence. The signal peptide sequence identified with SignalP-5.0 (http://www.cbs.dtu.dk/services/SignalP/) and the BRICHOS domain sequence identified with MyHits Motif Scan (https://myhits.isb-sib.ch/cgi-bin/motif_scan) are highlighted with brown and blue, respectively. The putative natural processing site is indicated with scissors. (**B**) Primary structure of capitellacin in comparison with that of tachyplesin-1.

Table 1. Characteristics of the recombinant AMPs.

Peptide	Recombinant Peptide Final Yield, mg/L	RP-HPLC Retention Time, min	Hydrophobicity Index [1]/Hydrophobic Residues, % [2]	Calculated [M + H]⁺ Monoisotopic Molecular Mass, Da [3]	Measured Monoisotopic m/z Value [4]
Capitellacin	6.1	38.5	−0.215/45	2379.16	2379.30
Tachyplesin-1	7.2	37.5	−0.482/47	2264.10	2263.73

[1] Mean Kyte-Doolittle hydrophobicity index (GRAVY) calculated using the Expasy ProtParam tool. The maximum and minimum values of this index are +4.5 and −4.5 for poly-Ile and poly-Arg sequences, respectively. [2] Percentage of hydrophobic amino acids was calculated using the APD database. [3] Molecular masses were calculated by considering the presence of four Cys residues forming two disulfide bonds and [4] were determined experimentally using MALDI-TOF mass spectrometry.

2.2. Spatial Structure of the Capitellacin in Aqueous Solution

Analysis of the NMR spectra of capitellacin in water revealed the presence of two structural forms of the peptide (Figure 2A). The relative population of the two forms was about 1:5. Complete ¹H and partial ¹³C resonance assignments of both peptide forms were obtained at pH 5.2 and 30 °C.

A summary of the obtained NMR data is shown in Figure 2B. The $^{13}C^\beta$ resonances of Cys5, Cys9, Cys14, and Cys18 residues of the major form and $^{13}C^\beta$ resonances of Cys5 and Cys18 residues of the minor form were observed in the chemical shifts range from 47 to 49 ppm, which are characteristic for the oxidized Cys residues forming disulfide bonds. The chemical shifts of Cys9 and Cys14 residues in both forms were identical.

Large positive values of the secondary chemical shifts of $^1H^\alpha$ nuclei, characteristic pattern of medium- and long-range nuclear Overhauser effect (NOE) contacts, and the values of the $^3J_{H^N H^\alpha}$ coupling constants exceeding 8 Hz (Figure 2B) suggested the formation of an antiparallel β-structure in the major peptide form. The antiparallel arrangement is in agreement only with the laddered (Cys5-Cys18 and Cys9-Cys14) disulfide bond pattern. Thus, the major form of capitellacin in solution has the β-hairpin conformation with Arg10-Val13 residues on its tip. The observed values of temperature coefficients of amide protons ($\Delta\delta^1H^N/\Delta T$) revealed that HN groups of Ile6, Val8, Arg10, Tyr15, Arg17, and Trp19 residues could participate in the hydrogen bond formation. This pattern also agrees well with the β-hairpin conformation.

Comparison of the $^1H^N$ and $^1H^\alpha$ chemical shifts between both forms of capitellacin in solution showed that the structural differences between the forms are greater at the N- and C-termini of the peptide and decrease towards the tip of the β-hairpin (Figure 2D). Analysis of the chemical shifts of $^{13}C^\beta$ and $^{13}C^\gamma$ nuclei of the Pro2 residue (Figure 2C) revealed that Ser1-Pro2 peptide bond in the major form has a *trans*- configuration ($\delta^{13}C^\beta - \delta^{13}C^\gamma = 4.7$ ppm), while this bond in the minor form has *cis*- configuration ($\delta^{13}C^\beta - \delta^{13}C^\gamma = 10.1$ ppm). Thus, observed conformational heterogeneity of capitellacin in solution is the consequence of *cis-trans* isomerization of Ser1-Pro2 peptide bond. The characteristic time of corresponding exchange process exceeds 200 ms.

The set of 20 capitellacin structures was calculated in the CYANA from 200 random starts using upper NOE-based distance restraints, torsion angle restraints, hydrogen and disulfide bond restraints (Figure 3A and Table S1). The peptide represents β-hairpin, formed by two β-strands (Val4-Cys9 and Cys14-Trp19). The tip of the β-hairpin (Arg10-Val13) is folded in type IV β-turn (Figure 2B). The disulfide bridges (Cys5-Cys18 and Cys9-Cys14) join residues opposite one another on the antiparallel β-strands and have a "short right-handed hook" or g+npng+ conformation (see the Material and Methods for the definition). The capitellacin structure is additionally stabilized by six backbone-backbone hydrogen bonds. The structure is well defined in the region enclosed by Cys5-Cys18 disulfide, while N- and C-terminal fragments show some disorder (Figure 3A).

The two-stranded β-sheet in the capitellacin structure has a pronounced right-handed twist (Figure 3A,B). The primary structure of the peptide basically contains two types of amino acid residues: hydrophobic/aromatic and positively charged. In spite of this, analysis of the surface properties (Figure 3C,D) did not reveal significant amphipathicity of the capitellacin molecule in aqueous solution. The charged moieties have an almost uniform distribution on the peptide surface (Figure 3C), leaving only one hydrophobic cluster formed by the side-chains of Pro2, Val4, Ile6, Val8, and Trp18 (Figure 3D).

Several AMPs from annelids having β-hairpin structure were previously studied by NMR spectroscopy in aqueous solution. The structures of arenicin-2 from *A. marina* and alvinellacin from *A. pompejana* are shown in the Figure 3E,F. Similar to capitellacin, both peptides contain disulfide-stabilized two-stranded antiparallel β-sheet. Interestingly, all the three peptides demonstrate right-handed twist of the β-structure. The arenicin-2 molecule has the largest twist of 213 ± 8° (per 8 residues, ~27°/res) [14], while the twist angles in the alvinellacin and capitellacin structures are smaller 98 ± 34° (per 6 residues, ~17°/res) and 127 ± 10° (per 7 residues, ~18°/res), respectively. This can be connected with larger degree of β-structure stabilization provided by two disulfides present in the alvinellacin and capitellacin molecules, as compared with only one disulfide in the arenicin-2 molecule (Figure 3B,E,F). In line with this, other β-hairpin AMPs with two disulfide bridges, protegrin-1 and tachyplesin-1 (Figure 3G,H), also demonstrate relatively small right-handed twist ~14° and ~7° per residue, respectively.

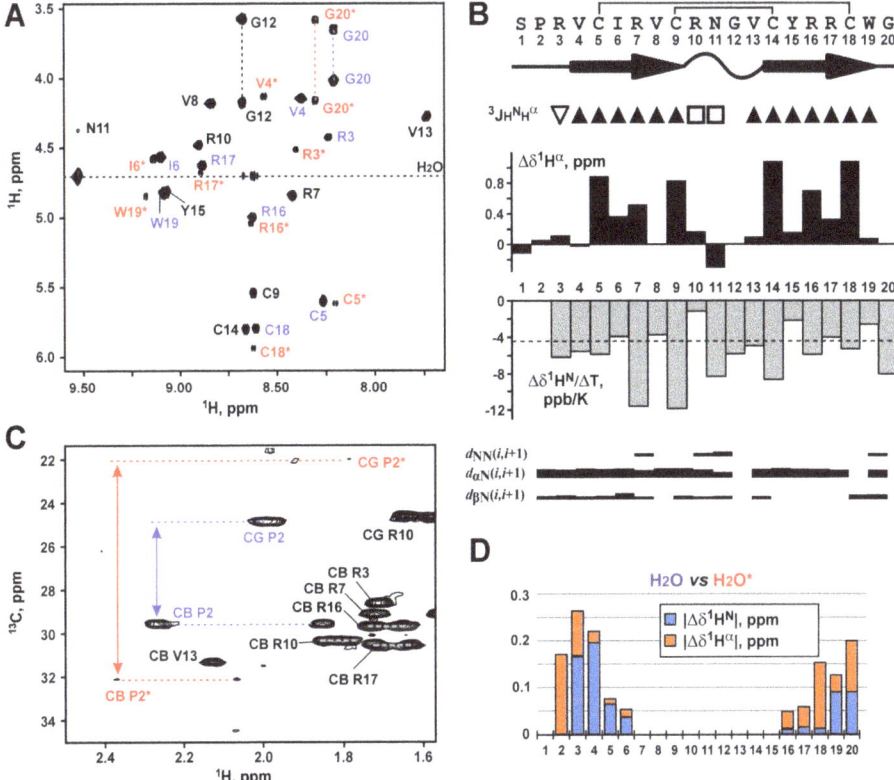

Figure 2. NMR data define the secondary structure and conformational heterogeneity of capitellacin in solution. (**A**). The fragment of the 2D ^{1}H-TOCSY spectrum of 1.5 mM capitellacin (5% D$_2$O, pH 5.2, 30 °C). The resonance assignment of H^N-H$^\alpha$ cross-peaks is shown. The signals of the major and minor forms of the peptide are marked in blue and red, respectively. The signals of the minor form are additionally marked with asterisks. The signals common to both forms are marked in black. (**B**). Overview of obtained NMR data. (From top to bottom) Secondary structure of capitellacin. The β-sheets are denoted by arrows and tight β-turn by wavy line. ($^3J_H{}^N{}_H{}^\alpha$) Large (>8 Hz), small (<6 Hz), and medium (others) coupling constants are indicated by the filled triangles, open triangles, and open squares, respectively. (Δδ^{1}H$^\alpha$) Secondary chemical shifts of ^{1}H$^\alpha$ nuclei. The positive values revealed formation of β-structure. (Δδ^{1}H^N/ΔT) Temperature gradients of amide protons. The values with amplitude <4.5 ppb/K (dashed line) indicated possible participation of HN group in the hydrogen bond formation. The NOE connectivities are shown as usual. The width of the lines corresponds to the relative intensity of the cross-peak in the 150 ms NOESY spectrum. (**C**). The fragment of the 2D ^{13}C-HSQC spectrum of capitellacin at natural isotope abundance. The resonance assignment of the signals of H$_2$C$^\beta$ and H$_2$C$^\gamma$ groups of Pro2 residue for the major and minor form of the peptide are marked in blue and red, respectively. The difference of chemical shifts between ^{13}C$^\beta$ and ^{13}C$^\gamma$ nuclei in both forms are shown. (**D**). Difference (absolute value) of ^{1}H^N (blue) and ^{1}H$^\alpha$ (orange) chemical shifts between the two forms of capitellacin in solution.

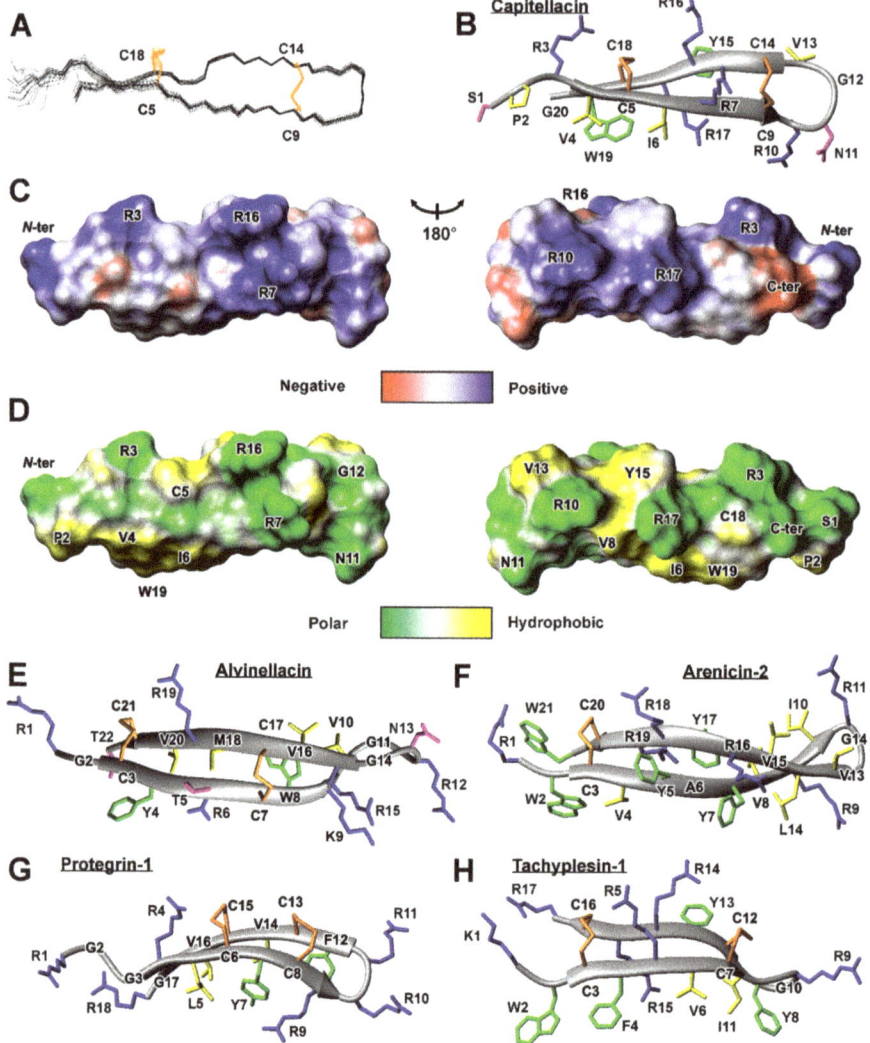

Figure 3. Spatial structure of capitellacin in comparison with other animal β-hairpin antimicrobial peptides. (**A**). The set of the best 20 capitellacin structures superimposed over the backbone atoms. Disulfide bonds are shown in orange. (**B**). The representative conformer of capitellacin in ribbon representation. The disulfide bonds, positively charged, hydrophobic, aromatic, and polar residues are colored in orange, blue, yellow, green, and magenta, respectively. (**C,D**) Two-sided view of molecular surface of capitellacin. Electrostatic (**C**) and molecular hydrophobicity (**D**) potentials are shown [13]. Red, blue, green, and yellow areas denote negative, positive, polar, and hydrophobic regions, respectively. Spatial structure of β-hairpin antimicrobial peptides alvinellacin (**E**), arenicin-2 (**F**), protegrin-1 (**G**), and tachyplesin-1 (**H**). PDB codes 7ALD, 2LLR, 2JNI, 1PG1, and 2RTV for capitellacin, alvinellacin, arenicin-2, protegrin-1, and tachyplesin-1, respectively.

Presently, it is generally accepted that a cellular membrane is the main target of the β-hairpin AMPs [11]. Previous NMR studies of arenicin-2 [15] and porcine protegrin-1 [16] revealed that β-hairpin AMPs can form dimers in the membrane environment which combines into the larger ion-conducting oligomeric pores. Significant untwisting of the arenicin-2 β-sheet was observed upon the dimer formation in the membrane mimicking media of detergent micelles; this results in the almost flat β-structural dimers [15]. Despite differences in the dimer structures (CN↑↑NC type of association for arenicin-2 and NC↑↑CN type of association for protegrin-1) in both cases β-strands predominantly composed of hydrophobic residues (and not containing charged or polar ones) are involved in the dimerization interface. Notably, the capitellacin sequence lacks such structural elements. The longest hydrophobic fragments (Val4-Ile6 and Val13-Tyr15) are composed of three residues which is insufficient for dimerization. Thus, it can be assumed that capitellacin dimerization is unlikely upon interaction with cell membranes. Indeed, for a number of β-hairpin peptides, it has been shown that the ability to form dimers is not a necessary condition for both membranolytic action and high antibacterial activity. Recently, we obtained the arenicin-1 analogue Val8Arg which had significantly lower dimerization propensity and cytotoxicity against mammalian cells [17]. At the same time, this analogue exhibited similar antibacterial activities and kinetics of bacterial membrane permeabilization as compared with wild-type arenicin.

2.3. Capitellacin Interaction with Model Membranes

To characterize capitellacin interaction with lipid bilayers we used several technics: circular dichroism (CD), FTIR, and Trp fluorescence spectroscopy. In this study, PE/PG (2:1) lipids mimicking plasma membrane of *E. coli* were utilized. As presented in Figure 4A, the CD spectra of capitellacin dissolved in water showed a negative peak at 207 nm and a positive one at 230 nm. It is known that the backbone structure has a basic influence on the n→π* and π→π* rotational strengths. The negative CD band at ~210 nm is typical for β-turns [18]. The addition of PE/PG lipids resulted in a significant increase in the intensity that indicates the formation of more rigid structure in lipid bilayer (Figure 4A). The same spectrum overall shape with negative band at 205 nm and positive band at 230 nm was earlier shown for another structurally related β-hairpin AMP gomesin from the spider *Acanthoscurria gomesiana* [19]. Notably, the increase in the intensity was also observed in the presence of POPG or POPC lipids [19]. Gomesin is known as non-dimerizing 18-residue peptide with highly rigid structure stabilized with two disulfide bridges and the flexible Arg-Gly-Arg C-termini [20].

While the CD spectra of capitellacin point only to formation of β-structure, the FTIR spectra provide more precise information. The spectra measured in amide I (C = O stretch) region (Figure 4B) have three peaks: band at 1630–1636 cm^{-1} and ~1650 cm^{-1} corresponds to the absorbance of the backbone CO groups in the β-structure, and another one at 1670–1678 cm^{-1} is attributed to free amide carbonyls which are not involved in intramolecular H-bonds [21,22]. Similarity of the FTIR spectra of the peptide in water and in PE/PG membrane indicates stability of its structure when passing into the lipid bilayer. This is in a sharp contrast to arenicins, dimerization of which in membrane-mimicking environments was shown to lead to significant changes in the appearance of FTIR spectra [21,22].

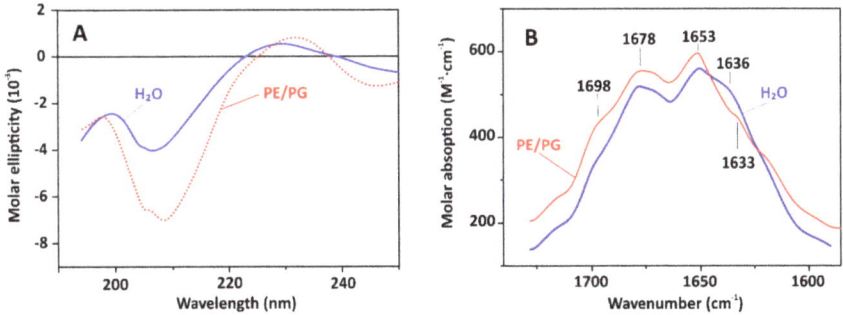

Figure 4. CD spectra (**A**) and FTIR spectra in amide I region (**B**) of capitellacin in water and in soybean PE/PG (2:1) liposomes.

Localization of capitellacin in PE/PG (2:1) lipid bilayer was studied by Trp fluorescence (Table 2). The peptide contains only one Trp19 residue located in the C-terminal part of the molecule. It is well known that change of polarity of the indole ring microenvironment led to blue shift from λ_{max} ~350 nm in an aqueous solution to λ_{max} ~330 nm in a hydrophobic environment. Intermediate position of the emission peak at 335–340 nm corresponds to an interface localization of Trp side chain or intermediate polarity of the solvent. In line with it, the λ_{max} values of 350 and 335 nm were observed for capitellacin in water and methanol (Table 2). The value of 332 nm observed in PE/PG bilayer indicates that the Trp residue of capitellacin is located in the hydrophobic acyl chain region of the membrane. Stern-Volmer constants (K_{sv}) of the Trp fluorescence quenching by iodide ions which do not penetrate into the hydrophobic region of bilayer are shown in Table 2. The K_{sv} value obtained for capitellacin in water (9.9 M^{-1}) was slightly higher than K_{sv} for isolated Trp in water (9.1 M^{-1}). Probably the quenching is enhanced by positive charges of the neighboring arginine residues. More than 3-times decrease of K_{sv} upon the peptide transfer from water to the lipid membrane confirms incorporation of capitellacin into PE/PG bilayer.

Table 2. Capitellacin Trp fluorescence parameters in different environments.

Environment	Dielectric Constant	λmax (nm)	K_{sv} (M^{-1})
H_2O	80.4	350	9.9
CH_3OH	33.6	335	-
PE/PG	~2 *	332	3.1

* The dielectric constant $\varepsilon = 2$ characteristic for hydrocarbons is usually used for the hydrophobic part of the membrane.

2.4. Conformation of Capitellacin in Membrane-Mimicking Detergent Micelles

To confirm the absence of capitellacin dimerization in the membrane-mimicking environment we studied its structure by NMR spectroscopy in solution of dodecyl-phosphocholine (DPC) micelles. This environment was previously used for structural NMR studies of the arenicin-1 and arenicin-2 dimers [15–17]. Two sets of the capitellacin signals was observed upon addition of DPC to the capitellacin sample to the detergent-to-peptide molar ratio (D:P) of 10:1 (Figure 5A, two upper traces, $H^{\varepsilon 1}$ signal of Trp19). These sets corresponded to the peptide molecules being free in solution and bound to the micelles. Further increase in the DPC concentration to D:P of 30:1 led to disappearance of the free peptide signal, thus indicating complete micelle binding. At the same time, at D:P of 70:1 the second micelle-bound form of capitellacin became apparent in the spectra (Figure 5A). Further addition of DPC resulted in the narrowing of the signals of the second capitellacin form. To minimize an influence of this broadening, we used the D:P ratio of 130:1 for the structural study.

Analysis of integral intensities in the 1D ^1H NMR spectrum and intensities of exchange cross-peaks observed in the 2D ^1H-NOESY spectrum (Figure 5B) revealed that the relative population of two capitellacin forms was of 3:1 and the rate of exchange between them was of ~130 ms. The presence of exchange cross-peaks and relative broadening of the signals of the second peptide form significantly complicated the resonance assignment procedure. Nevertheless, the complete backbone resonance assignment and partial side-chain assignments were obtained for the both structural forms (Figure 5C). The examples of arenicin-1 and -2 showed that formation of the asymmetric peptide dimers should result in the doubling of backbone resonances. The presence of single resonance sets for both micelle-bound forms of capitellacin indicated that they corresponded either to the monomeric state of the peptide or to symmetric dimers. A thorough analysis of NOESY spectra did not reveal any NOE cross-peaks, which could support the presence of symmetric peptide dimers. At the same time, the observed NOE connectivity patterns revealed that both forms of capitellacin in micelles have a β-hairpin conformation similar to that observed in water. Thus, present data do not give any evidence of capitellacin dimerization in the membrane-mimicking environment.

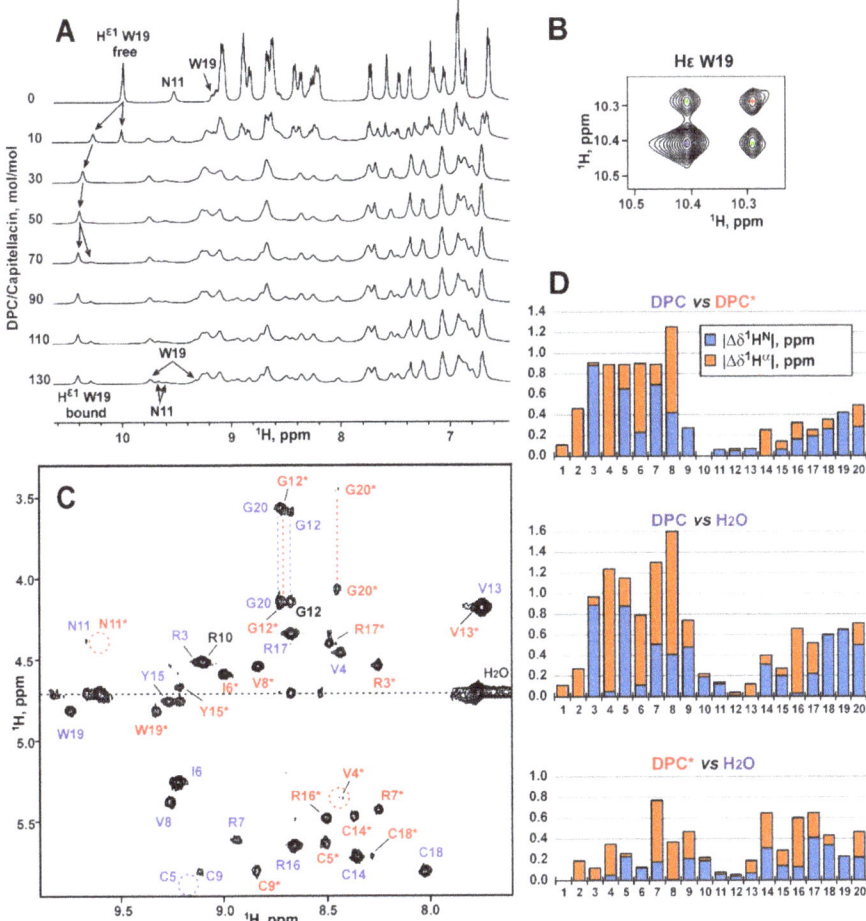

Figure 5. NMR data define the conformational heterogeneity of the micelle-bound capitellacin. (**A**). Titration of 0.5 mM capitellacin with DPC (5% D_2O, pH 5.2, 30 °C). The HN-aromatic region of 1D ^1H NMR spectrum at different DPC/capitellacin molar ratio is shown. (**B**). The fragment of 150 ms 2D ^1H-NOESY spectrum showing exchange $H^{\varepsilon 1}$-$H^{\varepsilon 1}$ cross-peaks between the signals of Trp19 belonging to two structural forms of capitellacin in DPC micelles. The diagonal cross-peaks are marked by blue and red crosses. The exchange cross-peaks are marked by green crosses. (**C**). The fragment of the 2D ^1H-TOCSY spectrum of capitellacin in DPC micelles (D:P = 130:1). The resonance assignment of H^N-H^α cross-peaks is shown. The signals of the major and minor forms of the peptide are marked in blue and red, respectively. The signals of the minor form are additionally marked with asterisks. The signal common to both forms (Arg10) is marked in black. (**D**). Difference (absolute value) of $^1H^N$ (blue) and $^1H^\alpha$ (orange) chemical shifts between the two forms of capitellacin in DPC micelles and major form of the peptide in water.

The comparison of $^1H^N$ and $^1H^\alpha$ chemical shifts (Figure 5D) revealed that two micelle-bound forms differed from each other by conformation of the N-terminal β-strand (Pro2-Val8). Thus, we suggest that these forms differ by the conformation of Ser1-Pro2 peptide bond or represent the peptide monomers with different degree of incorporation into the hydrophobic region of micelle (and this incorporation goes via the N-terminal β-strand). Interestingly, the chemical shifts of the second (minor) capitellacin form are much closer to the chemical shifts of the major peptide form in water (Figure 5D). Therefore, the minor form of the peptide in micelles either contains a *trans*-Ser1-Pro2 bond or corresponds to the peptide loosely associated with the micelle. At present, we cannot discriminate between these two possibilities. The low quality of NMR spectra in the micellar environment did not allow to analyze ^{13}C chemical shifts for the Pro2 residue and study a topology of the peptide-micelle interaction. Development of special protocols for production of stable isotope (^{13}C, ^{15}N) labeled capitellacin variants are needed for the detailed structural study.

2.5. Proton Transfer Activity of Capitellacin

Most amphipathic β-hairpin AMPs are known to penetrate bacterial membranes and at high concentrations induce pore-formation and/or cell lysis. To characterize the possible mechanism of capitellacin action, lipid-dependent pore formation was monitored by measurements of the proton transfer activity (PTA). Protonophore activity was analyzed using proteoliposomes containing a proton pump–bacteriorhodopsin from *Exiguobacterium sibiricum* (ESR). After incorporation into liposomes, ESR exhibits light-induced proton translocation, which causes a moderate decrease in the pH of the bulk solution corresponding to the proton pumping from the inside to the outside of liposomes [23]. The added peptide can dissipate the proton gradient across the liposomal membranes, increasing the pH value of the bulk solution to a certain level. Figure 6A shows the dependence of bulk pH values on the concentration of added capitellacin for two membrane systems. The absence of PTA in DMPC/DMPG (2:1) membranes and sigmoidal concentration dependence of ΔpH value in soybean PE/PG (2:1) liposomes were observed. This observation was rather unexpected, since both lipid systems contain the same proportion (~30%) of the anionic phosphatidylglycerol (PG) lipids. Thus, the observed difference in the PTA is primarily related to the difference in fluidity and cumulative curvature strain of the membranes. It is known that phosphatidylethanolamine (PE) lipids possess significant negative spontaneous curvature, while soybean lipids contain ≥ 50% unsaturated lipids (18:2 and 18:3) [24], which provide larger membrane fluidity. Both of these factors can enhance the peptide binding to the PE/PG bilayer surface as compared to the more rigid DMPC/DMPG membrane, which consists of the saturated lipids with almost zero spontaneous curvature.

Sigmoidal concentration dependence of PTA (Figure 6A) revealed cooperativity in the pore formation by capitellacin. The inflection point of the graph indicates the pore-forming concentration of ~6 μM. Activity of capitellacin in membranes of various lipid composition and at different salt concentrations is shown in Figure 6B. Interestingly, the proton transfer was observed only in the PE/PG lipid system and only at low ionic strength (10 mM NaCl). This indicates that electrostatic interactions of the positively charged peptide (overall charge +5) with the negatively charged component (PG) of the membrane are essential for the pore formation. In contrast, our experiments carried out under identical conditions revealed the pore formation by 5 μM tachyplesin-1 in soybean PE/PG liposomes at much larger (close to physiological) NaCl concentration (154 mM). Thus, two conditions are necessary for PTA manifestation by capitellacin: (1) the presence of negatively charged lipid (PG) and low salt concentration; (2) the presence of PE—the lipid with a negative spontaneous curvature. Although the interactions of AMPs with PE-containing bilayers was discussed in detail earlier [25,26], the dependence of the β-hairpin peptide activity on phosphatidylethanolamine lipids was discovered for the first time.

Bactericidal effect of the majority of AMPs is often considered to be due to their action on the lipid matrix with disruption of the bacterial cell membranes. Investigation of multiple AMPs by single bacteria cell imaging has allowed to detect local and stable pores at regions of high membrane curvature without uniform membrane coverage [27]. The PE/PG lipid system used in our study is considered as a good mimetic for the plasma membrane of Gram-negative bacteria. Thus, the pore formation observed in our study can be relevant also for perturbation of bacterial membranes. On the other hand, there are a variety of data indicating that β-structural AMPs can act via non–membranolytic mechanism. Indeed, in all our experiments liposomes were absolutely stable for many days after capitellacin collapsed the membrane potential. Previous studies of interaction of the β-hairpin AMP tachyplesin-1 and its analogs with lipids by solid-state NMR showed that membrane disruption is not correlated with antimicrobial activity of these peptides [28].

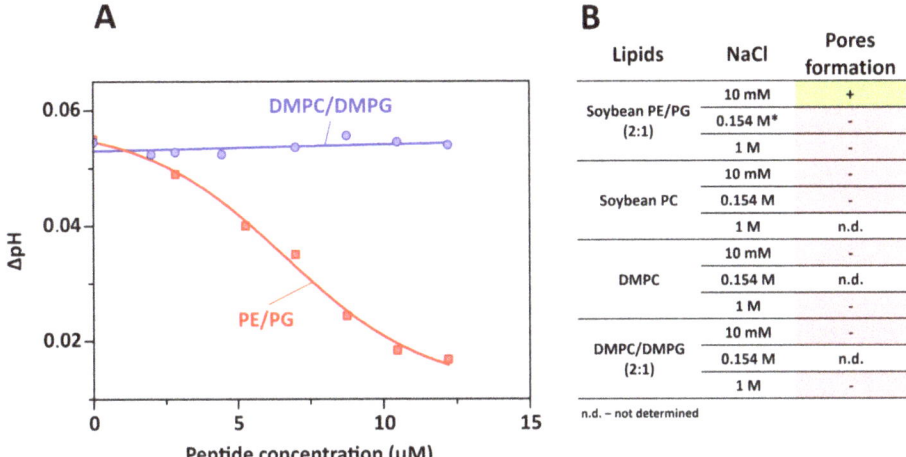

Figure 6. Proton transport measurements. (**A**) Dependence of the light-induced acidification of the bulk solution on the capitellacin concentration in the system with ESR proteoliposomes composed of DMPC/DMPG (2:1) or soybean PE/PG (2:1) lipids at 10 mM NaCl. (**B**) Comparative analysis of capitellacin pore-forming activity in different environment. * 5 µM tachyplesin-1 demonstrated proton transfer activity in this lipid system at 0.154 M NaCl.

Bacteria maintain cytoplasmic pH which is compatible with optimal function and structural integrity of the cytoplasmic proteins supporting growth. Most non-extremophilic bacteria grow over the broad range of external pH values from 5.5 to 9.0 and maintain cytoplasmic pH within the narrow range of 7.4 ÷ 7.8. Hence, they are able to acidify or alkalinize the cytoplasm relative to the external medium. Acid and alkaline pH homeostasis have been extensively studied and reviewed [29]. Therefore, capitellacin can break the H+ circulation required for pH homeostasis and work of the Na^+/H^+ antiport system. At the same time, the strong dependence of proton transfer activity on ionic strength implies that the pore formation and dissipation of the pH gradient are not the main mechanism of the capitellacin antimicrobial action.

2.6. Biological Activity and Mechanism of Antibacterial Action

Antimicrobial activity of capitellacin, tachyplesin-1, and the reference antibiotic polymyxin B was assessed by broth microdilution assay determining minimum inhibitory concentrations (MICs) against a panel of clinically isolated and reference ATCC strains of Gram-negative and Gram-positive bacteria (Table 3). To minimize interactions of amphiphilic AMPs with polystyrene plate, serial dilutions of the peptides were performed in the presence of bovine serum albumin (BSA). To estimate therapeutic potential of tested peptides we used Mueller-Hinton medium with 0.9% NaCl, which might constrain an absorption of the peptides to the bacterial surface.

Capitellacin exhibited high potency against most tested bacteria including XDR and metallo-β-lactamase producing strains which belong to ESKAPE pathogens; however, it was at least 2- to 8-fold lower than that of tachyplesin-1 (Table 3). This is not surprising, because tachyplesin-1 is known as one of the most active known AMPs, and its activity against Gram-negative bacteria is comparable to that for the last line antibiotic polymyxin B. Notably, all the peptides and polymyxin B were inactive against MDR *S. marcescens* at the tested concentrations—up to 32 µM. It is known, that *Serratia* spp. possess a natural (intrinsic) resistance to cationic AMPs because of the specific lipid composition of their membrane, which lacks an appropriate density of anionic binding sites [30]. The minimal difference in antimicrobial activity of the peptides against the panel of *E. coli* strains was shown with the median MIC values of 0.25 µM for capitellacin and 0.125 µM for tachyplesin-1. Next, the comparative analysis of kinetics of changes in *E. coli* cytoplasmic membrane permeability in the presence of the peptides was performed (Figure 7A).

Table 3. Antibacterial activity of capitellacin and known antimicrobial peptides.

Bacteria	Minimum Inhibitory Concentration (µM)		
	Capitellacin	Tachyplesin-1	Polymyxin B
Gram-positive			
S. aureus ATCC 6538P	8	1	n.d.
M. luteus B-1314	4	2	n.d.
B. subtilis B-886	16	2	n.d.
Gram-negative			
E. coli ATTC 25922	0.5	0.25	0.06
E. coli ML-35p	0.25	0.125	0.06
E. coli CI 214	0.125	0.06	0.03
E. coli (MDR CI 1057)	0.25	0.125	0.06
E. coli (MDR CI 3600)	0.5	0.06	0.06
E. cloacae (XDR CI 4172)	4	0.25	0.5
A. baumanii (XDR CI 2675)	0.25	0.016	0.5
A. baumanii (XDR CI 450)	0.5	0.06	0.03
K. pneumonia ATCC 700603	4	1	0.125
K. pneumonia (MDR CI 358)	2	1	0.06
K. pneumonia (XDR CI 1056)	4	0.5	0.5
K. pneumonia (XDR CI 3395)	2	0.5	0.125
P. aeruginosa ATCC 27853	2	0.25	0.125
P. aeruginosa PAO1	2	0.25	0.25
P. aeruginosa (MDR CI 223 *)	8	1	0.5
P. aeruginosa (XDR CI 236 *)	4	0.5	0.5
P. aeruginosa (XDR CI 1049 *)	4	1	0.25
P. aeruginosa (XDR CI 1995 *)	8	1	0.125
S. marcescens (MDR CI 1689)	>32	>32	>32

n.d., not determined. CI, clinical isolate. MDR, multidrug resistant strain. XDR, extensively drug resistant strain. * metallo-beta-lactamase (MβL) producing strain.

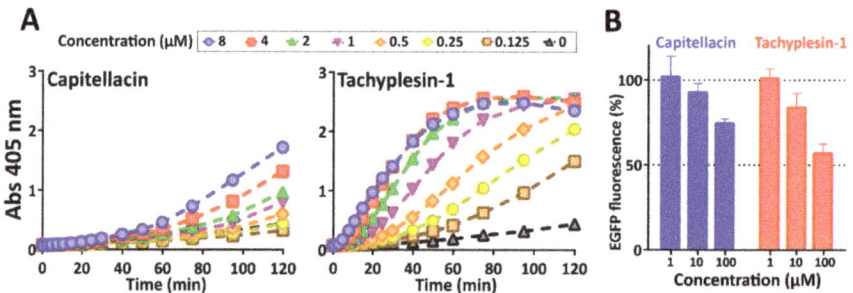

Figure 7. Comparative analysis of capitellacin and tachyplesin-1 antibacterial mechanism of action. (**A**) Kinetics of changes in *E. coli* ML-35p cytoplasmic membrane permeability at various peptide concentrations (from 0.125 to 8 µM, highlighted with colors) measured with the use of chromogenic marker—the product of ONPG (Abs 405 nm) hydrolysis. (**B**) Effects of the peptides on the fluorescence resulting from the in vitro translation of EGFP using *E. coli* BL21 (DE3) Star cell extract. The data are presented as the mean ± SD of three independent experiments.

Data on possible modes of tachyplesins action are quite controversial. The first proposed mechanism of tachyplesin-1 action on bacterial membrane suggested formation of anion-selective pores according to the "barrel-stave" model [31]. On the other hand, tachyplesin-1 does not aggregate and is too short for bilayer spanning and inducing transmembrane pores. Thus, tachyplesin-1-like AMPs were proposed to adopt the "in-plane diffusion" mechanism. In accordance with this model, AMPs are localized in parallel manner at the membrane surface and then exhibit significant segmental and global motions, causing membrane thinning and transient pores formation [32,33]. Our data confirm the pronounced membranolytic effect of tachyplesin-1 against *E. coli* at MIC and higher concentrations. Despite the longer hairpin length, capitellacin did not damage membrane at MIC. Moreover, even at the concentration of 32 × MIC (8 μM) a partial effect of cell membrane permeabilization was achieved after 2 h exposure. Similar effects were shown for some proline-rich antimicrobial peptide targeting bacterial 70S ribosome [34]. On the other hand, at higher concentrations some peptides like amyloid-beta (Aβ) can form oligomers and act via pore formation and subsequent membrane damage [35]. However, this finding contradicts the low amphiphilicity of the capitellacin structure and the absence of the peptide dimerization in model membranes even at the concentration of 3 mM that is far above the MIC value (Figures 4B and 5C).

Considering the inefficiency of capitellacin to disrupt cytoplasmic membrane integrity at concentrations near the MIC value, we tested the ability of this peptide to inhibit protein biosynthesis in vitro (Figure 7B). The experiment was carried out using the bacterial cell-free protein synthesis system expressing the enhanced green fluorescent protein (EGFP). Streptomycin served as the positive control inhibiting EGFP synthesis at 1 μM that is in line with our previous data [34]. Both capitellacin and tachyplesin-1 only slightly inhibited this process at concentrations far above the MIC value (100 μM). This effect likely results from a non-specific interaction of cationic AMPs with nucleic acids that is known for a number of peptides [34,36]. The mechanism of capitellacin action does not seem to be related to the inhibition of bacterial translation therefore other molecular targets are possible. It seems that at concentrations near the MIC value, the peptide can cross the membrane without its rupture and interacts with some intracellular targets. Putative targets may be suggested when studying the mechanism of action of structurally similar β-hairpin AMPs arenicin-3 and tachyplesin-3. The first one was hypothesized to dysregulate the Gram-negative bacteria phospholipid transport pathways via the MlaC protein binding [37]. This pathway maintains lipid asymmetry in the outer membrane by retrograde trafficking of phospholipids from the outer membrane to the inner membrane. The tachyplesin-3 was found to bind both *E. coli* and *S. aureus* FabG, the conserved β-ketoacyl-acyl carrier protein reductase, thus targeting bacterial pathway for unsaturated fatty acid biosynthesis [38].

Considering a low propensity of capitellacin to induce membrane disruption, next we analyzed its cytotoxic effects against adherent cell lines of human embryonic fibroblasts (HEF) as well as toward human red blood cells (hRBC). Tachyplesin-1 possesses a pronounced hemolytic activity with the HC_{50} value of 128 μM (Figure 8B). The obtained cytotoxicity data are in good agreement with those shown for hemolytic activity (Figure 8C). Tachyplesin-1 lysed 75% of the hRBC cells at the concentration of 64 μM. Noteworthy, capitellacin did not significantly affect both viability of fibroblasts and membrane integrity of erythrocytes at the concentration of 64 μM, which was 10–100-fold higher than antibacterial MICs measured *in vitro*. Interestingly, according to both calculated hydrophobicity index and experimental HPLC retention time, capitellacin is even more hydrophobic peptide as compared with tachyplesin-1 (Table 1, Figure 8A).

In the case of capitellacin, a low amphipathicity rather than hydrophobicity could be a key reason of the decreased cytotoxicity and overall membrane-active properties. One of the key structural differences between these peptides is the presence of Arg10 (capitellacin) and Tyr8 (tachyplesin-1) in the equivalent position of β-turn. We have previously shown that the replacement of Tyr8 by arginine in tachyplesin-1 minimizes cytotoxicity while decreasing antibacterial activity at least by 2–4-fold [39]. Interestingly, this analogue had a reduced potency to compromise *E. coli* ML-35p cytoplasmic membranes (unpublished data). A slight reduction of hydrophobicity by replacing Phe4 or Ile10 residues with alanine led to a sharp decrease in hemolytic activity as well [40]. The absence of key residues in the *N*- and *C*-terminal parts of the peptide, which are necessary for binding to lipopolysaccharide (LPS) as was shown for tachyplesin-1 [41], could be another reason of reduced activity of capitellacin against Gram-negative bacteria. Taking into account a low cytotoxicity of capitellacin, it is planned to improve its antimicrobial activity by designing a set of chimeric molecules that carry some structural elements of tachyplesin-1, in particular, the LPS-binding site.

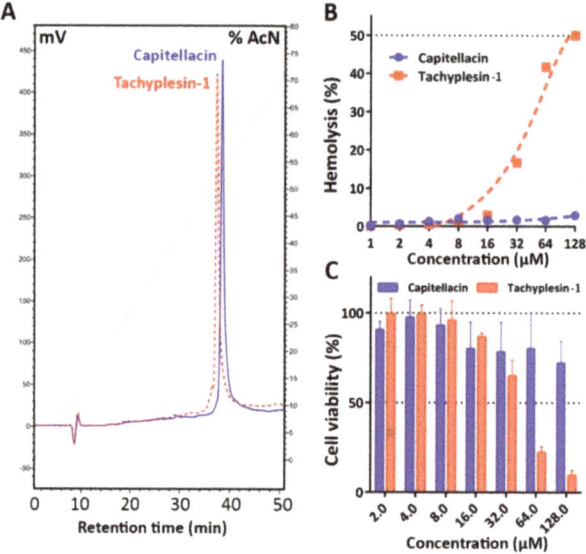

Figure 8. (A) Reversed-phase HPLC of recombinant capitellacin and tachyplesin-1 performed with a linear gradient of acetonitrile in water containing 0.1% TFA with the use of semi-preparative C18 column and detection at 214 nm. (B) Hemolytic activity of capitellacin and tachyplesin-1 after 1.5 h incubation (hemoglobin release assay). (C) Cytotoxicity of capitellacin and tachyplesin-1 against human embryonic fibroblasts (HEF) cell lines cells after 24 h incubation (3-(4,5-dimethylthiazol-2-yl)-2,5-diphenyltetrazolium bromide (MTT) dye reduction assay). The data are presented as the mean ± SD of at least three independent experiments.

3. Materials and Methods

3.1. Recombinant Production of the Peptides

Capitellacin and tachyplesin-1 were produced in a bacterial expression system as described previously [34]. Thioredoxin (Trx) was used as the fusion partner to ensure high yield of the peptide in the native conformation. The gene encoding capitellacin was obtained by annealing of two primers followed by one-round DNA-polymerase extension and then cloned into pET-based vector as described previously [39]. All the oligonucleotides used in this work were designed on the basis of *E. coli* K-12 codon usage bias. The target peptides were expressed in *E. coli* BL21 (DE3) as chimeric proteins that included 8×His tag, the *E. coli* thioredoxin A with the M37L substitution (TrxL), methionine residue, and a mature peptide. The cells transformed with the corresponding plasmid were grown at 37 °C in Lysogeny broth (LB) medium supplemented with 100 μg/mL ampicillin, 1 mM magnesium sulfate, 20 mM glucose, and were induced at OD_{600} 1.0 with 0.2 mM isopropyl β-D-1-thiogalactopyranoside (IPTG) for 5 h at 30 °C and 220 rpm. After centrifugation the pelleted cells were suspended and sonicated in the 100 mM phosphate buffer (pH 7.8) containing 20 mM imidazole and 6 M guanidine hydrochloride to fully solubilize the fusion protein. Purification of the peptide involved immobilized metal affinity chromatography (IMAC) of cell lysate with the use of Ni Sepharose (GE Healthcare),

CNBr cleavage of the fusion protein, and reversed-phase HPLC (RP-HPLC) with the use of Reprosil-pur C18-AQ column (Dr. Maisch GmbH) as described in [34]. The collected fractions were analyzed by MALDI-TOF mass-spectrometry using Reflex III instrument (Bruker Daltonics). The fractions containing the target peptides were lyophilized and dissolved in water. The peptides concentrations were estimated using UV absorbance. The fractions with confirmed masses were dried in vacuo and repurified to estimate exact RP-HPLC retention times. RP-HPLC was performed using the same column at a flow rate of 2 mL/min in a linear gradient of solution B2 (80% acetonitrile, 0.1% TFA) in solution A2 (5% acetonitrile, 0.1% TFA): 0–100% for 70 min (Figure 4A).

3.2. NMR Spectroscopy and 3D Structure Calculation

NMR study was performed using a 1.5 mM sample of the recombinant capitellacin in 5% D_2O at pH 5.2. The pH value of NMR sample was adjusted using concentrated HCl or NaOH solutions. For the NMR measurements in detergent micelles, d38-DPC (Anatrace) was added to the 0.5 mM peptide sample using aliquots of a concentrated water solution until the detergent-to-peptide molar ratio (D:P) of 130:1 was reached. The NMR spectra were measured at AVANCE 700 spectrometer equipped with room-temperature triple-resonance probe and at AVANCE-III 800 spectrometer equipped with cryoprobe (Bruker, Karlsruhe, Germany). The backbone and side chains resonance assignments were obtained by a standard approach using a combination of 2D ^{1}H-TOCSY, ^{1}H-NOESY, and ^{13}C-Heteronuclear Single Quantum Coherence spectroscopy (HSQC) spectra in the CARA (version 1.84, Zurich, Switzerland) program. The $^3J_{H^N H^\alpha}$ coupling constants were determined from line shape analysis of NOESY and TOCSY cross peaks in the Mathematica program (version 8.0, Wolfram Research, Champaign, IL, USA). The $^3J_{H^\alpha H^\beta}$ coupling constants were estimated from the multiplet patterns in 2D TOCSY spectrum. The spatial structure calculations were performed in the CYANA (version 3.97) program [42]. Upper interproton distance constraints were derived from the intensities of NOESY (τ_m = 150 ms) cross-peaks via a "1/r^6" calibration. Comparison of the intensities of the HN-HB2/3 cross-peaks showed that at this mixing time, the spin-diffusion effect does not strongly affect the signal intensities. Secondary structure of capitellacin was calculated from ^{1}H and ^{13}C chemical shifts using TALOS-N [43]. The φ and χ_1 dihedral angles restraints and stereospecific assignments were obtained from J-couplings, NOE, and TALOS data. Hydrogen bonds were introduced using temperature gradients of amide protons ($\Delta\delta^1H^N/\Delta T$), measured in the 20–45 °C temperature range in the 2D TOCSY and NOESY spectra. It was assumed that an amide proton with $\Delta\delta^1H^N/\Delta T >$ −4.5 ppb/K could participate in the hydrogen bond formation. Additional upper/lower distance restraints were applied to restrain disulfide connectivity.

The secondary structure assignment was performed with STRIDE [44]. Visual analysis of the structures and figure drawings were performed using the MOLMOL program [45]. The disulfide conformation was described analogously to [46]. The χ^1 and $\chi^{1\prime}$ angles of the disulfide were classified as usual: (−30°−−90°) – *g*+, (+30°−+90°) – *g*-, (−150° – +150°) – *t*, the χ^2, χ^3 and $\chi^{2\prime}$ angles were loosely classified as *p* for positive values and *n* for negative ones. The geometry of the β-hairpin peptides was analyzed as described in [14].

3.3. Accessing Codes

Experimental restraints, atomic coordinates, and chemical shifts of capitellacin in water solution have been deposited in PDB and BMRB databases under accession codes 7ALD and 34564, respectively.

3.4. Preparation of the Peptide-Containing Small Unilamellar Vesicles

The capitellacin (0.15–1.3 mg) was dissolved in methanol (0.6 mL) and mixed with required amounts of lipids in chloroform (0.6 mL) at 1:60 molar ratios. Then solvents were removed in rotary evaporator at 45 °C, and the samples were dried for 1 h under ~10^{-3} Torr. The peptide-lipid film was dissolved in 10 mM phosphate buffer (pH 7.2) to the final peptide concentration of 3 mM for FTIR, and 0.3 mM for CD measurements. The samples were incubated for 30 min at 20 °C and then were sonicated on ice for 1.5 min. Soybean phosphatidylethanolamine (PE), soybean phosphatidylglycerol (PG), and dimyristoylphosphatidylcholine (DMPC) were purchased from Sigma (St. Louis, MO, USA). Soybean phosphatidylcholine (PC) was purchased from Avanti Polar Lipids Inc. (Albaster, AL, USA). Dimyristoylphosphatidylglycerol (DMPG) was from Lipoid GmbH (Ludwigshafen, Germany).

3.5. Circular Dichroism Spectroscopy

Far-UV CD spectra were measured using a Jasco J-810 spectropolarimeter (Jasco, Tokyo, Japan) in demountable cells (Hellma Analytics, Müllheim/Baden, Germany) with 100 µm path length. Four scans were averaged.

3.6. Fourier-Transform Infrared Spectroscopy

FTIR spectra were measured on a Perkin-Elmer 1725 X Spectrometer (Perkin-Elmer, Beaconsfield, UK) with TGS detector and with hermetic interferometer area, which was sealed and fitted with two boxes of molecular sieves. The sieve boxes were baked at 250 °C for 8 h before measurements. Spectra in water and in aqueous suspension of liposomes were measured in very thin (12 µm) homemade demountable CaF_2 cuvettes. 150 scans were averaged with a resolution of 4 cm^{-1}.

3.7. Tryptophan Fluorescence and Quenching

Tryptophan fluorescence was measured by means of RF-5301PC spectrofluorophotometer (Shimadzu, Tokyo, Japan) fluorescence spectrophotometer using 1 × 0.4 cm quartz cuvettes (Hellma Analytics, Müllheim/Baden, Germany). Emission and excitation slits were 5 nm wide. The excitation wavelength was 280 nm. Fluorescence was quenched by addition of increasing amounts of 4 M potassium iodide.

3.8. Proton Transport Measurements

Protein expression, purification and spectroscopic characterization of the functional proton pump from *Exiguobacterium sibiricum* (ESR) was performed as described previously [23]. Reconstitution of ESR (from DDM) and formation of phospholipid proteoliposomes was carried out by cholate dialysis [47]. The protein to lipid molar ratio was 1:1700. 200 µL of proteoliposome suspension (protein concentration 0.25 mg/mL) was added to 2 mL salt solution so that lipid concentration in the cell was 2.5 mM. The peptide solution was added to the proteoliposomes with rapid stirring so that peptide to lipid molar ratio was in order of 1:500. The measurements were conducted in a thermostated cell at 25 °C with rapid stirring. Samples were illuminated with 500–Watt halogen lamp (OSRAM). pH was monitored with Cole-Parmer RZ-05658-65 electrode (Beverly, MA, USA) carefully shielded from radiation by foil.

3.9. Antimicrobial Assays

Gram-positive bacteria *Bacillus subtilis* B-886, *Micrococcus luteus* B-1314, *Staphylococcus aureus* 209P (ATCC 6538P) were obtained from All-Russian Collection of Microorganisms (Pushchino, Russia). The bacterial clinical isolates of Gram-negative bacteria (*Escherichia coli, Enterobacter cloacae, Acinetobacter baumanii, Klebsiella pneumoniae, Pseudomonas aeruginosa, Serratia marcescens*) were collected and provided by Solixant LLC (Solixant LLC, Moscow, Russia) and Sechenov First Moscow State Medical University hospital. The strains were characterized in our previous studies [17–34]. Other strains were obtained from American Type Culture Collection (ATCC, Manassas, VA, USA). Antimicrobial tests were performed as described previously [34]. Briefly, mid-log phase bacteria were diluted with the 2× Mueller-Hinton broth (MH, Sigma, St. Louis, MO, USA) supplemented with 1.8% NaCl or without it so that to reach a final cell concentration of 10^6 CFU/mL. Fifty microliter aliquots of the obtained suspension were added to the same volume of the peptide solutions serially diluted with 0.1% water solution of bovine serum albumin (BSA) in 96-well flat-bottom polystyrene microplates

(#0030730011, Eppendorf, Hamburg, Germany). After incubation for 24 h at 37 °C and 1000 rpm on the plate thermo-shaker (Biosan, Riga, Latvia), the minimum inhibitory concentrations (MICs) were calculated as the lowest concentration of peptide that prevented visible turbidity. To verify MIC values the respiratory activity of the bacteria was determined. Briefly, 20 µL of 0.1 mg/mL redox indicator resazurin (Sigma, St. Louis, MO, USA) was added to the wells, and the plate was incubated for an additional 2 h. The reduction of resazurin to resorufin was measured as the color change from blue to pink. The results were expressed as the median values of three experiments performed in duplicate. In all experiment series, no significant divergence was observed (within ±1 dilution step).

3.10. Bacterial Membranes Permeability Assay

The ability of the peptides to permeabilize the cytoplasmic bacterial membrane was accessed using a colorimetric assay with o-nitrophenyl-β-D-galactoside (ONPG, AppliChem, Darmstadt, Germany) and *E. coli* ML-35p strain constitutively expressing β-galactosidase. The final concentration of ONPG was of 2.5 mM. The concentration of the bacteria in each cell was of 2×10^7 CFU/mL. Peptide samples were placed in a 96-well plate with a non-binding surface (NBS, Corning #3641, Corning, NY, USA), and the optical density of the solution was measured at 405 nm using the Multiskan EX microplate reader (Thermo Fisher Scientific, Waltham, MA, USA). The assay was performed in phosphate buffered saline (PBS) at 32 °C under stirring at 400 rpm. Control experiments were performed under the same conditions without the addition of peptide. Three independent experiments were performed, and the curve patterns were similar for all three series.

3.11. Hemolysis and Cytotoxicity Assay

The hemolytic activity of antimicrobial peptides was estimated against fresh human red blood cells (hRBC) using the hemoglobin release assay as described previously [39]. Four experiments were performed with hRBC from blood samples of independent donors. The colorimetric 3-(4,5-dimethylthiazol-2-yl)-2,5-diphenyltetrazolium bromide (MTT) dye reduction assay was used to determine the cytotoxicity of the peptides against human embryonic fibroblasts (HEF) cell line as described previously [48]. The experimental data were obtained from at least three independent experiments. The data are represented as average means ± standard deviations (SD).

3.12. Cell-Free Protein Expression Assay

In order to investigate effects of AMPs on the translation process, the peptides were added to a cell-free protein synthesis (CFPS) reaction mix with a plasmid encoding EGFP under the control of the T7 promoter. The *E. coli* BL21 Star (DE3) lysate required for the translation inhibition assay and reaction mixtures were prepared as described previously with some modifications [34]. In particular, the final concentration of plasmid DNA encoding EGFP was of 2 ng/µL. The peptides were dissolved in water with the addition of 0.05% BSA. The reaction volume was of 50 µL. Streptomycin was used as a positive control antibiotic. Fluorescence of the sample without peptide/antibiotic was set to 100%. The reaction proceeded for 60 min in a 96-well V-bottom black polypropylene microplates (#00306019043340, Eppendorf, Hamburg, Germany) in a plate shaker (30 °C, 1000 rpm). EGFP fluorescence (λ_{Exc} = 488 nm, λ_{Em} = 510 nm) was measured with a AF2200 microplate reader (Eppendorf, Hamburg, Germany). The experimental data were obtained from two independent experiments performed in triplicate.

4. Conclusions

This study extends the knowledge of the structure and biological functions of animal β-hairpin AMPs, in particular, of BRICHOS domain-related ones. In aqueous solution capitellacin exists as monomeric right-handed twisted β-hairpin and its structure does not reveal significant amphipathicity. Moreover, the peptide retains a monomeric conformation in membrane environments when incorporating into lipid bilayers. The obtained results suggest a potential medical application of capitellacin. The pronounced bactericidal activity against drug-resistant ESKAPE bacteria as well as a wider therapeutic window as compared with tachyplesin-1 makes capitellacin a promising broad-spectrum antibacterial agent. In contrast to other known β-hairpin AMPs, like arenicins, protegrins and tachyplesins, this peptide likely acts via non-membranolytic mechanism at concentrations inhibiting bacterial growth. An ability of capitellacin to compromise biological membranes was shown only at concentrations far above its MIC value measured in vitro against bacteria. As the translation inhibition was excluded, it is necessary to perform further in-depth study on searching possible intracellular targets of capitellacin, which can be identified by selection and investigation of resistant bacterial strains.

Supplementary Materials: The following are available online at http://www.mdpi.com/1660-3397/18/12/620/s1, Figure S1: MALDI-MS analysis of the recombinant capitellacin, Table S1: Statistics for the best CYANA structures of capitellacin.

Author Contributions: P.V.P., A.V.T., S.V.S., Z.O.S., T.V.O. designed the experiments, analyzed data and wrote the paper; P.V.P., A.V.T., V.N.S., O.V.R., I.A.B., S.V.S. performed the experiments; P.V.P., T.V.O. contributed to the conception of the work; T.V.O. supervised the whole project. All authors have read and agreed to the published version of the manuscript.

Funding: This work was supported by the Russian Foundation for Basic Research (RFBR project No. 18-54-80026) and partially by The National Technological Initiative (NTI) project within the "BIOORGANICA" Consortium. NMR study was supported by the Russian Science Foundation (RSF project № 19-74-30014).

Acknowledgments: The authors thank Lada E. Petrovskaya for providing the ESR sample and A.A. Emelianova for assistance in running the experiments with mammalian cells.

Conflicts of Interest: The authors declare no conflict of interest.

References

1. Mookherjee, N.; Anderson, M.A.; Haagsman, H.P.; Davidson, D.J. Antimicrobial host defence peptides: Functions and clinical potential. *Nat. Rev. Drug Discov.* **2020**, *19*, 311–332. [CrossRef]
2. Ovchinnikova, T.V.; Aleshina, G.M.; Balandin, S.V.; Krasnosdembskaya, A.D.; Markelov, M.L.; Frolova, E.I.; Leonova, Y.F.; Tagaev, A.A.; Krasnodembsky, E.G.; Kokryakov, V.N. Purification and primary structure of two isoforms of arenicin, a novel antimicrobial peptide from marine polychaeta *Arenicola marina*. *FEBS Lett.* **2004**, *577*, 209–214. [CrossRef] [PubMed]
3. Tasiemski, A.; Jung, S.; Boidin-Wichlacz, C.; Jollivet, D.; Cuvillier-Hot, V.; Pradillon, F.; Vetriani, C.; Hecht, O.; Sönnichsen, F.D.; Gelhaus, C.; et al. Characterization and function of the first antibiotic isolated from a vent organism: The extremophile metazoan *Alvinella pompejana*. *PLoS ONE* **2014**, *9*, e95737. [CrossRef] [PubMed]
4. Panteleev, P.; Tsarev, A.; Bolosov, I.; Paramonov, A.; Marggraf, M.; Sychev, S.; Shenkarev, Z.; Ovchinnikova, T. Novel antimicrobial peptides from the arctic polychaeta *Nicomache minor* provide new molecular insight into biological role of the BRICHOS domain. *Mar. Drugs* **2018**, *16*, 401. [CrossRef] [PubMed]
5. Tasiemski, A.; Schikorski, D.; Le Marrec-Croq, F.; Pontoire-Van Camp, C.; Boidin-Wichlacz, C.; Sautière, P.-E. Hedistin: A novel antimicrobial peptide containing bromotryptophan constitutively expressed in the NK cells-like of the marine annelid, *Nereis diversicolor*. *Dev. Comp. Immunol.* **2007**, *31*, 749–762. [CrossRef]
6. Joo, M.-S.; Choi, K.-M.; Cho, D.-H.; Choi, H.-S.; Min, E.Y.; Han, H.-J.; Cho, M.Y.; Bae, J.-S.; Park, C.-I. The molecular characterization, expression analysis and antimicrobial activity of theromacin from Asian polychaeta (*Perinereis linea*). *Dev. Comp. Immunol.* **2020**, *112*, 103773. [CrossRef]
7. Seaver, E.C. Annelid models I: *Capitella teleta*. *Curr. Opin. Genet. Dev.* **2016**, *39*, 35–41. [CrossRef]
8. De Jong, D.M.; Seaver, E.C. Investigation into the cellular origins of posterior regeneration in the annelid *Capitella teleta*. *Regeneration* **2018**, *5*, 61–77. [CrossRef]
9. Nakamura, T.; Furunaka, H.; Miyata, T.; Tokunaga, F.; Muta, T.; Iwanaga, S.; Niwa, M.; Takao, T.; Shimonishi, Y. Tachyplesin, a class of antimicrobial peptide from the hemocytes of the horseshoe crab (*Tachypleus tridentatus*). Isolation and chemical structure. *J. Biol. Chem.* **1988**, *263*, 16709–16713.
10. Leppert, A.; Chen, G.; Johansson, J. BRICHOS: A chaperone with different activities depending on quaternary structure and cellular location? *Amyloid* **2019**, *26*, 152–153. [CrossRef]
11. Panteleev, P.V.; Balandin, S.V.; Ivanov, V.T.; Ovchinnikova, T.V. A therapeutic potential of animal β-hairpin antimicrobial peptides. *Curr. Med. Chem.* **2017**, *24*. [CrossRef] [PubMed]

12. Panteleev, P.V.; Balandin, S.V.; Ovchinnikova, T.V. Effect of arenicins and other β-hairpin antimicrobial peptides on *Pseudomonas aeruginosa* PAO1 biofilms. *Pharm. Chem. J.* **2017**, *50*, 715–720. [CrossRef]
13. Pyrkov, T.V.; Chugunov, A.O.; Krylov, N.A.; Nolde, D.E.; Efremov, R.G. PLATINUM: A web tool for analysis of hydrophobic/hydrophilic organization of biomolecular complexes. *Bioinformatics* **2009**, *25*, 1201–1202. [CrossRef] [PubMed]
14. Stavrakoudis, A.; Tsoulos, I.G.; Shenkarev, Z.O.; Ovchinnikova, T.V. Molecular dynamics simulation of antimicrobial peptide arenicin-2: β-Hairpin stabilization by noncovalent interactions. *Biopolymers* **2009**, *92*, 143–155. [CrossRef]
15. Shenkarev, Z.O.; Balandin, S.V.; Trunov, K.I.; Paramonov, A.S.; Sukhanov, S.V.; Barsukov, L.I.; Arseniev, A.S.; Ovchinnikova, T.V. Molecular mechanism of action of β-hairpin antimicrobial peptide arenicin: Oligomeric structure in dodecylphosphocholine micelles and pore formation in planar lipid bilayers. *Biochemistry* **2011**, *50*, 6255–6265. [CrossRef]
16. Mani, R.; Cady, S.D.; Tang, M.; Waring, A.J.; Lehrer, R.I.; Hong, M. Membrane-dependent oligomeric structure and pore formation of a beta-hairpin antimicrobial peptide in lipid bilayers from solid-state NMR. *Proc. Natl. Acad. Sci. USA* **2006**, *103*, 16242–16247. [CrossRef]
17. Panteleev, P.V.; Myshkin, M.Y.; Shenkarev, Z.O.; Ovchinnikova, T.V. Dimerization of the antimicrobial peptide arenicin plays a key role in the cytotoxicity but not in the antibacterial activity. *Biochem. Biophys. Res. Commun.* **2017**, *482*, 1320–1326. [CrossRef]
18. Perczel, A.; Hollosi, M.; Foxman, B.M.; Fasman, G.D. Conformational analysis of pseudocyclic hexapeptides based on quantitative circular dichroism (CD), NOE, and X-ray data. The pure CD spectra of type I and type II.beta.-turns. *J. Am. Chem. Soc.* **1991**, *113*, 9772–9784. [CrossRef]
19. Domingues, T.M.; Perez, K.R.; Miranda, A.; Riske, K.A. Comparative study of the mechanism of action of the antimicrobial peptide gomesin and its linear analogue: The role of the β-hairpin structure. *Biochim. Biophys. Acta BBA Biomembr.* **2015**, *1848*, 2414–2421. [CrossRef]
20. Deplazes, E.; Chin, Y.K.-Y.; King, G.F.; Mancera, R.L. The unusual conformation of cross-strand disulfide bonds is critical to the stability of β-hairpin peptides. *Proteins Struct. Funct. Bioinform.* **2020**, *88*, 485–502. [CrossRef]
21. Sychev, S.V.; Panteleev, P.V.; Ovchinnikova, T.V. Structural study of the β-hairpin marine antimicrobial peptide arenicin-2 in PC/PG lipid bilayers by fourier transform infrared spectroscopy. *Russ. J. Bioorganic Chem.* **2017**, *43*, 502–508. [CrossRef]
22. Sychev, S.V.; Sukhanov, S.V.; Panteleev, P.V.; Shenkarev, Z.O.; Ovchinnikova, T.V. Marine antimicrobial peptide arenicin adopts a monomeric twisted β-hairpin structure and forms low conductivity pores in zwitterionic lipid bilayers. *Pept. Sci.* **2018**, *110*, e23093. [CrossRef] [PubMed]
23. Petrovskaya, L.E.; Lukashev, E.P.; Chupin, V.V.; Sychev, S.V.; Lyukmanova, E.N.; Kryukova, E.A.; Ziganshin, R.H.; Spirina, E.V.; Rivkina, E.M.; Khatypov, R.A.; et al. Predicted bacteriorhodopsin from *Exiguobacterium sibiricum* is a functional proton pump. *FEBS Lett.* **2010**, *584*, 4193–4196. [CrossRef] [PubMed]
24. Galliard, T. Phospholipid metabolism in photosynthetic plants. In *Form and Function of Phospholipids*, 2nd ed.; Ansell, G.B., Hawthorne, J.N., Dawson, R.M.C., Eds.; Elsevier: New York, NY, USA, 1973; pp. 253–288.
25. Teixeira, V.; Feio, M.J.; Bastos, M. Role of lipids in the interaction of antimicrobial peptides with membranes. *Prog. Lipid Res.* **2012**, *51*, 149–177. [CrossRef] [PubMed]
26. Schmidt, N.W.; Wong, G.C.L. Antimicrobial peptides and induced membrane curvature: Geometry, coordination chemistry, and molecular engineering. *Curr. Opin. Solid State Mater. Sci.* **2013**, *17*, 151–163. [CrossRef] [PubMed]
27. Savini, F.; Bobone, S.; Roversi, D.; Mangoni, M.L.; Stella, L. From liposomes to cells: Filling the gap between physicochemical and microbiological studies of the activity and selectivity of host-defense peptides. *Pept. Sci.* **2018**, *110*, e24041. [CrossRef]
28. Doherty, T.; Waring, A.J.; Hong, M. Peptide–lipid interactions of the β-hairpin antimicrobial peptide tachyplesin and its linear derivatives from solid-state NMR. *Biochim. Biophys. Acta BBA Biomembr.* **2006**, *1758*, 1285–1291. [CrossRef]
29. Padan, E.; Bibi, E.; Ito, M.; Krulwich, T.A. Alkaline pH homeostasis in bacteria: New insights. *Biochim. Biophys. Acta BBA Biomembr.* **2005**, *1717*, 67–88. [CrossRef]
30. Méndez-Vilas, A. *Science Against Microbial Pathogens: Communicating Current Research and Technological Advances*; Formatex Research Center: Badajoz, Spain, 2011; ISBN 978-84-939843-1-1.

31. Matsuzaki, K.; Yoneyama, S.; Fujii, N.; Miyajima, K.; Yamada, K.; Kirino, Y.; Anzai, K. Membrane permeabilization mechanisms of a cyclic antimicrobial peptide, tachyplesin I, and its linear analog. *Biochemistry* **1997**, *36*, 9799–9806. [CrossRef]
32. Doherty, T.; Waring, A.J.; Hong, M. Dynamic structure of disulfide-removed linear analogs of tachyplesin-I in the lipid Bilayer from solid-state NMR. *Biochemistry* **2008**, *47*, 1105–1116. [CrossRef]
33. Su, Y.; Li, S.; Hong, M. Cationic membrane peptides: Atomic-level insight of structure–activity relationships from solid-state NMR. *Amino Acids* **2013**, *44*, 821–833. [CrossRef] [PubMed]
34. Panteleev, P.V.; Bolosov, I.A.; Kalashnikov, A.À.; Kokryakov, V.N.; Shamova, O.V.; Emelianova, A.A.; Balandin, S.V.; Ovchinnikova, T.V. Combined antibacterial effects of goat cathelicidins with different mechanisms of action. *Front. Microbiol.* **2018**, *9*, 2983. [CrossRef] [PubMed]
35. Ciudad, S.; Puig, E.; Botzanowski, T.; Meigooni, M.; Arango, A.S.; Do, J.; Mayzel, M.; Bayoumi, M.; Chaignepain, S.; Maglia, G.; et al. Aβ(1-42) tetramer and octamer structures reveal edge conductivity pores as a mechanism for membrane damage. *Nat. Commun.* **2020**, *11*, 3014. [CrossRef] [PubMed]
36. Yonezawa, A.; Kuwahara, J.; Fujii, N.; Sugiura, Y. Binding of tachyplesin I to DNA revealed by footprinting analysis: Significant contribution of secondary structure to DNA binding and implication for biological action. *Biochemistry* **1992**, *31*, 2998–3004. [CrossRef] [PubMed]
37. Elliott, A.G.; Huang, J.X.; Neve, S.; Zuegg, J.; Edwards, I.A.; Cain, A.K.; Boinett, C.J.; Barquist, L.; Lundberg, C.V.; Steen, J.; et al. An amphipathic peptide with antibiotic activity against multidrug-resistant Gram-negative bacteria. *Nat. Commun.* **2020**, *11*, 3184. [CrossRef] [PubMed]
38. Liu, C.; Qi, J.; Shan, B.; Ma, Y. Tachyplesin causes membrane instability that kills multidrug-resistant bacteria by inhibiting the 3-ketoacyl carrier protein reductase FabG. *Front. Microbiol.* **2018**, *9*, 825. [CrossRef] [PubMed]
39. Panteleev, P.V.; Ovchinnikova, T.V. Improved strategy for recombinant production and purification of antimicrobial peptide tachyplesin I and its analogs with high cell selectivity. *Biotechnol. Appl. Biochem.* **2017**, *64*, 35–42. [CrossRef]
40. Edwards, I.A.; Elliott, A.G.; Kavanagh, A.M.; Blaskovich, M.A.T.; Cooper, M.A. Structure–activity and −toxicity relationships of the antimicrobial peptide tachyplesin-1. *ACS Infect. Dis.* **2017**, *3*, 917–926. [CrossRef]
41. Kushibiki, T.; Kamiya, M.; Aizawa, T.; Kumaki, Y.; Kikukawa, T.; Mizuguchi, M.; Demura, M.; Kawabata, S.; Kawano, K. Interaction between tachyplesin I, an antimicrobial peptide derived from horseshoe crab, and lipopolysaccharide. *Biochim. Biophys. Acta BBA Proteins Proteom.* **2014**, *1844*, 527–534. [CrossRef]
42. Schmidt, E.; Güntert, P. Automated structure determination from NMR spectra. In *Structural Proteomics*; Owens, R.J., Ed.; Springer: New York, NY, USA, 2015; Volume 1261, pp. 303–329, ISBN 978-1-4939-2229-1.
43. Shen, Y.; Bax, A. Protein backbone and sidechain torsion angles predicted from NMR chemical shifts using artificial neural networks. *J. Biomol. NMR* **2013**, *56*, 227–241. [CrossRef]
44. Frishman, D.; Argos, P. Knowledge-based protein secondary structure assignment. *Proteins Struct. Funct. Genet.* **1995**, *23*, 566–579. [CrossRef] [PubMed]
45. Koradi, R.; Billeter, M.; Wüthrich, K. MOLMOL: A program for display and analysis of macromolecular structures. *J. Mol. Graph.* **1996**, *14*, 51–55. [CrossRef]
46. Shenkarev, Z.O.; Nadezhdin, K.D.; Sobol, V.A.; Sobol, A.G.; Skjeldal, L.; Arseniev, A.S. Conformation and mode of membrane interaction in cyclotides. *FEBS J.* **2006**, *273*, 2658–2672. [CrossRef]
47. Huang, K.S.; Bayley, H.; Liao, M.J.; London, E.; Khorana, H.G. Refolding of an integral membrane protein. Denaturation, renaturation, and reconstitution of intact bacteriorhodopsin and two proteolytic fragments. *J. Biol. Chem.* **1981**, *256*, 3802–3809. [PubMed]
48. Kuzmin, D.V.; Emelianova, A.A.; Kalashnikova, M.B.; Panteleev, P.V.; Balandin, S.V.; Serebrovskaya, E.O.; Belogurova-Ovchinnikova, O.Y.; Ovchinnikova, T.V. Comparative in vitro study on cytotoxicity of recombinant β-hairpin peptides. *Chem. Biol. Drug Des.* **2018**, *91*, 294–303. [CrossRef]

Publisher's Note: MDPI stays neutral with regard to jurisdictional claims in published maps and institutional affiliations.

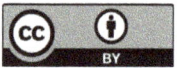

© 2020 by the authors. Licensee MDPI, Basel, Switzerland. This article is an open access article distributed under the terms and conditions of the Creative Commons Attribution (CC BY) license (http://creativecommons.org/licenses/by/4.0/).

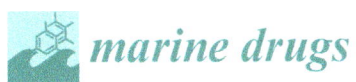

Article

Antimicrobial Peptide Arenicin-1 Derivative Ar-1-(C/A) as Complement System Modulator

Ilia A. Krenev [1,2], Ekaterina S. Umnyakova [1,*], Igor E. Eliseev [3], Yaroslav A. Dubrovskii [2,4], Nikolay P. Gorbunov [1], Vladislav A. Pozolotin [1], Alexei S. Komlev [1], Pavel V. Panteleev [5], Sergey V. Balandin [5], Tatiana V. Ovchinnikova [5,6], Olga V. Shamova [1] and Mikhail N. Berlov [1]

1. Department of General Pathology and Pathological Physiology, Institute of Experimental Medicine, Acad. Pavlov Str. 12, 197376 Saint Petersburg, Russia; il.krenevv13@yandex.ru (I.A.K.); niko_laygo@mail.ru (N.P.G.); vlad.yugra.nyagan@gmail.com (V.A.P.); witcher-lex@yandex.ru (A.S.K.); oshamova@yandex.ru (O.V.S.); berlov.mn@iemspb.ru (M.N.B.)
2. Faculty of Chemistry, Saint Petersburg State University, Universitetskaya Emb, 7/9, 199034 Saint Petersburg, Russia; dubrovskiy.ya@gmail.com
3. Nanobiotechnology Laboratory, Alferov University, Khlopin Str. 8/3, 194021 Saint Petersburg, Russia; eliseev@spbau.ru
4. Almazov National Medical Research Centre, Akkuratov Str, 2, 197341 Saint Petersburg, Russia
5. M.M. Shemyakin and Yu. A. Ovchinnikov Institute of Bioorganic Chemistry, Russian Academy of Sciences, Miklukho-Maklaya Str., 16/10, 117997 Moscow, Russia; alarm14@gmail.com (P.V.P.); serb@ibch.ru (S.V.B.); ovch@ibch.ru (T.V.O.)
6. Department of Biotechnology, I.M. Sechenov First Moscow State Medical University, Trubetskaya Str., 8-2, 119991 Moscow, Russia
* Correspondence: umnyakova.es@iemspb.ru; Tel.: +7-981-971-4975

Received: 3 November 2020; Accepted: 8 December 2020; Published: 10 December 2020

Abstract: Antimicrobial peptides (AMPs) are not only cytotoxic towards host pathogens or cancer cells but also are able to act as immunomodulators. It was shown that some human and non-human AMPs can interact with complement proteins and thereby modulate complement activity. Thus, AMPs could be considered as the base for complement-targeted therapeutics development. Arenicins from the sea polychaete *Arenicola marina*, the classical example of peptides with a β-hairpin structure stabilized by a disulfide bond, were shown earlier to be among the most prospective regulators. Here, we investigate the link between arenicins' structure and their antimicrobial, hemolytic and complement-modulating activities using the derivative Ar-1-(C/A) without a disulfide bond. Despite the absence of this bond, the peptide retains all important functional activities and also appears less hemolytic in comparison with the natural forms. These findings could help to investigate new complement drugs for regulation using arenicin derivatives.

Keywords: antimicrobial peptide; arenicin; complement system; complement regulation

1. Introduction

Antimicrobial peptides (AMPs) are short, predominantly cationic polypeptide molecules that possess toxic activity against different pathogens: bacteria, enveloped viruses, fungi, parasites, etc. These peptides were first discovered to be cytotoxic agents against bacteria but later more and more data appeared about the immunoregulatory and wound-healing activities of different AMPs. For example, human defensins possess chemotactic activities for some immune cells [1–4] and stimulate angiogenesis [5] and collagen synthesis in fibroblasts [6]. They also participate in autoimmune processes [7]. All these findings give evidence that AMPs could be used as a promising basis for the development of new generations of antibiotic and anticancer drugs [8–10]. These substances not only participate in host defense against pathogens but they also possess immunomodulatory activity [11].

In particular, human and non-human AMPs were found to bind complement proteins and to modulate human complement system activity [12–18].

The complement system is a network containing more than 30 soluble and membrane-associated proteins that consistently activate each other through limited proteolysis reactions. This leads to anaphylatoxin (C3a and C5a) formation, to opsonization of the target surfaces by derivatives of the complement proteins and to membrane attack complex (MAC) assembly, which could provoke the complement-mediated lysis of target cells that is mainly typical of Gram-negative bacteria [19]. The dysregulation of the complement can cause different dangerous inflammatory diseases. They can be directly associated with excessive activation of the complement system (age-related macular degeneration, atypical hemolytic uremic syndrome, type II membranoproliferative glomerulonephritis, paroxysmal nocturnal hemoglobinuria), as well as with insufficient complement activation [20]. One of the most severe problems of modern medicine is the absence of available therapeutic agents that regulate complement activation. Thus, we are searching for such substances among AMPs.

We showed earlier that one of the most promising candidates appeared to be arenicin-1 (Ar-1), the antimicrobial peptide from *Arenicola marina*, that is able to modulate complement activity [18]. Arenicins were discovered by Ovchinnikova and co-workers [21], and there are three isoforms in total, of which two, Ar-1 and Ar-2, differ in a single amino acid residue [22]. Our next aim was to modify the primary structure of this peptide to achieve the following goals: (1) to improve the ability to inhibit complement activity to treat diseases caused by hyperactivation of this system; (2) to lower cytotoxic activity towards the host cells decrease undesirable side effects; (3) to save the antimicrobial activity of the peptide for the host defense against bacteria while the complement is inhibited. Here, we made an Ar-1 derivative without the intramolecular disulfide bond, where Cys3 and Cys20 were replaced by Ala and thus we named this peptide Ar-1-(C/A). This design was developed to check whether this bond is critical for the structural stability and biological activity, i.e., antimicrobial activity against Gram-positive and Gram-negative bacteria, cytotoxic activity toward human erythrocytes and the ability to regulate the human complement system. The main goal of this investigation was to identify the differences in the action of natural arenicins Ar-1, Ar-2 and analog Ar-1-(C/A).

2. Results

We performed successful peptide synthesis of a new derivative of natural Ar-1. Our variant contains two alanine residues (Ala^3 and Ala^{20}) instead of two cysteines, thus, it is not stabilized by a disulfide bond. The mass spectrum of Ar-1-(C/A) is presented in Figure 1.

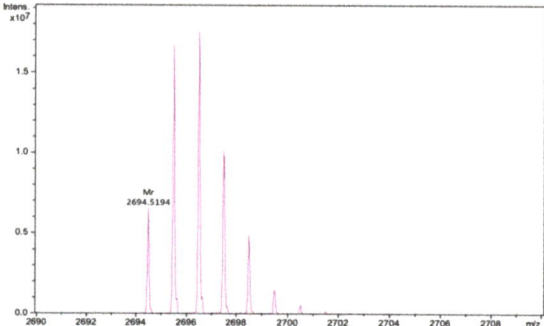

Figure 1. Fragment of the mass spectrum of Ar-1(C/A) after deconvolution for neutral molecule. The calculated monoisotopic mass of the peptide is 2694.525, the experimentally determined *m/z* value is 2694.519.

We studied the spatial structure of Ar-1-(C/A) and its conformational transitions upon membrane binding by circular dichroism spectroscopy in aqueous solution and in a lipid environment modeled by anionic SDS micelles. To allow the direct comparison with homologs, we analyzed experimental CD data previously collected for wild-type Ar-1 [23] and Ar-2 [24] in similar experimental conditions. The CD spectrum of Ar-1-(C/A) in aqueous solution, shown in Figure 2A, is quite uncommon and has two positive bands at approximately 205 and 230 nm and two negative bands at 195 and 215 nm. This spectrum is remarkably similar to that of wild-type Ar-1 and Ar-2, which are highly right-twisted and kinked β-hairpin molecules in aqueous solution [23–26], yet the amplitude of the CD signal for Ar-1-(C/A) is lower.

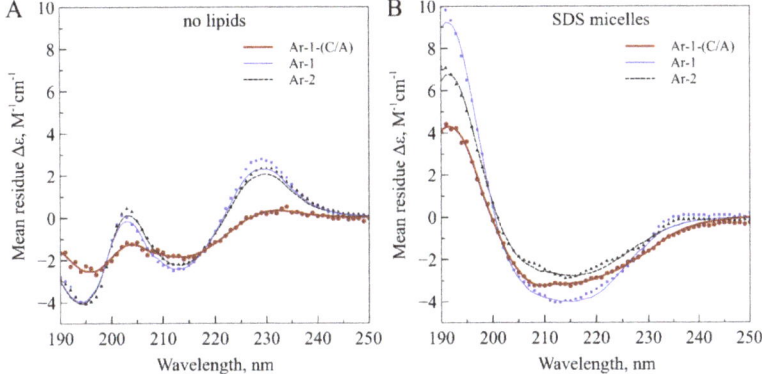

Figure 2. Circular dichroism spectra of Ar-1-(C/A) variant, Ar-1 and Ar-2 in (**A**) aqueous solution and in (**B**) complex with anionic SDS micelles (P:D = 1:350). Experimental data points are shown with symbols and fitted curves calculated with *BeStSel* are pictured as lines. Data for Ar-1 are taken from Panteleev et al. [23] and data for Ar-2 are from Ovchinnikova et al. [24].

For a more detailed structural analysis, we performed spectra deconvolution using the β-structure selection method [27] recently implemented in the BeStSel web server [28]. As seen from Table 1, BeStSel produced a good fit to the experimental data according to normalized root mean square deviations (NRMSDs), and its estimates of the secondary structure components are given in Table 1.

Table 1. The content of secondary structure elements in Ar-1-(C/A), Ar-1 and Ar-2 estimated by the deconvolution of CD spectra with *BeStSel*.

Peptide		α-Helix, %		β-Sheet, %				Turn, %	Other, %	NRMSD
				Antiparallel						
		Regular	Distorted	Left-Twisted	Relaxed	Right-Twisted	Parallel			
Ar-1-(C/A)	aqueous solution	1.5	1.5	1.4	12.2	45.2	7.8	9.0	44.2	0.034
		0.0				23.8				
	SDS micelles	11.8	5.4	0.0	9.1	22.5	8.4	11.9	53.7	0.015
		6.5				5.0				
Ar-1	aqueous solution	0.0	0.0	3.6	24.0	66.0	0.0	0.0	34.0	0.034
		0.0				38.4				
	SDS micelles	15.5	0.0	4.5	22.9	41.7	0.0	8.3	34.5	0.018
		15.5				14.3				
Ar-2	aqueous solution	0.0	0.0	3.9	24.6	67.4	0.0	0.0	32.6	0.027
		0.0				38.9				
	SDS micelles	7.8	0.4	5.0	22.9	44.8	0.0	11.7	35.7	0.016
		7.5				16.8				

According to this analysis, Ar-1-(C/A) adopts a predominantly antiparallel β-sheet structure with a considerable right twist in aqueous solution. The experimentally observed propensity of

Ar-1-(C/A) to form a β-hairpin structure even without the disulfide bond supports the previous molecular dynamics simulations showing the rapid folding of linear Ar-1 with alkylated cysteines into its native conformation [29]. Indeed, the average content of β-sheet structures in Ar-1-(C/A) is lower than in wild-type arenicins, where disulfide bonds restrict the conformational space and confer additional stability to the β-hairpin.

Upon binding to anionic micelles, Ar-1-(C/A) undergoes a conformational transition which partly transforms the CD spectrum (Figure 2B). The spectrum of micelle-bound Ar-1-(C/A) again resembles that of arenicins in complex with anionic SDS or zwitterionic dodecylphosphocholine (DPC) micelles [23–26]. The deconvolution of the CD spectrum also gives prevalent β-sheets and turns, however some α-helical characteristics are also detected. Although the helical content is relatively low in all three peptides, the stronger dichroism signal from the α-helices leads to significant transformation of CD spectra of micelle-bound peptides.

Another interesting structural feature of the micelle-bound Ar-1-(C/A) is the decrease in right-twisted antiparallel β-sheet content and a simultaneous increase in the proportion of relaxed antiparallel and parallel β-sheets. We anticipate that these changes in the distribution of various β-sheet types evidence the formation of a more planar structure, which was previously observed for membrane-bound Ar-2 dimers by NMR [25].

We measured antimicrobial activity for arenicins using the radial diffusion assay (Figure 3) for measuring the minimum inhibitory concentration (MIC). This method is not very canonical but it provides the data about the antimicrobial activity in solid media. According to the results presented in Table 2, the MICs of Ar-1, Ar-2 and Ar-1-(C/A) against *Escherihia coli* ML-35p are 3.3 ± 1.3, 1.7 ± 0.3 and 4.0 ± 0.5 µM, respectively. The MICs of Ar-1, Ar-2 and Ar-1-(C/A) against *Listeria monocytogenes* EGD are 2.2 ± 0.8, 2.0 ± 0.01 and 3.6 ± 0.8 µM, respectively (see Table 2). Therefore, Ar-1-(C/A) has a slightly but insignificantly weaker activity against both Gram-negative and Gram-positive bacteria than the natural peptides.

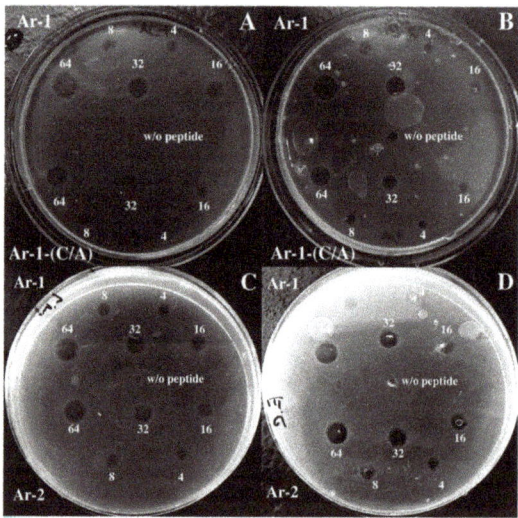

Figure 3. Results of radial diffusion antimicrobial assay against (**A,C**) *L. monocytogenes* EGD, (**B,D**) *E. coli* ML-35p. Ar-1, Ar-2 and Ar-1-(C/A) were added at concentrations 64, 32, 16, 8 and 4 µM. As a negative control (w/o peptide), deionized water was used.

The studied peptides possess different hemolytic activity against human erythrocytes (Table 2). The two naturally occurring peptides, Ar-1 and Ar-2, appeared to be more hemolytic (MHC 2.9 ± 1.2

and 1.8 ± 0.9 µM, respectively) than the modification lacking the disulfide bond, Ar-1-(C/A) (MHC 11.1 ± 2.3 µM).

In the assay with antibody-sensitized sheep erythrocytes (Er^{sh}), which was the model of the classical pathway (CP) activation, the dose-dependent modulation of the complement-mediated hemolysis by the peptides was observed. In Figure 4A, we see in the graph that if the line is above zero, there is complement activation and when it is below zero, that means inhibition of the hemolysis in this test system. As we can see from Figure 4A, Ar-1 led to a significant augmentation of the hemolysis at lower concentrations, but almost abolished Er^{sh} lysis at higher concentrations. Almost the same picture was observed for Ar-2 and Ar-1-(C/A) but the concentrations were slightly different from Ar-1.

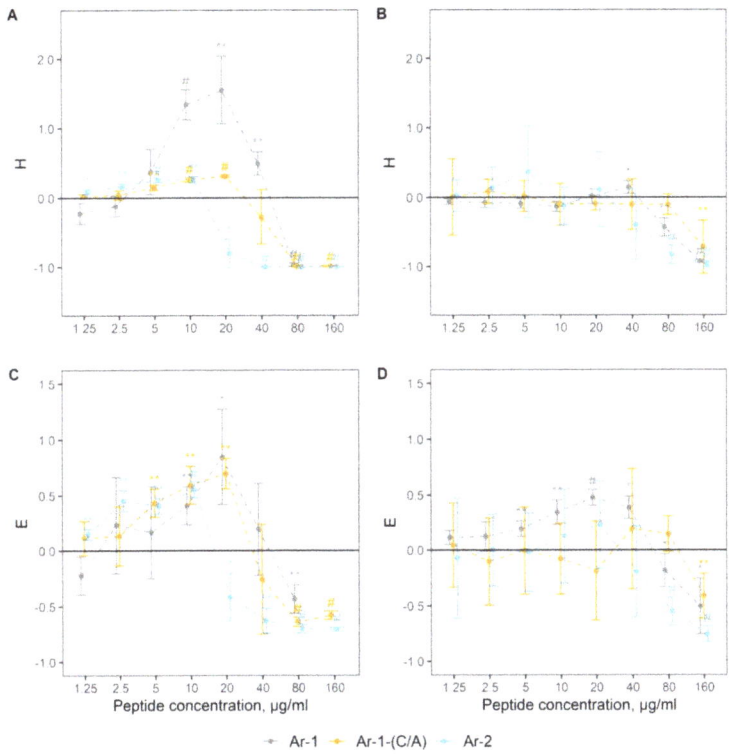

Figure 4. The action of arenicins on complement activation, expressed in H and E coefficients. Data are represented as mean ± standard deviation (n = 5). * p < 0.05; ** < 0.01; # p < 0.001 (H- and E-values vs. zero). (**A**) Alterations in lysis of antibody-sensitized sheep erythrocytes (E^{sh}) (CP model); (**B**) alterations in lysis of rabbit erythrocytes (E^{rab}) (AP model); (**C**) C3a accumulation in the model with E^{sh}; (**D**) C3a accumulation in the model with E^{rab}.

To confirm the contribution of complement to the hemolysis, we utilized an ELISA system for human anaphylatoxin C3a detection. In Figure 4C, there is a graph that is similar to that in Figure 4A: a line above zero means active C3a accumulation and complement activation and a line below zero means complement inhibition. Thus, from Figure 4C, we can easily see that in the Er^{sh} hemolytic assay, the elevation of C3a production was observed in the presence of Ar-1, Ar-2 and Ar-1-(C/A) at relatively low concentrations. It was diminished by all arenicin peptides at concentrations corresponding to those at which they abolished hemolysis.

The hemolytic assay with rabbit erythrocytes (Er^{rab}) was used as the model of the alternative pathway (AP) activation. It was similar to that for the Er^{sh} lysis assessment and the graph in Figure 4B has the same features. As we can see in Figure 4B, all arenicins demonstrated a strong inhibitory activity at high concentrations. However, it was also shown for Ar-1 that it could slightly activate the complement at a lower concentration. This effect was not detected for Ar-2 and Ar-1-(C/A).

In the E^{rab} hemolytic assay, ELISA revealed a slight C3a elevation in the presence of Ar-1 at lower concentrations but this was not observed for Ar-2 and Ar-1-(C/A). The C3a level was significantly reduced by the peptides at the concentrations at which they diminished E^{rab} lysis (Figure 4D).

Importantly, none of the peptides themselves led to hemolysis in experimental models since the lysis level did not differ from the baseline when active serum was replaced by heat-inactivated serum and none of the peptides per se generated a signal in the ELISA system.

In experiments modeling complement activation either via CP or via AP, we observed a good correlation between the level of erythrocyte lysis and C3a accumulation (Figure 5).

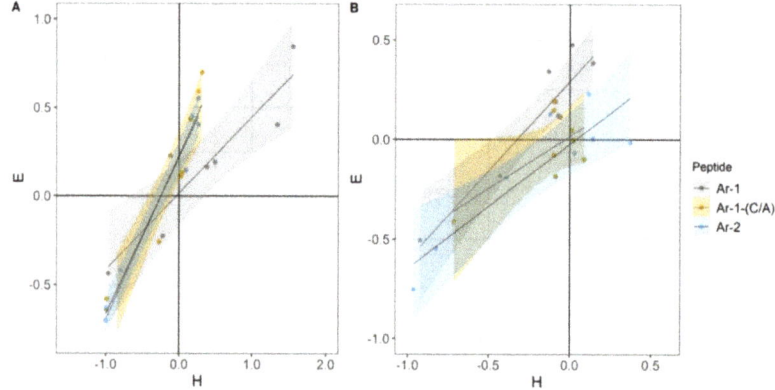

Figure 5. Correlation between H- and E-indexes. These coefficients were used for evaluation of the hemolytic activity of complement (H) and of complement-dependent C3a accumulation (E). (**A**) Correlation between the indexes in the E^{sh} CP model. Pearson correlation coefficient values were calculated as 0.92 for Ar-1, 0.96 for Ar-1-(C/A) and 0.99 for Ar-2. (**B**) Correlation between the indexes in the E^{rab} AP model. Pearson correlation coefficient values were calculated as 0.93 for Ar-1, 0.68 for Ar-1-(C/A) and 0.89 for Ar-2.

Thus, all three peptides demonstrated the ability to modulate complement activation via both pathways. For more details, see Table 2.

Table 2. Biological action of Ar-1, Ar-2 and Ar-1-(C/A). ↑—activation; ↓—inhibition; MHC—minimal hemolytic concentration; MIC—minimal inhibitory concentration. All the concentrations are in µM.

Peptide	Modulation of Human Complement System				MHC	MIC	
	Classical Pathway		Alternative Pathway			E. coli	L. monocytogenes
	Hemolysis	C3a	Hemolysis	C3a			
Ar-1	↑3.6—14.5 ↓29	↑3.6—7.2 ↓29	↑14.5 ↓29—58	↑1.8—14.5 ↓29—58	2.9 ± 1.2	3.3	2.2
Ar-2	↑0.5—3.6 ↓7.2—57.7	↑0.5—3.6 ↓7.2—57.7	↑no ↓28.8—57.7	↑no ↓28.8—57.7	1.8 ± 0.9	1.7	2.0
Ar-1-(C/A)	↑1.9—7.4 ↓29.7—59.3	↑1.9—7.4 ↓29.7—59.3	↑no ↓59.3	↑no ↓59.3	11.1 ± 2.3	4.0	3.6

3. Discussion

One of the main difficulties in using AMPs as therapeutic agents is that they often display high cytotoxic activity towards the host cells and especially erythrocytes. It is possible to lower this effect by modifying the primary structure of AMPs.

We created the arenicin derivative Ar-1-(C/A) to check whether the cysteine bond is critical for (1) the structural stability, (2) biological activity, i.e., antimicrobial function, (3) cytotoxic activity (hemolysis) and (4) the ability to regulate the human complement system. Despite the absence of the disulfide bond, the peptide Ar-1-(C/A) retains the β-hairpin structure, as was shown using CD spectrometry: the spectrum is remarkably similar to that of wild-type Ar-1 and Ar-2 [23–25]. However, the average content of β-strand structures in Ar-1-(C/A) is lower than in natural arenicins.

The antimicrobial activity of Ar-1-(C/A) also remained at the level of natural analogs, but the hemolytic activity became 3.5 times lower according to our results. A similar effect was observed earlier by Panteleev and colleagues though they had performed a different modification [30]. It is known that natural Ar-1 and Ar-2 peptides form dimers under membrane-mimicking conditions that usually lead to high cytotoxicity [26]. They created the arenicin derivative Ar-1[V8R] that was less predisposed to form dimers. It was shown to be less cytotoxic for erythrocytes but not for bacterial cells [30].

Another approach was proposed by Lee and co-authors [31]. They demonstrated that one of the ways that could lead to lower cytotoxicity is to replace in the Ar-1 structure Cys3 and Cys20 that form the intramolecular disulfide bond. This modification of Ar-1 without a disulfide bond demonstrated lower antimicrobial and hemolytic activity compared to the natural peptide [31].

Thus, it should be considered that a lower hemolytic activity may correlate with a lower antimicrobial activity due to reduced membranolytic capacity. In this work, we also created an arenicin without a disulfide bond but it appeared that it is not really linear: it is able to form a twisted β-hairpin structure despite the absence of a disulfide bond and it saved the main features that are typical for natural arenicins, except cytotoxic activity against erythrocytes. We anticipate that the lower cytotoxicity is due to the lower stability of the β-hairpin structure in Ar-1-(C/A).

The derivative Ar-1-(C/A) also was shown to retain the ability to modulate the complement system.

In our experiments, we previously observed opposite effects of Ar-1 on complement activation, expressed in the up-regulated or down-regulated hemolysis level and/or up-regulated or down-regulated C3a level that depended on the tested concentration [18]. Here, we found that a similar mode of action is shared by other structurally related peptides, Ar-2 and Ar-1-(C/A).

Natural Ar-1 and Ar-2 differ in a single amino acid residue and both adopt a right-twisted β-hairpin conformation. Nevertheless, a comparison of 3D structures of Ar-1 [32] and Ar-2 [24] determined by NMR suggests that some inequality may exist. The overall conformation of Ar-1 can be described as more compact compared with the more elongated Ar-2 conformation [32]. It remains to be established whether this subtle difference can explain why the effects of Ar-1 and Ar-2 on complement activity are not completely identical.

In our previous works, we showed the ability of Ar-1 to bind C1q [17] and demonstrated its strong inhibitory effect in hemolytic assays for the CP [18]. This fact could serve as evidence that arenicins can lead, through the interaction with C1q, to complement-dependent lysis inhibition and low C3a production. We also found that high doses of Ar-1 inhibit classical and alternative pathways, and the latter cannot be explained only by the interaction of arenicins with C1q. This effect must be related to the action on the common point of both pathways, i.e., C3 cleavage. It is highly probable that arenicins bind the C3 component that leads to its protection from cleavage, although interactions of arenicins with C3 convertases are also possible. Using surface plasmon resonance, we showed that Ar-1 is able to bind C3b protein [33]. Thus, we can suggest that arenicins can bind C1q and C3 or/and C3b and, in some cases, this can lead to complement inhibition.

The ability of arenicins to interact with different complement proteins could be adopted to explain their opposite effects on complement activation. However, there is one more presumable mechanism for complement activation that does not imply direct interaction of the peptides with complement proteins. This effect may be connected with the electrostatic interaction due to which a potent complement inhibitor, heparin (or maybe other GAGs), can be neutralized by peptides that contain the heparin-binding motif XBBXBX, where X—hydrophobic residue, B—basic residue [34].

Indeed, all arenicins contain such motifs, as we can see from Figure 6. A similar mechanism was described for the heparin-binding polypeptide PF4 (platelet factor 4). Although heparin itself is a complement inhibitor [35,36], at the same time, heparin in complex with PF4 was described as activating the complement cascade [37].

The approach involving the use of AMPs as new complement modulators has several advantages. Firstly, these molecules are relatively small, which means that the immune response to these substances will be limited. Secondly, these peptides do not resemble human antimicrobial peptides, which means that these substances would not demonstrate any cross-reactivity and we can avoid a number of side effects. Thirdly, this approach will also help to provide microbicidal or at least bacteriostatic conditions, considering the inhibited complement system. This point is extremely important because using complement inhibitors usually leads to recurrent bacterial infections [38].

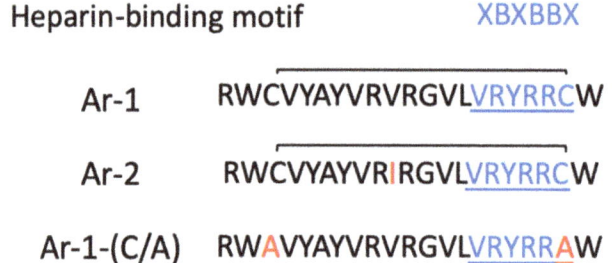

Figure 6. The primary structure of arenicins. Residues in red differ Ar-2 and Ar-1-(C/A) from Ar-1. Underlined residues in blue form a heparin-binding motif.

4. Materials and Methods

4.1. Arenicin Peptides

The primary structures of Ar-1, Ar-2 and Ar-1-(C/A) are demonstrated in Figure 6.

The Ar-1 peptide was synthesized using solid phase based on the 9-fluorenylmethoxycarbonyl (Fmoc) protocol with O-(benzotriazol-1-yl)-N,N,N′,N′-tetramethyluronium tetrafluoroborate/N,N diisopropylethylamine (TBTU/DIEA) activation, using Wang resin as the solid phase and triphenylmethyl-protecting groups for cysteines, as described previously [24].

The Ar-2 recombinant peptide was expressed in *Escherichia coli* and then purified as described earlier [24].

The Ar-1-(C/A) peptide was assembled utilizing SymphonyX UV/IR peptide synthesizer (Protein Technologies Inc., Tucson, AZ, USA) running the Fmoc SPPS protocol at a 0.1 mmol scale on Fmoc-Rink amide resin. Side-chain functionalities were protected with tert-butyl (Tyr) groups for tyrosine and a 2,2,4,6,7-pentamethyldihydrobenzofuran-5-sulfonyl group for arginine. Fivefold excess of Fmoc-L-amino acids (Oxyma Pure and DIC), purchased from Iris Biotech (Marktredwitz, Germany), was used for the coupling steps, with NMP as a solvent. After chain assembly, the full deprotection and cleavage were carried out with TFA/H2O/thioanisole/TIS (92.5:2.5:2.5:2.5 v/v, 120 min, rt). Initial steps of peptide isolation were performed according to the standard procedure in Fmoc chemistry: precipitation with cold diethyl ether, dissolution of the peptide in 0.1 M acetic acid and lyophilization.

Analytical reversed-phase HPLC was performed on C18 columns (4.6 × 100 mm, 3.5 µm, Waters, Milford, MA, USA) in a System Gold 125/166 (Beckman coulter, Pasadena, CA, USA). As solvent A, 0.1% TFA in water was used and as solvent B, 0.1% TFA in acetonitrile. The elution was held using a linear gradient of 5–70% of solvent B to solvent A over 65 min at a 1 mL/min flow rate with UV detection at 235 nm. For the peptide Ar-1-(C/A), identification mass spectrometry was used. Mass spectra were obtained on the maXis impact Q-TOF mass spectrometer (Bruker Daltonics GmbH, Bremen, Germany), equipped with an electrospray ionization (ESI) source (Bruker Daltonics GmbH, Bremen, Germany), operated in positive ionization mode. Mass calibration was carried out with a sodium formate solution (Calibration Mode HPC, standard deviation: 0.336 ppm). Flow injection mode was used for peptide analysis, mass range from 50 to 2000 m/z. Mass spectra were analyzed and created for a neutral molecule using DataAnalysis® software (Bruker Daltonics GmbH, Bremen, Germany).

All peptides were stored lyophilized and were reconstituted using deionized water before use.

4.2. Serum and Erythrocytes

Normal human serum used as a source of complement was collected from 30 healthy volunteers, pooled, aliquoted and stored at −70 °C. Erythrocytes were purified from whole blood of rabbit, sheep and healthy donors. The fresh blood was mixed with Alsever's solution (1:2) and stored at 4 °C for no more than 5 days. Before use, we obtained erythrocytes from the blood and washed them with an appropriate buffer: DGVB^{++} (dextrose gelatin veronal buffer with Ca^{2+} and Mg^{2+}: 5 mM sodium barbital buffer containing 150 mM NaCl, 15 mM glucose, 1 mM MgCl$_2$, 0.15 mM CaCl$_2$, 0.05% gelatin; pH 7.35) for sheep erythrocytes (E^{sh}); GVB$^+$ (gelatin veronal buffer with Mg^{2+}: 5 mM sodium barbital buffer containing 150 mM NaCl, 10 mM Mg-EGTA, 0.05% gelatin; pH 7.35) for rabbit erythrocytes (E^{rab}) and PBS (phosphate buffered saline; pH 7.4) for human erythrocytes (E^{hum}). Sheep erythrocytes were sensitized with antibodies (anti-sheep red blood cell stroma antibodies produced in rabbits, S1389, Sigma, St. Louis, MO, USA) before use in experiments; we used a 1:1600 dilution of these antibodies and incubated sheep erythrocytes for 30 min at 37 °C.

4.3. Circular Dichroism Spectroscopy

The secondary structure of Ar-1-(C/A) was studied by CD spectroscopy. To the estimate conformational transition of the peptide under membrane-mimicking conditions, spectra were obtained either in a buffer alone or one containing anionic SDS micelles. Samples were prepared in 5 mM sodium phosphate buffer (pH 7.5) with 100 mM NaF. Peptide and detergent solutions were mixed, giving final peptide and sodium dodecyl sulfate (SDS) concentrations of 87 µM and 30 mM (P:D ≈ 1:350) and incubated for 1 h at room temperature before the data collection. Circular dichroism spectra were acquired on a Chirascan instrument (Applied Photophysics, Leatherhead, Surrey, UK) in the range 190–250 nm with a 1 nm step size and bandwidth at a 1 s per nm scan rate. The spectra were averaged over five measurements, converted to Δε units and analyzed using the BeStSel web server [24,25].

4.4. Antimicrobial Assay

To compare the antimicrobial activity of Ar-1, its modification Ar-1-(C/A) and Ar-2, we used the radial diffusion assay that identifies the antimicrobial activity in the solid medium [39]. For the experiment, the log-phase cultures of *Escherichia coli* ML-35p and *Listeria monocytogenes* EGD were prepared in 3% tryptone soya broth (TSB) at 37 °C for 2.5 h. After this incubation, bacteria were centrifuged at 760× *g* for 12 min at 4 °C to purify them from the medium, then they were washed in 10 mM sodium phosphate buffer (pH 7.4) and centrifuged in the same conditions. After this preparation, bacteria were mixed with warm (43 °C) melted 1% agarose to a final concentration of 4×10^5 CFU/mL. This suspension was poured in Petri dishes and they were left till the agarose became solid. Several wells were cut in this solid agarose layer (4 mm), then peptides were added to these wells at concentrations of 64, 32, 16, 8 and 4 µM. After a 2 h incubation at 37 °C, the mixture of 1% melted agarose and 6% TSB was added onto the Petri dishes to form another layer with nutrients. Three independent experiments were performed.

After the overnight incubation, the diameters of the wells and the zones of growth inhibition were measured. The antimicrobial activity (AMA) was counted as:

$$AMA = (D - d) \times 10$$

where "D" is the diameter of the zone of inhibition, "d" is the diameter of the well. Minimal inhibitory concentration (MIC) was measured using the dependence of AMA on a peptide concentration, where lg[$C_{peptide}$] is its decimal logarithm. Using a linear regression method, a line was drawn through the points, and the intersection point of this line with the abscissa axis was found. The concentration value for this point was taken as the MIC.

4.5. Hemolytic Activity of Peptides

For the evaluation of hemolytic activity, fresh human erythrocytes (E^{hum}) were used at a final concentration of 1.25%. They were mixed with the peptides that were diluted consistently in PBS. The final concentrations of each peptide were 100, 25, 5 and 1 µg/mL. These samples were incubated for 30 min at 37 °C. The reaction was stopped by the addition of ice-cold PBS in a ratio of 4:1. Then the samples were centrifuged at 500× g for 5 min at room temperature. The optical density of the hemoglobin-containing supernatants was measured at 414 nm (OD_{414}). As a negative control, we used the sample with E^{hum} in PBS. As a positive control (100% hemolysis), we took the sample with the E^{hum} but the reaction was stopped by the addition of distilled water instead of PBS.

Hemolytic activity was calculated as:

$$(OD_{414(sample)} - OD_{414(neg.contr.)}) \times 100\% / (OD_{414(pos.contr.)} - OD_{414(neg.contr.)})$$

The minimal hemolytic concentration (MHC) was the concentration of the peptide leading to 10% hemolysis. Three independent experiments were performed.

4.6. Complement Activation

The ability of peptides to modulate the human complement system was evaluated in hemolytic assay systems and by ELISA, as previously described [18], except that we slightly modified the buffer composition for the hemolytic assay in the model of the classical pathway activation and introduced a novel way for the analysis and visualization of results. For these purposes, we utilized coefficients for the evaluation of the hemolytic activity of complement (H) and of complement-dependent C3a accumulation (E). The hemolytic activity of serum in a sample was measured as

$$H = (OD_{414(sample)} - OD_{414(control)}) / OD_{414(control)}$$

The control was a sample with no peptides added. H values above zero indicate augmentation of complement-mediated hemolysis, while H values below zero mean inhibition. H = −1 corresponds to the complete inhibition of complement-mediated hemolysis and H = 1 corresponds to its two-fold augmentation. The alterations in C3a accumulation were expressed as

$$E = (OD_{450(sample)} - OD_{450(control)}) / OD_{450(control)}$$

As the control, a sample with no peptides added was used. As with the H coefficient, E values above zero indicate an increase in C3a accumulation and E values below zero show a decrease in C3a accumulation. E = −1 corresponds to abolished C3a generation. In practice, reaching this value seems elusive as a small amount of C3a pre-exists in serum due to the spontaneous complement activation. E = 1 corresponds to the two-fold augmentation of C3a accumulation.

4.7. Statistical Analysis

Statistical analysis was done using the R language (v4.0.2) in an RStudio environment (R Core Team, R Foundation for Statistical Computing, Vienna, Austria). The significance of H- and E-indexes' deviation from zero was evaluated by a one-sample t-test. The experiments on complement modulation were performed at least five times for each of the peptides. For both hemolytic and ELISA assays, p-values less than 0.05 were considered statistically significant. To confirm the link between hemolysis and complement activation, the Pearson correlation coefficient was used. The *p*-values less than 0.05 were considered statistically significant. The plots were drawn using the R language with ggplot2 (v3.3.2) and ggpubr (v.0.4.0) packages.

Author Contributions: M.N.B. and E.S.U. conceived and designed this study; V.A.P. and A.S.K. synthesized and purified the peptide Ar-1-(C/A), Y.A.D. provided mass spectrometry of this peptide and interpreted the MS results, I.E.E. obtained the CD spectrum of Ar-1-(C/A) and calculated the structure's parameters; P.V.P. and S.V.B. synthesized and purified peptides arenicin-1 and -2 for our experiments; N.P.G. developed the ELISA system for C3a and helped to interpret the data; E.S.U. and I.A.K. performed the experiments, analyzed the data and wrote the paper with M.N.B.; T.V.O. and O.V.S. analyzed all the experimental data, revised the manuscript critically and prepared it for publication. All authors contributed to manuscript preparation and approved the presented data. All authors have read and agreed to the published version of the manuscript.

Funding: This work was partially supported by the Russian Foundation for Basic Research (RFBR project No. 18-54-80026). The investigations provided by I.E.E. were supported by the Ministry of Science and Higher Education of the Russian Federation (project 0791-2020-0006).

Acknowledgments: We thank M.M. Firulyova for her help in preparation of graphs.

Conflicts of Interest: The authors declare no conflict of interest.

References

1. Niyonsaba, F.; Hirata, M.; Ogawa, H.; Nagaoka, I. Epithelial cell-derived antibacterial peptides human beta-defensins and cathelicidin: Multifunctional activities on mast cells. *Curr. Drug Targets Inflamm. Allergy* **2003**, *2*, 224–231. [CrossRef] [PubMed]
2. Yang, D.; Chertov, O.; Bykovskaia, S.N.; Chen, Q.; Buffo, M.J.; Shogan, J.; Anderson, M.; Schröder, M.J.; Wang, M.; Howard, O.M.Z.; et al. β-Defensins: Linking innate and adaptive immunity through dendritic and T cell CCR6. *Science* **1999**, *286*, 525–528. [CrossRef] [PubMed]
3. Yang, D.; Chen, Q.; Chertov, O.; Oppenheim, J.J. Human neutrophil defensins selectively chemoattract naive T and immature dendritic cells. *J. Leukoc. Biol.* **2000**, *68*, 9–14. [CrossRef]
4. Territo, M.C.; Ganz, T.; Selsted, M.E.; Lehrer, R. Monocyte-chemotactic activity of defensins from human neutrophils. *J. Clin. Investig.* **1989**, *84*, 2017–2020. [CrossRef] [PubMed]
5. Chavakis, T.; Cines, D.B.; Rhee, J.-S.; Liang, O.D.; Schubert, U.; Hammes, H.-P.; Higazi, A.A.-R.; Nawroth, P.P.; Preissner, K.T.; Bdeiret, K. Regulation of neovascularization by human neutrophil peptides (α-defensins): A link between inflammation and angiogenesis. *FASEB J.* **2004**, *18*, 1306–1308. [CrossRef]
6. Oono, T.; Shirafuji, Y.; Huh, W.K.; Akiyama, H.; Iwatsuki, K. Effects of human neutrophil peptide-1 on the expression of interstitial collagenase and type I collagen in human dermal fibroblasts. *Arch. Dermatol. Res.* **2002**, *294*, 185–189. [CrossRef]
7. Umnyakova, E.S.; Zharkova, M.S.; Berlov, M.N.; Shamova, O.V.; Kokryakov, V.N. Human antimicrobial peptides in autoimmunity. *Autoimmunity* **2020**, *53*, 137–147. [CrossRef] [PubMed]
8. Zharkova, M.S.; Orlov, D.S.; Golubeva, O.Y.; Chakchir, O.B.; Eliseev, I.E.; Grinchuk, T.M.; Shamova, O.V. Application of antimicrobial peptides of the innate immune system in combination with conventional antibiotics-a novel way to combat antibiotic resistance? *Front. Cell Infect. Microbiol.* **2019**, *9*, 128. [CrossRef] [PubMed]
9. Mahlapuu, M.; Håkansson, J.; Ringstad, L.; Björn, C. Antimicrobial peptides: An emerging category of therapeutic agents. *Front. Cell Infect. Microbiol.* **2016**, *6*, 1–12. [CrossRef]
10. Umnyakova, E.S.; Kudryavtsev, I.V.; Grudinina, N.A.; Balandin, S.V.; Bolosov, I.A.; Panteleev, P.V.; Filatenkova, T.A.; Orlov, D.S.; Tsvetkova, E.V.; Ovchinnikova, T.V.; et al. Internalization of antimicrobial peptide acipensin 1 into human tumor cells. *Med. Immunol.* **2016**, *18*, 575–582. [CrossRef]
11. Chessa, C.; Bodet, C.; Jousselin, C.; Wehbe, M.; Lévêque, N.; Garcia, M. Antiviral and immunomodulatory properties of antimicrobial peptides produced by human keratinocytes. *Front. Microbiol.* **2020**, *11*, 1155. [CrossRef] [PubMed]
12. Prohászka, Z.; Német, K.; Csermely, P.; Hudecz, F.; Mezõ, G.; Füst, G. Defensins purified from human granulocytes bind c1q and activate the classical complement pathway like the transmembrane glycoprotein gp41 of HIV-1. *Mol. Immunol.* **1997**, *34*, 809–816. [CrossRef]

13. van den Berg, R.H.; Faber-Krol, M.C.; van Wetering, S.; Hiemstra, P.S.; Daha, M.R. Inhibition of activation of the classical pathway of complement by human neutrophil defensins. *Blood* **1998**, *92*, 3898–3903. [CrossRef] [PubMed]
14. Groeneveld, T.W.L.; Ramwadhdoebé, T.H.; Trouw, L.A.; van den Ham, D.L.; van der Borden, V.; Drijfhout, J.W.; Hiemstra, P.S.; Daha, M.R.; Roos, A. Human neutrophil peptide-1 inhibits both the classical and the lectin pathway of complement activation. *Mol. Immunol.* **2007**, *44*, 3608–3614. [CrossRef]
15. Panyutich, A.V.; Szold, O.; Poon, P.H.; Tseng, Y.; Ganz, T. Identification of defensin binding to C1 complement. *FEBS Lett.* **1994**, *356*, 169–173. [CrossRef]
16. Chen, J.; Xu, X.-M.; Underhill, C.B.; Yang, S.; Wang, L. Tachyplesin activates the classical complement pathway to kill tumor cells. *Cancer Res.* **2005**, *65*, 4614–4622. [CrossRef]
17. Berlov, M.N.; Umnyakova, E.S.; Leonova, T.S.; Milman, B.L.; Krasnodembskaya, A.D.; Ovchinnikova, T.V.; Kokryakov, V.N. Interaction of arenicin-1 with C1q protein. *Russ. J. Bioorganic. Chem.* **2015**, *41*, 597–601. [CrossRef]
18. Umnyakova, E.S.; Gorbunov, N.P.; Zhakhov, A.V.; Krenev, I.A.; Ovchinnikova, T.V.; Kokryakov, V.N.; Berlov, M.N. Modulation of human complement system by antimicrobial peptide arenicin-1 from Arenicola marina. *Mar. Drugs* **2018**, *16*, 480. [CrossRef]
19. Merle, N.S.; Church, S.E.; Fremeaux-Bacchi, V.; Roumenina, L.T. Complement system part I—Molecular mechanisms of activation and regulation. *Front. Immunol.* **2015**, *6*, 262. [CrossRef]
20. Schröder-Braunstein, J.; Kirschfink, M. Complement deficiencies and dysregulation: Pathophysiological consequences, modern analysis, and clinical management. *Mol. Immunol.* **2019**, *114*, 299–311. [CrossRef]
21. Ovchinnikova, T.V.; Aleshina, G.M.; Balandin, S.V.; Krasnodembskaya, A.D.; Markelov, M.L.; Frolova, E.I.; Leonova, Y.F.; Tagaev, A.A.; Krasnodembsky, E.G.; Kokryakov, V.N. Purification and primary structure of two isoforms of arenicin, a novel antimicrobial peptide from marine polychaeta Arenicola marina. *FEBS Lett.* **2004**, *577*, 209–214. [CrossRef] [PubMed]
22. Berlov, M.N.; Maltseva, A.L. Immunity of the lugworm Arenicola marina: Cells and molecules. *Invertebr. Surviv. J.* **2016**, *13*, 247–256. [CrossRef]
23. Panteleev, P.V.; Bolosov, I.A.; Balandin, S.V.; Ovchinnikova, T.V. Design of antimicrobial peptide arenicin analogs with improved therapeutic indices. *J. Pep. Sci.* **2014**, *21*, 105–113. [CrossRef] [PubMed]
24. Ovchinnikova, T.V.; Shenkarev, Z.O.; Nadezhdin, K.D.; Balandin, S.V.; Zhmak, M.N.; Kudelina, I.A.; Finkina, E.I.; Arseniev, A.S. Recombinant expression, synthesis, purification, and solution structure of arenicin. *Biochem. Biophys. Res. Commun.* **2007**, *360*, 156–162. [CrossRef] [PubMed]
25. Shenkarev, Z.O.; Balandin, S.V.; Trunov, K.I.; Paramonov, A.S.; Sukhanov, S.V.; Barsukov, L.I.; Arseniev, A.S.; Ovchinnikova, T.V. Molecular mechanism of action of β-Hairpin antimicrobial peptide arenicin: Oligomeric structure in dodecylphosphocholine micelles and pore formation in planar lipid bilayers. *Biochemistry* **2011**, *50*, 6255–6265. [CrossRef] [PubMed]
26. Panteleev, P.V.; Myshkin, M.Y.; Shenkarev, Z.O.; Ovchinnikova, T.V. Dimerization of the antimicrobial peptide arenicin plays a key role in the cytotoxicity but not in the antibacterial activity. *Biochem. Biophys. Res. Commun.* **2017**, *482*, 1320–1326. [CrossRef]
27. Micsonai, A.; Wien, F.; Kernya, L.; Lee, Y.H.; Goto, Y.; Réfrégiers, M.; Kardos, J. Accurate secondary structure prediction and fold recognition for circular dichroism spectroscopy. *Proc. Natl. Acad. Sci. USA* **2015**, *112*, E3095–E3103. [CrossRef]
28. Micsonai, A.; Wien, F.; Bulyáki, É.; Kun, J.; Moussong, É.; Lee, Y.H.; Goto, Y.; Réfrégiers, M.; Kardos, J. BeStSel: A web server for accurate protein secondary structure prediction and fold recognition from the circular dichroism spectra. *Nucleic Acids Res.* **2018**, *46*, W315–W322. [CrossRef]

29. Orlov, D.S.; Shamova, O.V.; Eliseev, I.E.; Zharkova, M.S.; Chakchir, O.B.; Antcheva, N.; Zachariev, S.; Panteleev, P.V.; Kokryakov, V.N.; Ovchinnikova, T.V.; et al. Redesigning arenicin-1, an antimicrobial peptide from the marine polychaeta *Arenicola marina*, by strand rearrangement or branching, substitution of specific residues, and backbone linearization or cyclization. *Mar. Drugs* **2019**, *17*, 376. [CrossRef]
30. Ovchinnikova, T.V.; Shenkarev, Z.O.; Balandin, S.V.; Nadezhdin, K.D.; Paramonov, A.S.; Arseniev, A.S.; Kokryakov, V.N. Molecular insight into mechanism of antimicrobial action of the β-hairpin peptide arenicin: Specific oligomerization in detergent micelles. *Biopolymers* **2008**, *89*, 455–464. [CrossRef]
31. Lee, J.-U.; Kang, D.-I.; Zhu, W.L.; Shin, S.Y.; Hahm, K.-S.; Kim, Y. Solution structures and biological functions of the antimicrobial peptide, arenicin-1, and its linear derivative. *Pept. Sci.* **2006**, *88*, 208–216. [CrossRef] [PubMed]
32. Andrä, J.; Jakovkin, I.; Grötzinger, J.; Hecht, O.; Krasnosdembskaya, A.D.; Goldmann, T.; Thomas Gutsmann, T.; Leippe, M.; Andrä, J. Structure and mode of action of the antimicrobial peptide arenicin. *Biochem. J.* **2008**, *410*, 113–122. [CrossRef] [PubMed]
33. Umnyakova, E.S.; Krenev, I.A.; Legkovoy, S.V.; Sokolov, A.V.; Rogacheva, O.N.; Ovchinnikova, T.V.; Kokryakov, V.N.; Berlov, M.N. The interaction of arenicin-1 with C3b complement protein. *Med. Acad. J.* **2019**, *19*, 187–188. [CrossRef]
34. Capila, I.; Linhardt, J.R. Heparin-protein interactions. *Angew. Chem. Int. Ed.* **2002**, *41*, 390–412. [CrossRef]
35. Yu, H.; Muñoz, E.M.; Edens, R.E.; Linhardt, R.J. Heparin regulation of the complement system. *Chem. Biol. Heparin Heparan Sulfate* **2005**, 313–343. [CrossRef]
36. Zaferani, A.; Talsma, D.; Richter, M.K.S.; Daha, M.R.; Navis, G.J.; Seelen, M.A.; van den Born, J. Heparin/heparan sulphate interactions with complement—A possible target for reduction of renal function loss? *Nephrol. Dial. Transplant.* **2014**, *29*, 515–522. [CrossRef]
37. Khandelwal, S.; Johnson, A.M.; Liu, J.; Keire, D.; Sommers, C.; Ravi, J.; Lee, G.M.; Lambris, J.D.; Reis, E.S.; Arepally, G.M. Novel Immunoassay for Complement Activation by PF4/Heparin Complexes. *Thromb. Haemost.* **2018**, *118*, 1484–1487. [CrossRef]
38. Ricklin, D.; Lambris, J.D. Complement in immune and inflammatory disorders: Pathophysiological mechanisms. *J. Immunol.* **2013**, *190*, 3831–3838. [CrossRef]
39. Lehrer, R.I.; Rosenman, M.; Harwig, S.S.; Jackson, R.; Eisenhauer, P. Ultrasensitive assays for endogenous antimicrobial polypeptides. *J. Immunol. Methods* **1991**, *137*, 167–173. [CrossRef]

Publisher's Note: MDPI stays neutral with regard to jurisdictional claims in published maps and institutional affiliations.

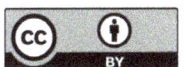

© 2020 by the authors. Licensee MDPI, Basel, Switzerland. This article is an open access article distributed under the terms and conditions of the Creative Commons Attribution (CC BY) license (http://creativecommons.org/licenses/by/4.0/).

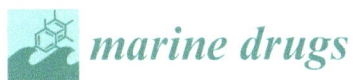 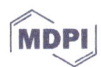

Article

Antioxidant Peptides from the Protein Hydrolysate of Spanish Mackerel (*Scomberomorous niphonius*) Muscle by in Vitro Gastrointestinal Digestion and Their In Vitro Activities

Guo-Xu Zhao [1], Xiu-Rong Yang [1], Yu-Mei Wang [2], Yu-Qin Zhao [2], Chang-Feng Chi [1,*] and Bin Wang [2,*]

1. National and Provincial Joint Laboratory of Exploration and Utilization of Marine Aquatic Genetic Resources, National Engineering Research Center of Marine Facilities Aquaculture, School of Marine Science and Technology, Zhejiang Ocean University, Zhoushan 316022, China; xuzhao1109@sina.com (G.-X.Z.); yxr1948008999@163.com (X.-R.Y.)
2. Zhejiang Provincial Engineering Technology Research Center of Marine Biomedical Products, School of Food and Pharmacy, Zhejiang Ocean University, Zhoushan 316022, China; wangym731@126.com (Y.-M.W.); zhaoy@hotmail.com (Y.-Q.Z.)
* Correspondence: chichangfeng@hotmail.com (C.-F.C.); wangbin4159@hotmail.com (B.W.); Tel./Fax: +86-580-255-4818 (C.-F.C.); +86-580-255-4781 (B.W.)

Received: 9 August 2019; Accepted: 11 September 2019; Published: 12 September 2019

Abstract: For the full use of Spanish mackerel (*Scomberomorous niphonius*) muscle to produce antioxidant peptides, the proteins of Spanish mackerel muscle were separately hydrolyzed under five kinds of enzymes and in vitro gastrointestinal digestion, and antioxidant peptides were isolated from the protein hydrolysate using ultrafiltration and multiple chromatography methods. The results showed that the hydrolysate (SMPH) prepared using in vitro GI digestion showed the highest degree of hydrolysis (27.45 ± 1.76%) and DPPH radical scavenging activity (52.58 ± 2.68%) at the concentration of 10 mg protein/mL among the six protein hydrolysates, and 12 peptides (SMP-1 to SMP-12) were prepared from SMPH. Among them, SMP-3, SMP-7, SMP-10, and SMP-11 showed the higher DPPH radical scavenging activities and were identified as Pro-Glu-Leu-Asp-Trp (PELDW), Trp-Pro-Asp-His-Trp (WPDHW), and Phe-Gly-Tyr-Asp-Trp-Trp (FGYDWW), and Tyr-Leu-His-Phe-Trp (YLHFW), respectively. PELDW, WPDHW, FGYDWW, and YLHFW showed high scavenging activities on DPPH radical (EC_{50} 1.53, 0.70, 0.53, and 0.97 mg/mL, respectively), hydroxyl radical (EC_{50} 1.12, 0.38, 0.26, and 0.67 mg/mL, respectively), and superoxide anion radical (EC_{50} 0.85, 0.49, 0.34, and 1.37 mg/mL, respectively). Moreover, PELDW, WPDHW, FGYDWW, and YLHFW could dose-dependently inhibit lipid peroxidation in the linoleic acid model system and protect plasmid DNA (pBR322DNA) against oxidative damage induced by H_2O_2 in the tested model systems. In addition, PELDW, WPDHW, FGYDWW, and YLHFW could retain their high activities when they were treated under a low temperature (<60 °C) and a moderate pH environment (pH 5–9). These present results indicate that the protein hydrolysate, fractions, and isolated peptides from Spanish mackerel muscle have strong antioxidant activity and might have the potential to be used in health food products.

Keywords: Spanish mackerel (*Scomberomorous niphonius*); muscle; peptide; antioxidant activity; stability

1. Introduction

Food nutrition is intricately linked with human health because they can provide the necessary bioactive substances and cause specific physiological responses in the human body [1]. Among all the biological nutrients, food proteins, hydrolysates, and peptides are believed to the most well researched biomolecules [1,2]. Bioactive peptides are encrypted in the protein sequences and released by the hydrolysis action of proteases or fermentation [3,4]. Over the last decade, there has been an explosion of scientific research on the topic of bioactive peptides, which display a broad scope of functions beyond basic nutritional benefits, such as antioxidant, immunomodulatory, antihypertensive, metal-chelation, cytomodulatory, antimicrobial, antithrombotic, and opiate activities [1,5,6]. Therefore, bioactive peptides have attracted a high amount of interest from researchers and consumers because of their huge potential of serving as functional components applied in foods and other dietary supplements [3,7].

Recently, antioxidant peptides (APs) from food resources, especially from aquatic products and their byproducts, have caused widespread attention because of their safety and strong capacities in regard to reactive oxygen species (ROS) scavenging, DNA protection, and lipid peroxidation inhibition [3,8–10]. Moreover, seafood-derived APs could upregulate the level of intracellular antioxidant enzymes, such as superoxide dismutase (SOD), catalase (CAT), glutathione (GSH) peroxidase (GSH-Px), and GSH reductase (GSH-Rx), to protect cells and organism from the damage of oxidative stress [3,11,12]. YGDEY isolated from the gelatin hydrolysate of tilapia skin could effectively prevent UVB-induced photoaging in human keratinocytes (HaCaT) cells through decreasing levels of intracellular ROS, MMP-1 (collagenase), and MMP-9 (gelatinase), increasing antioxidant factor (SOD and GSH) expression and type I procollagen production, maintaining a balance between GSH and GSSG, and preventing DNA from oxidative damage [13]. You et al. reported that loach peptide (500 < MW < 1000 Da) prepared using flavorzyme digestion could effectively increase the swimming time of mice and decrease levels of blood urea nitrogen (BUN) and liver malonaldehyde (MDA) in mice [14]. Himaya et al. reported that GGFDMG from the gelatin hydrolysate of Japanese flounder skin could protect leukemia cells in mouse macrophage (RAW 264.7) from ROS-mediated intracellular macromolecule damage through scavenging intracellular ROS by upregulating the expression levels of inherent antioxidative factors (SOD-1, GSH, and CAT) [15]. Lin et al. indicated that the gill hydrolysate of bighead carp had high Fe^{2+}-chelating and 2,2-diphenyl-1-picrylhydrazyl (DPPH) radical (DPPH·) scavenging activity. In addition, surimi with the gill hydrolysate had greater Ca^{2+}-ATPase activity, higher salt-soluble and sulfhydryl protein concentrations, lower disulfide bonds, carbonyls, and hydrophobicity, as well as better gel strength and texture [16]. Therefore, APs from food resources, especially from seafoods and their byproducts, have huge potential for use in functional foods and other dietary interventions of food preservation, disease control, and health promotion.

Spanish mackerel (*Scomberomorous niphonius*) is a subset of the mackerel family (Scombridae) and distributed in the Western North Pacific, including the East China Sea, the Yellow Sea, and the Bohai Sea of China. Recently, some bioactive ingredients have been prepared and identified from the skins and bones of Spanish mackerel [17]. Li et al. isolated acid and pepsin soluble collagens from Spanish mackerel skins and bones and characterized them as type I collagen [17]. Subsequently, the skin collagen hydrolysate and fractions of Spanish mackerel were prepared, and they showed strong antioxidant activities [18]. In addition, eight APs including GPY, GPTGE, PFGPD, GPTGAKG, PYGAKG, GATGPQG, GPFGPM, and YGPM were isolated from the skin collagen hydrolysate fraction (F7) [6]. Among them, PFGPD, PYGAKG, and YGPM could effectively inhibit lipid peroxidation, reduce Fe^{3+} to Fe^{2+}, and scavenge DPPH·, hydroxyl radical (HO·), superoxide anion radical (O_2^-·), and 2,2′-azino-bis(3-ethylbenzothiazoline-6-sulphonic acid) (ABTS) cation radical in a concentration-activity manner. However, no literature regarding APs from Spanish mackerel muscle has been reported. Thus, the objectives of this paper are to (i) isolate and characterize APs from protein hydrolysate of Spanish mackerel muscle by in vitro gastrointestinal (GI) digestion and (ii) evaluate the in vitro antioxidant and stability properties of the isolated APs.

2. Results and Discussion

2.1. Preparation of Protein Hydrolysate of Spanish Mackerel (S. niphonius) Muscle

The defatted Spanish mackerel muscles were separately hydrolyzed under five kinds of enzymes and in vitro GI digestion (pepsin-trypsin system). As shown in Table 1, the protein hydrolysate (SMPH) prepared using in vitro GI digestion showed the highest degree of hydrolysis (DH, 27.45 ± 1.76%) among the six protein hydrolysates. Similarly, DPPH· scavenging activity of SMPH (52.58 ± 2.68%) was significantly higher than those of the crude protein of defatted muscle (SMP) (14.26 ± 1.03%) and protein hydrolysates using pepsin (27.64 ± 1.48%), neutrase (34.28 ± 1.37%), papain (25.98 ± 1.55%), trypsin (32.96 ± 2.33%), and alcalase (41.53 ± 3.41%), respectively ($p < 0.05$).

Table 1. Degree of hydrolysis (%) and DPPH· scavenging activity (%) of protein hydrolysate of Spanish mackerel (S. niphonius) muscle using five kinds of enzymes and in vitro GI digestion.

Protease	Degree of Hydrolysis (%)	DPPH· Scavenging Activity (10.0 mg protein/mL, %)
Pepsin	16.58 ± 0.94 [a]	27.64 ± 1.48 [a]
Neutrase	20.48 ± 1.62 [b]	34.28 ± 1.37 [b]
Papain	17.29 ± 0.48 [a]	25.98 ± 1.55 [a]
Trypsin	20.12 ± 1.15 [b]	32.96 ± 2.33 [b]
Alcalase	23.47 ± 1.51 [c]	41.53 ± 3.41 [c]
in vitro gastrointestinal digestion	26.58 ± 1.25 [d]	52.58 ± 2.68 [d]

All data are presented as the mean ± standard deviation (SD, n = 3). [a–c] Values with the same letters in each column indicate no significant difference ($p > 0.05$).

The specificity of the protease applied for the hydrolysis process is the key factor for the production of APs because the protein hydrolysates displayed very different spectra of substrate specificity, such as DH, biological activity, and nutritive values [3]. Wang et al. reported that the neutrase hydrolysate of blue mussel (*Mytilus edulis*) protein showed the highest DPPH· scavenging activity compared to the hydrolysates prepared using alcalase, neutrase, pepsin, and papain [9]. Agrawal et al. reported that the DH (17.47 ± 0.63%) of trypsin hydrolysate of finger millet protein was higher than that of the pepsin hydrolysate (13.73 ± 0.18%) [19]. The EC_{50} value (0.945 mg/mL) of papain hydrolysate of purple sea urchin (*Strongylocentrotus nudus*) gonad on DPPH· was significantly higher than those of trypsin (1.699 mg/mL) and dual-enzymatic (papain + trypsin) hydrolysates (2.481 mg/mL) [20]. Fish gelatin hydrolysate (FSGH) of Nile tilapia skin using ginger protease exhibited higher DH (13.08%), lipid peroxidation (48.46%), and DPPH· scavenging activity (97.21%) than hydrolysate using pepsin-pancreatin did [21]. Therefore, the protein hydrolysate (SMPH) of Spanish mackerel muscles prepared using in vitro GI digestion showed the highest DH and DPPH· scavenging activity and was chosen for further experiment.

2.2. Purification of APs from SMPH

2.2.1. Fractionation of SMPH Using Membrane Ultrafiltration

SMPH was fractionated gradually by molecular weight (MW) Cut Off (MWCO) membranes of 3, 5, and 10 kDa, and four fractions including SMPH-I (MW < 3 kDa), SMPH-II (3 kDa < MW < 5 kDa), SMPH-III (5 kDa < MW < 10 kDa), and SMPH-II (>10 kDa) were prepared. As shown in Figure 1, DPPH· scavenging activity of SMPH-I was 68.24 ± 3.29% at the concentration of 10.0 mg protein/mL, and this was significantly higher than those of SMP (14.26 ± 1.03%), SMPH (52.58 ± 2.68%), SMPH-II (44.68 ± 3.65%), SMPH-III (28.74 ± 1.41%), and SMPH-IV (21.62 ± 1.52%), respectively ($p < 0.05$). The differences in the activities among SMPH and its fractions are mainly because of the chain length, and the amino acid composition and sequence, which led to the diversity in the mechanisms of action [3]. The data agreed with the reports that the MW distribution of protein hydrolysates was negative relative to their antioxidant activity [18,22]. In addition, the lowest MW fractions from protein hydrolysates of blue-spotted stingray [23], buffalo and bovine casein [24], and *Tergillarca granosa* [25] showed the highest antioxidant activity. Therefore, SMPH-I with small MW was selected for the subsequent separation.

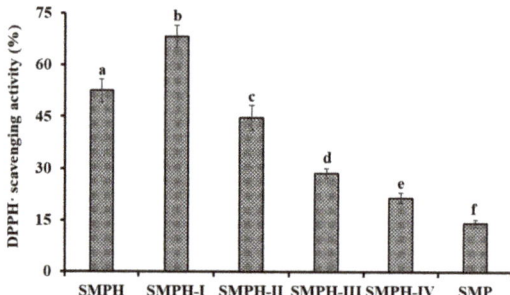

Figure 1. DPPH· scavenging activity of SMPH and its fractions by ultrafiltration at the concentration of 10.0 mg protein/mL. All data are presented as the mean ± SD (n = 3). $^{a-e}$ Values with the same superscripts indicate no significant difference ($p > 0.05$).

2.2.2. Anion-Exchange Chromatography of SMPH-I

According to the interaction strength between DEAE-52 cellulose and the hydrophobic/acidic amino acid residues in peptide sequences, five fractions (SMPH-I-1 to SMPH-I-5) were separated from SMPH-I fraction (Figure 2A). Amongst those fractions, SMPH-I-1 was eluted using deionized water (DW), SMPH-I-2 and SMPH-I-3 were eluted using 0.1 M NaCl, SMPH-I-4 was eluted using 0.5 M NaCl, and SMPH-I-5 was eluted using 1.0 M NaCl. DPPH· scavenging activities of SMPH-I and five fractions are shown in Figure 2B, and the data indicate that the DPPH· scavenging activity of SMPH-I-3 was 82.29 ± 4.37% at the concentration of 10.0 mg protein/mL, which was significantly higher than those of SMP (14.26 ± 1.03%), SMPH-I (68.24 ± 3.28%), SMPH-I-1 (26.35 ± 1.67%), SMPH-I-2 (49.43 ± 3.25%), SMPH-I-4 (73.11 ± 2.98%), and SMPH-I-5 (37.21 ± 1.69%), respectively ($p < 0.05$). Therefore, SMPH-I-3 was selected for the following experiment.

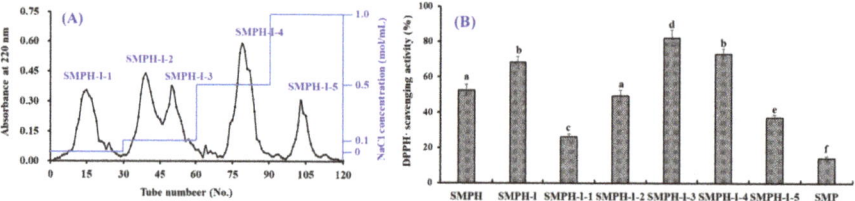

Figure 2. Elution profile of SMPH-I in DEAE-52 cellulose anion-exchange chromatography (A) and DPPH· scavenging activity of SMPH-I and its fractions at the concentration of 10.0 mg protein/mL (B). All data are presented as the mean ± SD (n = 3). $^{a-f}$ Values with the same superscripts of this type indicate no significant difference ($p > 0.05$).

2.2.3. Gel Filtration Chromatography of SMPH-I-3

APs separated by gel filtration depend on their molecular size, which does not directly influence their structures and bioactivities [3,6]. Therefore, gel filtration chromatography has become a popular method to concentrate and fractionate APs from different protein hydrolysates, such as croaker muscle [26], flounder fish [27], purple sea urchin gonad [20], hairtail muscle [28], and blue-spotted stingray [23]. As shown in Figure 3A, SMPH-I-3 was separated into three fractions (SMPH-I-3a,

SMPH-I-3b, and SMPH-I-3c) using a Sephadex G-25 column. Figure 3B indicates that the DPPH·
scavenging activity of SMPH-I-3c was 48.36 ± 2.28% at the concentration of 5.0 mg protein/mL,
which was significantly higher than those of SMP (8.57 ± 0.95%), SMPH-I (31.29 ± 2.05%), SMPH-I-3
(31.29 ± 2.05%), SMPH-I-3a (20.15 ± 0.98%), and SMPH-I-3a (35.24 ± 2.31%) ($p < 0.05$). Therefore,
SMPH-I-3c was selected for the following isolation process.

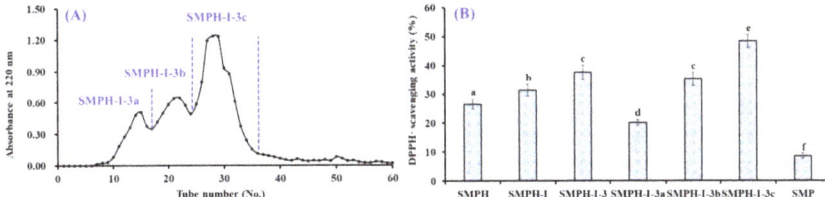

Figure 3. Elution profile of SMPH-I-3 in Sephadex G-25 chromatography (**A**) and DPPH· scavenging activities of SMPH-I-3 and its fractions at 5.0 mg protein/mL concentration (**B**). All data are presented as the mean ± SD of triplicate results. $^{a-f}$ Values with the same superscripts indicate no significant difference ($p > 0.05$).

2.2.4. Isolation of APs from SMPH-I-3c by RP-HPLC

As shown in Figure 4, 12 major peaks (SMP-1 to SMP-12) were isolated from SMPH-I-3c using
the RP-HPLC system on their retention time (RT), and their DPPH· scavenging activities are shown
in Figure 5. The data indicate that the DPPH· scavenging activities of SMP-3 (76.91 ± 2.36%), SMP-7
(81.09 ± 3.56%), SMP-10 (86.52 ± 4.06%), and SMP-11 (78.54 ± 3.55%) at the concentration of 5.0 mg
protein/mL were significantly higher than those of other eight APs. Therefore, SMP-3, SMP-7, SMP-10,
and SMP-11 with retention times of 11.02, 14.74, 17.58, and 19.83 min, respectively, were collected and
lyophilized for amino acid sequence identification and activity evaluation.

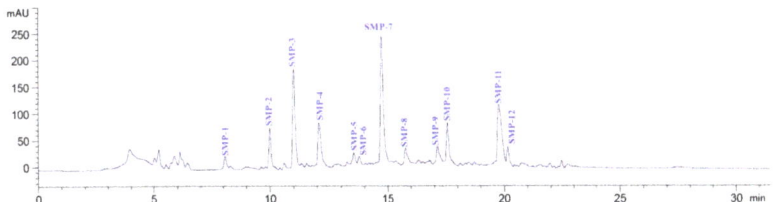

Figure 4. Elution profile of SMPH-I-3c separated by RP-HPLC system on a Zorbax, SB C-18 column (4.6 × 250 mm) from 0 to 30 min.

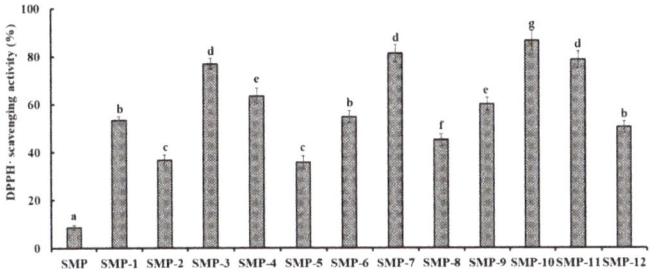

Figure 5. DPPH· scavenging activities of twelve major sub-fractions (SMP-1 to SMP-12) of SMPH-I-3c at the concentration of 5.0 mg protein/mL. All data are presented as the mean ± SD ($n = 3$). $^{a-g}$ Values with the same superscripts indicate no significant difference ($p > 0.05$).

2.3. Amino Acid Sequence and Molecular Mass Analysis of APs

The amino acid sequences and molecular mass of four APs (SMP-3, SMP-7, SMP-10, and SMP-11) were determined using a protein sequencer and a quadrupole time-of-flight mass spectrometer (MS) coupled with an electrospray ionization (ESI) source, and the results are shown in Table 2 and Figure 6. The amino acid sequences of four APs were identified as Pro-Glu-Leu-Asp-Trp (PELDW, SMP-3), Trp-Pro-Asp-His-Trp (WPDHW, SMP-7), Phe-Gly-Tyr-Asp-Trp-Trp (FGYDWW, SMP-10), and Tyr-Leu-His-Phe-Trp (YLHFW, SMP-11). The detected MWs of SMP-3, SMP-7, SMP-10, and SMP-11 agreed well with their theoretical masses (Table 2).

Table 2. Retention time, amino acid sequences, and molecular weights of four isolated peptides (SMP-3, SMP-7, SMP-10, and SMP-11) from protein hydrolysate of Spanish mackerel (*S. niphonius*) muscle.

No.	Retention Time (min)	Amino Acid Sequence	Theoretical Mass/Observed Mass (Da)
SMP-3	11.02	PELDW	658.70/658.72
SMP-7	14.74	WPDHW	739.78/739.81
SMP-10	17.58	FGYDWW	872.92/872.93
SMP-11	19.83	YLHFW	764.87/764.90

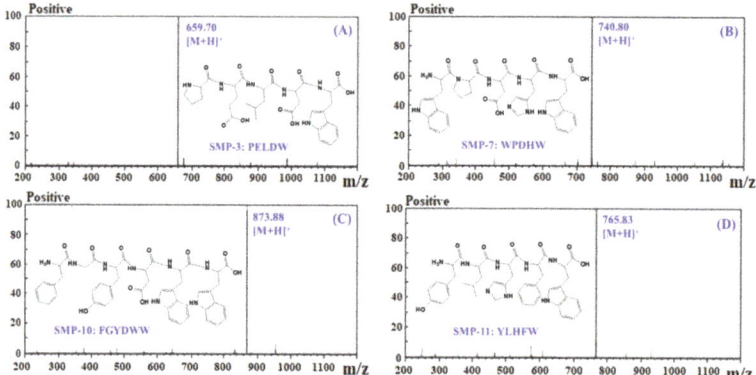

Figure 6. Mass spectra of four APs (SMP-3 (**A**), SMP-7 (**B**), SMP-10 (**C**), and SMP-11 (**D**)) from protein hydrolysate of Spanish mackerel (*S. niphonius*) muscle.

2.4. Antioxidant Activity

Three kinds of radical (DPPH·, HO·, and O_2^-·) scavenging, lipid peroxidation inhibition, and plasmid DNA protective assays were used to evaluate the activity of four APs (SMP-3, SMP-7, SMP-10, and SMP-11), and the results are presented in Table 3 and Figures 7–9.

Table 3. EC_{50} vales of four APs (SMP-3, SMP-7, SMP-10, and SMP-11) and the positive control of glutathione (GSH) on DPPH·, HO·, and O·.

No.	Half Elimination Ratio (EC_{50}, mg/mL)		
	DPPH·	HO·	O_2^-·
SMP3	1.53 ± 0.12 [a]	1.12 ± 0.09 [a]	0.85 ± 0.07 [a]
SMP7	0.70 ± 0.04 [b]	0.38 ± 0.02 [b]	0.49 ± 0.04 [b]
SMP10	0.53 ± 0.03 [c]	0.26 ± 0.02 [c]	0.34 ± 0.05 [c]
SMP11	0.97 ± 0.06 [d]	0.67 ± 0.05 [d]	1.37 ± 0.11 [d]
GSH	0.22 ± 0.01 [e]	0.12 ± 0.01 [e]	0.09 ± 0.01 [e]

All data are presented as the mean ± SD (n = 3). [a–f] Values with the same letters indicate no significant difference of different samples at the same radicals ($p > 0.05$).

2.4.1. Radical Scavenging Activity

DPPH· Scavenging Activity

As shown in Figure 7A, four APs (SMP-3, SMP-7, SMP-10, and SMP-11) could dose-dependently scavenge DPPH· when the concentration ranged from 0.25 to 10.0 mg/mL. The half elimination ratio (EC_{50}) values of SMP-3, SMP-7, SMP-10, and SMP-11 were 1.53, 0.70, 0.53, and 0.97 mg/mL, respectively, which were less effective than the positive control of GSH (0.22 mg/mL) ($p < 0.05$) (Table 3). The EC_{50} value of SMP-10 was significantly lower than those of SMP-3, SMP-7, SMP-11, and other APs from the protein hydrolysates of *Tergillarca granosa* muscle (MDLFTE: 0.53 mg/mL; WPPD: 0.36 mg/mL) [25], red stingray cartilages (IEPH: 1.90 mg/mL; LEEEE: 3.69 mg/mL; IEEEQ: 4.01 mg/mL; VPR: 4.61 mg/mL) [28], loach (PSYV: 17.0 mg/mL) [14], spotless smoothhound cartilages (GAERP: 3.73 mg/mL; GEREANVM: 1.87 mg/mL; AEVG: 2.30 mg/mL) [11], salmon pectoral fin (TTANIEDRR: 2.50 mg/mL) [29], Spanish mackerel skins (PFGPD: 0.80 mg/mL; PYGAKG: 3.02 mg/mL; YGPM: 0.72 mg/mL) [6], croceine croaker scales (GFRGTIGLVG: 1.271 mg/mL; GPAGPAG: 0.675 mg/mL) [30], *Sphyrna lewini* muscle (WDR: 3.63 mg/mL; PYFNK: 4.11 mg/mL) [31], and skipjack tuna bones (GADIVA: 0.57 mg/mL) [10]. Therefore, four APs (SMP-3, SMP-7, SMP-10, and SMP-11) could act as a contributor of electrons or hydrogen radicals to strongly inhibit the DPPH· reaction.

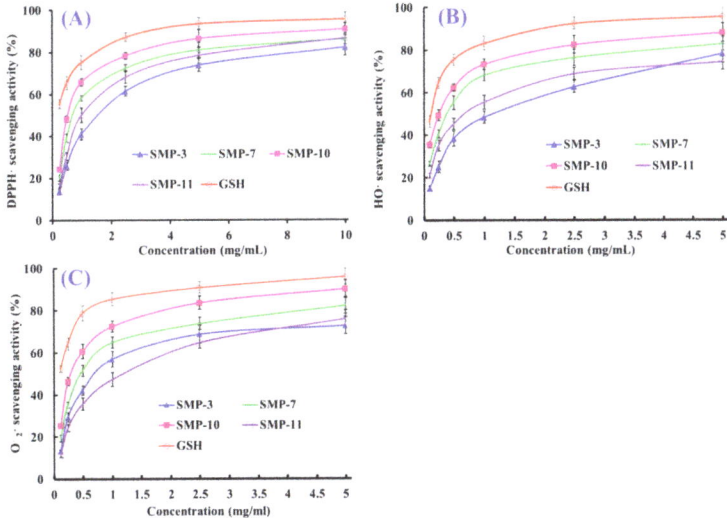

Figure 7. DPPH· (**A**), HO· (**B**), and $O_2^-·$ (**C**) scavenging activities of four APs (SMP-3, SMP-7, SMP-10, and SMP-11) from protein hydrolysate of Spanish mackerel (*S. niphonius*) muscle. Glutathione (GSH) was used as the positive control. All data are presented as the mean ± SD ($n = 3$).

HO· Scavenging Activity

The scavenging activities of SMP-3, SMP-7, SMP-10, and SMP-11 on HO· are presented in Figure 7B and Table 3. The data indicate that SMP-3, SMP-7, SMP-10, and SMP-11 could effectively scavenge HO· in a concentration-dependent manner. The EC_{50} value of SMP-10 was 0.26 mg/mL, which was significantly lower than those of SMP-3 (1.12 mg/mL), SMP-7 (0.38 mg/mL), and SMP-11 (0.67 mg/mL), respectively, but significantly higher than that of GSH (0.12 mg/mL). Moreover, the EC_{50} value of SMP-10 was less than those of APs from croceine croaker scales (GFRGTIGLVG: 0.29 mg/mL) [30], weatherfish loach (PSYV: 2.64 mg/mL) [14], hairtail muscle (KA: 1.74 mg/mL; AKG: 2.38 mg/mL; IYG: 2.50 mg/mL) [32], grass carp skin (PYSFK: 2.283mg/mL; VGGRP: 2.055 mg/mL) [33], red stingray cartilages (VPR: 0.77 mg/mL; IEPH: 0.46 mg/mL; LEEEE: 0.70 mg/mL; IEEEQ: 1.30 mg/mL) [28], bluefin leatherjacket heads (GPP: 2.385 mg/mL; WEGPK: 5.567 mg/mL; GVPLT: 4.149 mg/mL) [8], Spanish mackerel skins (PFGPD: 0.81 mg/mL, PYGAKG: 0.66 mg/mL, and YGPM: 0.88 mg/mL) [6], and spotless smoothhound cartilages (GEREANVM: 0.34 mg/mL) [11] and muscle (GVV: 1.63 mg/mL; GFVG: 0.89 mg/mL) [34]. Superfluous HO· generated from the decomposition of hydroperoxides have highly destructive effects on key biological macromolecules and cause serial chronic diseases related to oxidative stress in organisms [4,9]. The present results indicate that four APs (SMP-3, SMP-7, SMP-10, and SMP-11) might be used as HO· scavenging agent to help the organisms from the damage of oxidative stress.

O_2^-· Scavenging Activity

Figure 7C indicates the O_2^-· scavenging activities of four APs (SMP-3, SMP-7, SMP-10, and SMP-11) increased significantly when their concentrations increased from 0.125 to 5.0 mg/mL, but their activities were less than that of GSH at the same concentration. The EC_{50} values of SMP-3, SMP-7, SMP-10, and SMP-11 were 0.85, 0.49, 0.34, and 1.37 mg/mL, respectively. The EC_{50} value of SMP-10 was significantly less than those of SMP-3, SMP-7, SMP-11 and other APs from skipjack tuna bones (GADIVA: 0.52 mg/mL) [25], Spanish mackerel skins (PFGPD: 0.91 mg/mL; PYGAKG: 0.80 mg/mL; YGPM: 0.73 mg/mL) [6], giant squid (LNGLEGLA: 0.864 mg/mL; NGLEGLK: 0.419 mg/mL) [35], bluefin leatherjacket heads (WEGPK: 3.223 mg/mL; GPP: 4.668 mg/mL; GVPLT: 2.8819 mg/mL) [8], hairtail muscle (KA: 2.08 mg/mL; AKG: 2.54 mg/mL; IYG: 1.36 mg/mL) [32], miiuy croaker swim bladders (YLPYA:3.61 mg/mL; VPDDD:4.11 mg/mL) [4], spotless smoothhound muscle (GVV: 0.67 mg/mL) [34], and croceine croaker scales (GFRGTIGLVG: 0.46 mg/mL) [30] and muscle (VLYEE: 0.693 mg/mL; MILMR: 0.993 mg/mL) [36]. Under harmful environmental factors, such as pollutants, γ-radiation, cigarette smoke, and UV light, the organisms will generate excessive O_2^-· and further be translated into HO· and peroxy radicals, which will destroy cytomembrane and key biomolecules [2,37]. Then, SMP-3, SMP-7, SMP-10, and SMP-11 can assist SOD in scavenging excess O_2^-· in biological systems.

2.4.2. Lipid Peroxidation Inhibition Activity

The inhibiting abilities of SMP-3, SMP-7, SMP-10, and SMP-11 on the lipid peroxidation system were expressed as the absorbance of 500 nm, and the higher absorbance of the sample group illustrated lower antioxidant capacity [31]. Figure 8 shows that the absorbance of the SMP-10 group was significantly lower than those of SMP-3, SMP-7, SMP-11, and the negative control (without antioxidant), but slightly higher than that of the positive control of GSH. The data indicate that SMP-10 had the highest ability of lipid peroxidation inhibition among four APs.

The peroxidation of the membrane lipids caused by ROS can lead to cell injury and eventually unprogrammed apoptosis, and it is a crucial step in the pathogenesis of several disease states in adult and infant patients [38–40]. In addition, lipid peroxidation is also an important factor in high-fat food spoilage [28,36]. Therefore, the lipid peroxidation inhibition assay in the linoleic acid model system has been widely applied to evaluate the comprehensive ability of APs from seafoods, such as bluefin leatherjacket [8,36], miiuy croaker [4,7], red stingray [28], and monkfish [41]. SMP-10 can dramatically inhibit the peroxidation of linoleic acid over 7 days of incubation and has significant potential applications in food and medicine.

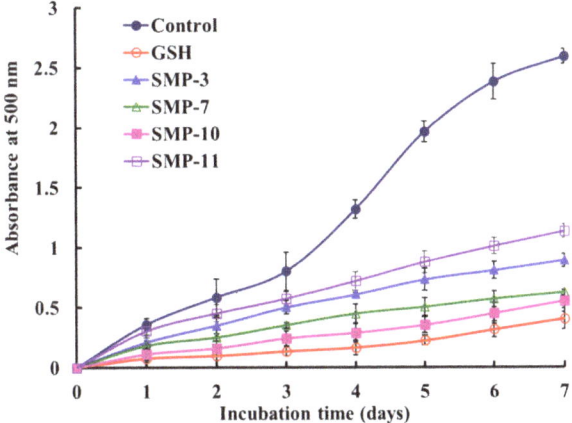

Figure 8. Lipid peroxidation inhibition activities of four APs (SMP-3, SMP-7, SMP-10, and SMP-11) from protein hydrolysate of Spanish mackerel (*S. niphonius*) muscle. Glutathione (GSH) was used as the positive control, and a solution without APs was used as the negative control. All data are presented as the mean ± SD ($n = 3$).

2.4.3. Protective Effect on Plasmid DNA Damaged by H_2O_2

In the assay, HO· was produced from the decomposition of H_2O_2 mediated by iron when $FeSO_4$ and H_2O_2 were added to the sample solutions, and the resulted HO· subsequently broke the supercoiled DNA and converted the supercoiled form into the open circular and/or linear form. Therefore, the protective effects of four APs (SMP-3, SMP-7, SMP-10, and SMP-11) on the oxidative damage of pBR322DNA induced by H_2O_2 were measured, and the results are shown in Figure 9. The results indicate that the plasmid DNA (pBR322DNA) was mainly of the supercoiled form under normal conditions (Figure 9A). An open circular form was generated when one phosphodiester chain of a supercoiled form of plasmid DNA was broken by HO· (Figure 9B). However, almost no linear form of DNA was found in Figure 9B, which indicates that the HO· produced from iron-mediated decomposition of H_2O_2 might be too little to break some double-strand of DNA in the assay. As shown in Figure 9C-E, the contents of the open circular form of DNA was obvious lower than that of Figure 9B, which indicates that four APs (SMP-3, SMP-7, SMP-10, and SMP-11) and the positive control of GSH have different protective effects on DNA damaged by oxidation, and the protective effect of SMP-10 was slightly higher than that of SMP-7 and significantly higher than those of SMP-3 and SMP-7. In addition, the image of SMP-10 and SMP-7 was similar to those of the positive control of GSH (Figure 9C) and the normal control (Figure 9A). Therefore, four APs (SMP-3, SMP-7, SMP-10, and SMP-11), especially SMP-10 and SMP-11, have high abilities to guard the supercoiled pBR322DNA against HO·-dependent strand breaks. In the organism, DNA damage is a key step in ROS-induced degenerative processes, such as premature aging, hepatopathy, and diabetes, cancer, atherosclerosis, and neurodegenerative diseases [42,43]. The present results indicate that SMP-10 had a potential ability to protect pBR322DNA from oxidative damage, and our future experiment will be performed on the cell and in vivo.

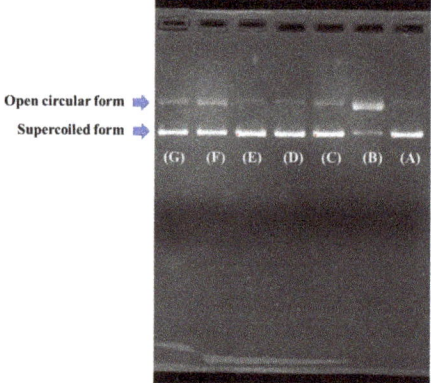

Figure 9. Protective effects of four APs (SMP-3, SMP-7, SMP-10, and SMP-11) on plasmid DNA damaged by H_2O_2. (**A**) The native pBR322DNA; (**B**) pBR322DNA treated with $FeSO_4$ and H_2O_2; (**C**) pBR322DNA treated with $FeSO_4$, H_2O_2, and the positive control of glutathione (GSH) (1.0 mg/mL); (**D**) pBR322DNA treated with $FeSO_4$, H_2O_2, and SMP-11 (3.0 mg/mL); (**E**) pBR322DNA treated with $FeSO_4$, H_2O_2, and SMP-10 (3.0 mg/mL); (**F**) pBR322DNA treated with $FeSO_4$, H_2O_2, and SMP-7 (3.0 mg/mL); (**G**) pBR322DNA treated with $FeSO_4$, H_2O_2, and SMP-3 (3.0 mg/mL).

2.5. Effects of Thermal and pH Treatments on the Stability of SMP-3, SMP-7, SMP-10, and SMP-11

Figure 10A shows that the effects of temperature on HO· scavenging activity of SMP-3, SMP-7, SMP-10, and SMP-11 (expressed as an EC_{50} value). No significant difference in EC_{50} values of SMP-3 and SMP-11 was found when the treated temperature was 20, 40, and 60 °C ($p > 0.05$), but their EC_{50} values significantly increased when the treated temperatures increased to 80 and 100 °C ($p < 0.05$). Compared with SMP-3 and SMP-11, thermal treatment had stronger effects on SMP-7 and SMP-10 because their EC_{50} values treated at 60 °C were significantly ($p > 0.05$) higher than those of SMP-7 and SMP-10 treated at 20 and 40 °C ($p < 0.05$). The results indicate that SMP-3 and SMP-11 could retain their antioxidant activity when the treated temperature was lower than 60 °C, but SMP-7 and SMP-10 would lose their function at the same processing temperature. Figure 10B shows the EC_{50} values of SMP-3, SMP-7, SMP-10, and SMP-11 on HO· when they were treated at a pH value ranging from 3 to 11. No significant difference on EC_{50} values of SMP-3, SMP-7, SMP-10, or SMP-11 was found when pH value ranged from 5 to 9, but pH values of 3 and 11 significantly affected the EC_{50} values of SMP-3, SMP-7, SMP-10, and SMP-11 ($p < 0.05$).

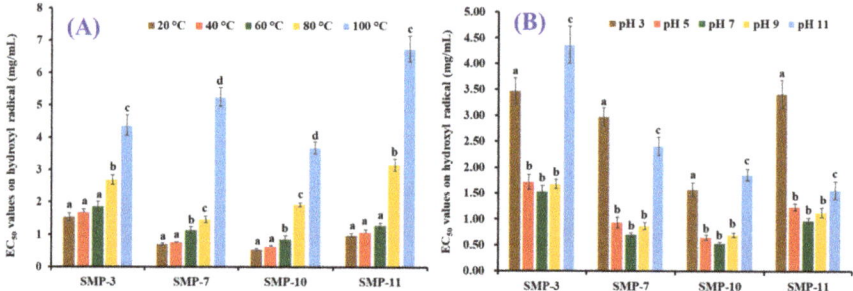

Figure 10. EC_{50} values of SMP-3, SMP-7, SMP-10, and SMP-11 on HO· scavenging activities when they were treated at different temperatures (**A**) and pH values (**B**). All data are expressed as mean ± SD ($n = 3$). [a–d] Values with the same letters indicate no significant difference of same sample ($p > 0.05$).

Thermal and pH treatments are popular processing methods of food products for altering their taste, physicochemical properties, nutritional ingredients, and safety. Therefore, the stability of APs on thermal and pH treatments is closely related to their application scopes [32,44,45]. Thermal treatment can eliminate the majority of spoilage and pathogenic microorganisms, and APs can effectively inhibit lipid peroxidation if they have strong heat-resistant properties. A combination of APs and heat treatment will significantly prolong the shelf life of products. In addition, APs with broad acid-alkali tolerance properties can be used in more food products [23]. Two antioxidant hexapeptides (WAFAPA and MYPGLA) from the hydrolysate of blue-spotted stingray showed high stability because their EC_{50} values on HO· were not significantly different when they were treated at 25–100 °C or at pH values of 3–11 ($p > 0.05$) [23]. Yang et al. reported that MDLFTE and WPPD from protein hydrolysate of *Tergillarca granosa* could not stand the high-temperature (>80 °C) and strong basic (pH > 9.0) processing [25]. Similarly, Jang et al. reported that ATSHH from hydrolysate of sandfish incubated at 50–90 °C reduced its partial DPPH· scavenging activity. In addition, ATSHH lost some biological activity when it was treated at strong basicity (pH 10–12) or acidity (pH 2) [46]. Our results indicate that SMP-3 (PELDW), SMP-7 (WPDHW), SMP-10 (FGYDWW), and SMP-11 (YLHFW) had similar thermal and pH stability with MDLFTE, WPPD, and ATSHH because they could only keep their high activity when they were treated under a low temperature (<60 °C) and a moderate pH environment (pH 5–9).

3. Experimental Section

3.1. Materials

Spanish mackerel (*S. niphonius*) was purchased from Fengmao Market in Zhoushan city of China. DEAE-52 cellulose and Sephadex G-15 were purchased from Shanghai Source Poly Biological Technology Co., Ltd. (Shanghai, China). Acetonitrile (ACN) and trifluoroacetic acid (TFA) were purchased from Thermo Fisher Scientific Co., Ltd. (Shanghai, China). DPPH and bovine serum albumin (BSA) were purchased from Sigma Aldrich Trading Co., Ltd. (Shanghai, China). Plasmid DNA (pBR322DNA) was purchased from TaKaRa Biotechnology Co., Ltd. (Dalian, China). SMP-3 (PELDW), SMP-7 (WPDHW), SMP-10 (FGYDWW), and SMP-11 (YLHFW) were synthesized in China Peptides Co., Ltd. (Suzhou, China) and used to evaluate their antioxidant activity and stability.

3.2. Preparation of Protein Hydrolysate from Spanish Mackerel Muscle

The Spanish mackerel muscle was homogenized and blended with isopropanol at a ratio of 1:4 (w/v) and stand at 30 ± 2 °C for 6 h, and the isopropanol was changed each 2.0 h. Finally, the solution was filtered using a cheesecloth and the solid precipitate was air-dried at 35 ± 2 °C.

The hydrolytic process of the defatted muscle using five proteases was performed following the previous methods [9]. The dispersions of the defatted muscle (1%, w/v) were ultrasonic for 15 min and hydrolyzed separately on their optimal hydrolysis parameters (Table 4).

Table 4. Hydrolysis parameters of different proteases and their combination.

Protease	Temperature (°C)	Enzyme Dosage (g Enzyme/100 g Defatted Muscle)	Time (h)	pH Value
Pepsin	37	2	4	2.0
Neutrase	60	2	4	7.0
Papain	50	2	4	6.0
Trypsin	37	2	4	7.0
Alcalase	50	2	4	8.0
In vitro gastrointestinal digestion	37	Trypsin 1	2	2.0
		Pepsin 1	2	7.0

The hydrolytic process of the defatted muscle using in vitro gastrointestinal (GI) digestion was performed on the method described by Yang et al. [10]. Briefly, the defatted muscle powders dispersed in DW (pH 1.5, 1%) were ultrasonic for 15 min and firstly hydrolyzed by pepsin with a dosage of 1 g pepsin/100 g defatted powder under the conditions of 37.0 ± 2 °C and pH 1.5. Two hours later, the pH of the degraded solution was adjusted to 7.0 using a 1.0 M NaOH solution and further hydrolyzed using trypsin with a dosage of 1 g trypsin/100 g defatted powder for 2 h.

After 4 h of hydrolysis, the hydrolysis solutions were heated at 90 ± 2 °C for 20 min and centrifuged at 8000 g for 25 min at −4 °C. The resulting supernatant were freeze-dried and kept at −20 °C. The dispersions of the defatted muscle (1%, w/v) were ultrasonic for 15 min and freeze-dried, and the freeze-dried powder was referred to as SMP. The protein hydrolysate of Spanish mackerel muscle prepared using in vitro GI digestion method was referred to as SMPH. The concentrations of hydrolysates and their fractions were expressed as mg protein/mL and measured by the dye binding method of Bradford [47], and BSA was used as the standard protein.

3.3. Isolation of APs from SMPH

3.3.1. Fractionation of SMPH

Figure 11 shows the flow diagram of isolating APs from SMPH. SMPH was fractionated using ultrafiltration with 3, 5, and 10 kDa MWCO membranes (Millipore, Hangzhou, China), and four fractions termed SMPH-I (MW < 3 kDa), SMPH-II (3 kDa < MW < 5 kDa), SMPH-III (5 kDa < MW < 10 kDa), and SMPH-IV (>10 kDa) were collected and lyophilized.

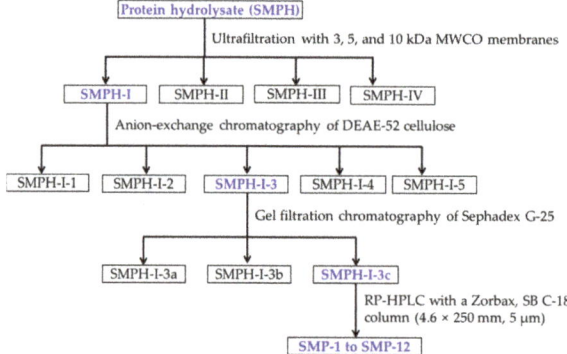

Figure 11. The flow diagram of isolating APs from the hydrolysate (SMPH) of Spanish mackerel muscle prepared using in vitro GI digestion.

3.3.2. Chromatography Isolation of APs from SMPH-I

The chromatography isolation process was performed according to previous methods [48,49]. Five milliliters of an SMPH-I solution (40.0 mg/mL) were injected into a pre-equilibrated DEAE-52 cellulose column (1.6 × 80 cm) and separately eluted with 150 mL of DW, 0.1 M NaCl, 0.5 M NaCl, and 1.0 M NaCl solution at a flow rate of 1.0 mL/min. Each eluate (5.0 mL) was collected and detected at 214 nm. Finally, five fractions (SMPH-I-1 to SMPH-I-5) were prepared on the chromatogram. Five milliliters of SMPH-I-3 were separated on a column of Sephadex G-25 (2.6 × 160 cm) eluted with DW at a flow rate of 0.6 mL/min. Each eluate (3.0 mL) was collected and measured at 214 nm. Three fractions (SMPH-I-3a to SMPH-I-3c) were prepared on the chromatogram. Five milliliters of SMPH-I-3c were further purified using RP-HPLC with a Zorbax, SB C-18 column (4.6 × 250 mm, 5 μm) on an Agilent 1260 (Santa Rosa, CA, USA). The sample was eluated with a linear gradient of ACN (0–40% in 0–30 min) in 0.1% TFA at a flow rate of 1.0 mL/min. Twelve major peaks (SMP-1 to SMP-12) were isolated on the absorbance at 214 nm.

3.4. Analysis of Amino Acid Sequence and Molecular Mass

The amino acid sequences of four APs (SMP-3, SMP-7, SMP-10, and SMP-11) were measured on an Applied Biosystems 494 protein sequencer (Perkin Elmer/Applied Biosystems Inc, Foster City, CA, USA). The molecular masses of four APs (SMP-3, SMP-7, SMP-10, and SMP-11) were measured using a Q-TOF mass spectrometer coupled with an ESI source (Waters, Los Angeles, CA, USA), respectively.

3.5. Antioxidant Activity

3.5.1. Radical Scavenging Assays

The DPPH·, HO·, and O_2^-· scavenging assays of four APs (SMP-3, SMP-7, SMP-10, and SMP-11) were performed according to the previous methods [28,31], and the EC_{50} was defined as the concentration where a sample caused a 50% decrease of the initial radical concentration.

DPPH· Scavenging Assay

Two milliliters of samples consisting of DW and different concentrations of the analytes were placed in cuvettes, and 500 µL of an ethanolic solution of DPPH (0.02%) and 1.0 mL of ethanol were added. A control sample containing the DPPH solution without the sample was also prepared. In the blank, the DPPH solution was substituted with ethanol. The DPPH· scavenging activity was calculated using the following formula:

$$\text{DPPH· scavenging activity (\%)} = (A_c + A_b - A_s)/A_c \times 100\%$$

where A_s is the absorbance rate of the sample, A_c is the control group absorbance, and A_b is the blank absorbance.

HO· Scavenging Assay

One milliliter of a 1.865 mM 1,10-phenanthroline solution and 2.0 mL of the sample were added to a screw-capped tube and mixed. Afterwards, 1.0 mL of a $FeSO_4 \cdot 7H_2O$ solution (1.865 mM) was added to the mixture. The reaction was initiated by adding 1.0 mL of H_2O_2 (0.03%, v/v). After incubating at 37 °C for 60 min in a water bath, the absorbance of the reaction mixture was measured at 536 nm against a reagent blank. The reaction mixture without any antioxidant was used as the negative control, and a mixture without H_2O_2 was used as the blank. The HO· scavenging activity was calculated using the following formula:

$$\text{HO· scavenging activity (\%)} = [(A_s - A_n)/(A_b - A_n)] \times 100\%$$

where A_s, A_n, and A_b are the absorbance values determined at 536 nm of the sample, the negative control, and the blank after the reaction, respectively.

O_2^-· Scavenging Assay

Superoxide anions were generated in 1.0 mL of nitrotetrazolium blue chloride (NBT) (2.52 mM), 1.0 mL of NADH (624 mM), and 1.0 mL of different sample concentrations. The reaction was initiated by adding 1.0 mL of phenazine methosulphate (PMS) solution (120 µM) to the reaction mixture. The absorbance was measured at 560 nm against the corresponding blank after 5 min incubation at 25 °C. The O_2^-· scavenging activity was calculated using the following equation:

$$O_2^- \text{·scavenging activity (\%)} = [(A_c - A_s)/A_c] \times 100\%$$

where A_c is the absorbance without sample, and A_s is the absorbance with sample.

3.5.2. Lipid Peroxidation Inhibition Assay

The lipid peroxidation inhibition activity of the APs was measured in the linoleic acid model system according to the method of Wang et al. [28]. Briefly, a sample (5.0 mg) was dissolved in 10.0 mL of 50.0 mM phosphate buffer solution (PBS, pH 7.0) and added to 0.13 mL of a solution of linoleic acid and 10.0 mL of 99.5% ethanol. The total volume was adjusted to 25 mL with DW. The mixture was incubated in a conical flask with a screw cap at 40 °C in a dark room, and the degree of oxidation was evaluated by measuring ferric thiocyanate values. The reaction solution (100 µL) incubated in the linoleic acid model system was mixed with 4.7 mL of 75% ethanol, 0.1 mL of 30% ammonium thiocyanate, and 0.1 mL of 20 mM ferrous chloride solution in 3.5% HCl. After 3 min, the thiocyanate value was measured at 500 nm following color development with $FeCl_2$ and thiocyanate at different intervals during the incubation period at 40 °C.

3.5.3. Protective Effect on Plasmid DNA

The protective effects of four APs (SMP-3, SMP-7, SMP-10, and SMP-11) on supercoiled plasmid DNA (pBR322) were measured according to the previous method [12]. In brief, 15 µL of reaction mixtures containing 5 µL of PBS (10 mM, pH 7.4), 2 µL of $FeSO_4$ (1.0 mM), 1 µL of pBR322 (0.5 µg), 5 µL of the AP (SMP-3, SMP-7, SMP-10, or SMP-11, respectively), and 2 µL of H_2O_2 (1.0 mM) were incubated at 37 °C. After 0.5 h of incubation, 2 µL of loading buffer containing glycerol (50%, v/v), EDTA (40 mM), and bromophenol blue (0.05%) were added to terminate the reaction. The resulted reaction mixtures were subsequently electrophoresed on 1% agarose gel containing 0.5 µg/mL EtBr for 50 min (60 V), and the DNA in the agarose gel was photographed under ultraviolet light.

3.6. Stability Properties

The stability of four APs (SMP-3, SMP-7, SMP-10, and SMP-11) were measured according to the previous methods [10,50]. The thermostability of four APs (SMP-3, SMP-7, SMP-10, and SMP-11) was determined using a water bath at 20, 40, 60, 80, or 100 °C for 0.5 h. pH values of 3, 5, 7, 9, or 11 were used to evaluate the pH stability of four APs (SMP-3, SMP-7, SMP-10, and SMP-11) at 25 °C for 2.5 h. HO· scavenging activities (EC_{50} value) of the treated four APs (SMP-3, SMP-7, SMP-10, and SMP-11) were measured according to the methods described in Section 2.5.

3.7. Statistical Analysis

The data are expressed as the mean ± SD (n = 3). ANOVA test for differences between means of each group was used to analyze data using SPSS 19.0 (SPSS Corporation, Chicago, IL, USA). A *p*-value of less than 0.05 was considered statistically significant.

4. Conclusions

In the experiment, the proteins of Spanish mackerel (*S. niphonius*) muscle were hydrolyzed under five kinds of enzymes and in vitro GI digestion, and four APs (SMP-3, SMP-7, SMP-10, and SMP-11) were isolated from the hydrolysate prepared using in vitro GI digestion and identified as PELDW, WPDHW, FGYDWW, and YLHFW, respectively. PELDW, WPDHW, FGYDWW, and YLHFW showed high radical scavenging activity, lipid peroxidation inhibition ability, and protective effects on plasmid DNA (pBR322DNA) against oxidative damage induced by H_2O_2. Moreover, four APs (PELDW, WPDHW, FGYDWW, and YLHFW) from protein hydrolysate of Spanish mackerel muscle might be applied as an ingredient in new functional foods and products under a normal temperature (<40 °C) and a moderate pH environment (pH 5–9).

Author Contributions: B.W. and Y.-Q.Z. conceived and designed the experiments. G.-X.Z., X.-R.Y., and Y.-M.W. performed the experiments and analyzed the data. C.-F.C. and B.W. contributed the reagents, materials, and analytical tools and wrote the paper.

Funding: This work was funded by the National Natural Science Foundation of China (NSFC) (No. 31872547), the International S&T Cooperation Program of China (No. 2012DFA30600), and the Zhejiang Province Public Technology Research Project (LGN18D060002).

Acknowledgments: The authors thank Zhao-Hui Zhang at the Beijing Agricultural Biological Testing Center for his technical support on the isolation and amino acid sequence identification of peptides from Spanish mackerel (*S. niphonius*) muscle.

Conflicts of Interest: The authors declare no conflict of interest.

References

1. Agyei, D.; Ongkudon, C.M.; Wei, C.Y.; Chan, A.S.; Danquah, M.K. Bioprocess challenges to the isolation and purification of bioactive peptides. *Food Bioprod. Process.* **2016**, *98*, 244–256. [CrossRef]
2. Pan, X.; Zhao, Y.Q.; Hu, F.Y.; Wang, B. Preparation and identification of antioxidant peptides from protein hydrolysate of skate (*Raja porosa*) cartilage. *J. Funct. Foods* **2016**, *25*, 220–230. [CrossRef]
3. Sila, A.; Bougatef, A. Antioxidant peptides from marine by-products: Isolation, identification and application in food systems. A review. *J. Funct. Foods* **2016**, *21*, 10–26. [CrossRef]
4. Zhao, W.H.; Luo, Q.B.; Pan, X.; Chi, C.F.; Sun, K.L.; Wang, B. Preparation, identification, and activity evaluation of ten antioxidant peptides from protein hydrolysate of swim bladders of miiuy croaker (*Miichthys miiuy*). *J. Funct. Foods* **2018**, *47*, 503–511. [CrossRef]
5. Lorenzo, J.M.; Munekata, P.E.S.; Gómez, B.; Barba, F.J.; Mora, L.; Pérez-Santaescolástica, C.; Toldrá, F. Bioactive peptides as natural antioxidants in food products—A review. *Trends Food Sci. Technol.* **2018**, *79*, 136–147. [CrossRef]
6. Zhang, J.B.; Wang, Y.M.; Chi, C.F.; Sun, K.L.; Wang, B. Eight peptides from collagen hydrolysate fraction of Spanish mackerel (*Scomberomorous niphonius*) skin: Isolation, identification, and antioxidant activity in vitro. *Mar. Drugs* **2019**, *17*, 224. [CrossRef] [PubMed]
7. He, Y.; Pan, X.; Chi, C.F.; Sun, K.L.; Wang, B. Ten new pentapeptides from protein hydrolysate of miiuy croaker (*Miichthys miiuy*) muscle: Preparation, identification, and antioxidant activity evaluation. *LWT Food Sci. Technol.* **2019**, *105*, 1–8. [CrossRef]
8. Chi, C.F.; Hu, F.Y.; Wang, B.; Li, Z.R.; Luo, H.Y. Influence of amino acid compositions and peptide profiles on antioxidant capacities of two protein hydrolysates from skipjack tuna (*Katsuwonus pelamis*) dark muscle. *Mar. Drugs* **2015**, *13*, 2580–2601. [CrossRef]
9. Wang, B.; Li, L.; Chi, C.F.; Ma, J.H.; Luo, H.Y.; Xu, Y.F. Purification and characterisation of a novel antioxidant peptide derived from blue mussel (*Mytilus edulis*) protein hydrolysate. *Food Chem.* **2013**, *138*, 1713–1719. [CrossRef]
10. Yang, X.R.; Zhao, Y.Q.; Qiu, Y.T.; Chi, C.F.; Wang, B. Preparation and characterization of gelatin and antioxidant peptides from gelatin hydrolysate of skipjack tuna (*Katsuwonus pelamis*) bone stimulated by in vitro gastrointestinal digestion. *Mar. Drugs* **2019**, *17*, 78. [CrossRef]
11. Tao, J.; Zhao, Y.Q.; Chi, C.F.; Wang, B. Bioactive peptides from cartilage protein hydrolysate of spotless smoothhound and their antioxidant activity in vitro. *Mar. Drugs* **2018**, *16*, 100. [CrossRef] [PubMed]
12. Zhao, Y.Q.; Zeng, L.; Yang, Z.S.; Huang, F.F.; Ding, G.F.; Wang, B. Anti-fatigue effect by peptide fraction from protein hydrolysate of croceine croaker (*Pseudosciaena crocea*) swim bladder through inhibiting the oxidative reactions including DNA damage. *Mar. Drugs* **2016**, *14*, 221. [CrossRef]
13. Xiao, Z.; Liang, P.; Chen, J.; Chen, M.F.; Gong, F.; Li, C.; Zhou, C.; Hong, P.; Yang, P.; Qian, Z.J. A peptide YGDEY from tilapia gelatin hydrolysates inhibits UVB-mediated skin photoaging by regulating MMP-1 and MMP-9 expression in HaCaT cells. *Photochem. Photobiol.* **2019**. [CrossRef] [PubMed]
14. You, L.; Ren, J.; Yang, B.; Regenstein, J.; Zhao, M. Antifatigue activities of loach protein hydrolysates with different antioxidant activities. *J. Agric. Food Chem.* **2012**, *60*, 12324–12331. [CrossRef] [PubMed]
15. Himaya, S.W.A.; Ryu, B.; Ngo, D.H.; Kim, S.K. Peptide Isolated from Japanese flounder skin gelatin protects against cellular oxidative damage. *J. Agric. Food Chem.* **2012**, *60*, 9112–9119. [CrossRef] [PubMed]
16. Lin, J.; Hong, H.; Zhang, L.; Zhang, C.; Luo, Y. Antioxidant and cryoprotective effects of hydrolysate from gill protein of bighead carp (*Hypophthalmichthys nobilis*) in preventing denaturation of frozen surimi. *Food Chem.* **2019**, *298*, 124868. [CrossRef] [PubMed]

17. Li, Z.R.; Wang, B.; Chi, C.F.; Zhang, Q.H.; Gong, Y.D.; Tang, J.J.; Luo, H.Y.; Ding, G.F. Isolation and characterization of acid soluble collagens and pepsin soluble collagens from the skin and bone of Spanish mackerel (*Scomberomorous niphonius*). *Food Hydrocoll.* **2013**, *3*, 103–113. [CrossRef]
18. Chi, C.F.; Cao, Z.H.; Wang, B.; Hu, F.Y.; Li, Z.R.; Zhang, B. Antioxidant and functional properties of collagen hydrolysates from spanish mackerel skin as influenced by average molecular weight. *Molecules* **2014**, *19*, 11211–11230. [CrossRef]
19. Agrawal, H.; Joshi, R.; Gupta, M. Purification, identification and characterization of two novel antioxidant peptides from finger millet (*Eleusine coracana*) protein hydrolysate. *Food Res. Int.* **2019**, *120*, 697–707. [CrossRef]
20. Zhao, S.; Cheng, Q.; Peng, Q.; Yu, X.; Yin, X.; Liang, M.; Ma, C.W.; Huang, Z.; Jia, W. Antioxidant peptides derived from the hydrolyzate of purple sea urchin (*Strongylocentrotus nudus*) gonad alleviate oxidative stress in Caenorhabditis elegans. *J. Funct. Foods* **2018**, *48*, 594–604. [CrossRef]
21. Zheng, L.; Yu, H.; Wei, H.; Xing, Q.; Zou, Y.; Zhou, Y.; Peng, J. Antioxidative peptides of hydrolysate prepared from fish skin gelatin using ginger protease activate antioxidant response element-mediated gene transcription in IPEC-J2 cells. *J. Funct. Foods* **2018**, *51*, 104–112. [CrossRef]
22. Li, Z.; Wang, B.; Chi, C.; Gong, Y.; Luo, H.; Ding, G. Influence of average molecular weight on antioxidant and functional properties of cartilage collagen hydrolysates from *Sphyrna lewini*, *Dasyatis akjei* and *Raja porosa*. *Food Res. Int.* **2013**, *51*, 283–293. [CrossRef]
23. Wong, F.C.; Xiao, J.; Ong, M.G.L.; Pang, M.J.; Wong, S.J.; The, L.K.; Chai, T.T. Identification and characterization of antioxidant peptides from hydrolysate of blue-spotted stingray and their stability against thermal, pH and simulated gastrointestinal digestion treatments. *Food Chem.* **2019**, *271*, 614–622. [CrossRef] [PubMed]
24. Shazly, A.B.; He, Z.; El-Aziz, M.A.; Zeng, M.; Zhang, S.; Qin, F.; Chen, J. Fractionation and identification of novel antioxidant peptides from buffalo and bovine casein hydrolysates. *Food Chem.* **2017**, *232*, 753–762. [CrossRef] [PubMed]
25. Yang, X.R.; Zhang, L.; Zhao, Y.Q.; Chi, C.F.; Wang, B. Purification and characterization of antioxidant peptides derived from protein hydrolysate of the marine bivalve mollusk *Tergillarca granosa*. *Mar. Drugs* **2019**, *17*, 251. [CrossRef] [PubMed]
26. Nazeer, R.A.; Sampath Kumar, N.S.; Jai Ganesh, R. In vitro and in vivo studies on the antioxidant activity of fish peptide isolated from the croaker (*Otolithes ruber*) muscle protein hydrolysate. *Peptides* **2012**, *35*, 261–268. [CrossRef] [PubMed]
27. Ko, J.Y.; Lee, J.H.; Samarakoon, K.; Kim, J.S.; Jeon, Y.J. Purification and determination of two novel antioxidant peptides from flounder fish (*Paralichthys olivaceus*) using digestive proteases. *Food Chem. Toxicol.* **2013**, *52*, 113–120. [CrossRef]
28. Pan, X.Y.; Wang, Y.M.; Li, L.; Chi, C.F.; Wang, B. Four antioxidant peptides from protein hydrolysate of red stingray (*Dasyatis akajei*) cartilages: Isolation, identification, and in vitro activity evaluation. *Mar. Drugs* **2019**, *17*, 263. [CrossRef]
29. Ahn, C.B.; Cho, Y.S.; Je, J.Y. Purification and anti-inflammatory action of tripeptide from salmon pectoral fin byproduct protein hydrolysate. *Food Chem.* **2015**, *168*, 151–156. [CrossRef]
30. Wang, B.; Wang, Y.M.; Chi, C.F.; Hu, F.Y.; Deng, S.G.; Ma, J.Y. Isolation and characterization of collagen and antioxidant collagen peptides from scales of croceine croaker (*Pseudosciaena crocea*). *Mar. Drugs* **2013**, *11*, 4641–4661. [CrossRef]
31. Wang, B.; Li, Z.R.; Chi, C.F.; Zhang, Q.H.; Luo, H.Y. Preparation and evaluation of antioxidant peptides from ethanol-soluble proteins hydrolysate of *Sphyrna lewini* muscle. *Peptides* **2012**, *36*, 240–250. [CrossRef] [PubMed]
32. Yang, X.R.; Zhang, L.; Ding, D.G.; Chi, C.F.; Wang, B.; Huo, J.C. Preparation, identification, and activity evaluation of eight antioxidant peptides from protein hydrolysate of hairtail (*Trichiurus japonicas*) muscle. *Mar. Drugs* **2019**, *17*, 23. [CrossRef] [PubMed]
33. Cai, L.; Wu, X.; Zhang, Y.; Li, X.; Ma, S.; Li, J. Purification and characterization of three antioxidant peptides from protein hydrolysate of grass carp (*Ctenopharyngodon idella*) skin. *J. Funct. Foods* **2015**, *16*, 234–242. [CrossRef]
34. Wang, B.; Gong, Y.D.; Li, Z.R.; Yu, D.; Chi, C.F.; Ma, J.Y. Isolation and characterisation of five novel antioxidant peptides from ethanol-soluble proteins hydrolysate of spotless smoothhound (*Mustelus griseus*) muscle. *J. Funct. Foods* **2014**, *6*, 176–185. [CrossRef]

35. Rajapakse, N.; Mendis, E.; Byun, H.G.; Kim, S.K. Purification and in vitro antioxidative effects of giant squid muscle peptides on free radical-mediated oxidative systems. *J. Nutr. Biochem.* **2005**, *9*, 562–569. [CrossRef]
36. Chi, C.F.; Wang, B.; Wang, Y.M.; Zhang, B.; Deng, S.G. Isolation and characterization of three antioxidant peptides from protein hydrolysate of bluefin leatherjacket (*Navodon septentrionalis*) heads. *J. Funct. Foods* **2015**, *12*, 1–10. [CrossRef]
37. Zhang, Q.; Tong, X.; Li, Y.; Wang, H.; Wang, Z.; Qi, B.; Sui, X.; Jiang, L. Purification and characterization of antioxidant peptides from alcalase-hydrolyzed soybean (*Glycine max* L.) hydrolysate and their cytoprotective effects in human intestinal Caco-2 cells. *J. Agric. Food Chem.* **2019**, *67*, 5772–5781. [CrossRef]
38. Mylonas, C.; Kouretas, D. Lipid peroxidation and tissue damage. *In Vivo* **1999**, *13*, 295–309.
39. Niki, E. Lipid peroxidation products as oxidative stress biomarkers. *Biofactors* **2008**, *34*, 171–180. [CrossRef]
40. Guéraud, F.; Atalay, M.; Bresgen, N.; Cipak, A.; Eckl, P.M.; Huc, L.; Jouanin, I.; Siems, W.; Uchida, K. Chemistry and biochemistry of lipid peroxidation products. *Free Radic. Res.* **2010**, *44*, 1098–1124. [CrossRef]
41. Chi, C.F.; Wang, B.; Wang, Y.M.; Deng, S.G.; Ma, J.Y. Isolation and characterization of three antioxidant pentapeptides from protein hydrolysate of monkfish (*Lophius litulon*) muscle. *Food Res. Int.* **2014**, *55*, 222–228. [CrossRef]
42. Agrawal, H.; Joshi, R.; Gupta, M. Isolation, purification and characterization of antioxidative peptide of pearl millet (*Pennisetum glaucum*) protein hydrolysate. *Food Chem.* **2016**, *204*, 365–372. [CrossRef] [PubMed]
43. Bougatef, A.; Balti, R.; Haddar, A.; Jellouli, K.; Souissi, N.; Nasri, M. Antioxidant and functional properties of protein hydrolysates of bluefin tuna (*Thunnus thynnus*) heads as influenced by the extent of enzymatic hydrolysis. *Biotechnol. Bioprocess Eng.* **2012**, *17*, 841–852. [CrossRef]
44. Ren, J.Y.; Zhao, M.M.; Shi, J.; Wang, J.S.; Jiang, Y.M.; Cui, C.; Kakuda, Y.; Xue, S.J. Purification and identification of antioxidant peptides from grass carp muscle hydrolysates by consecutive chromatography and electrospray ionization-mass spectrometry. *Food Chem.* **2008**, *108*, 727–736. [CrossRef] [PubMed]
45. Lafarga, T.; Hayes, M. Bioactive peptides from meat muscle and by-products: Generation, functionality and application as functional ingredients. *Meat Sci.* **2014**, *98*, 227–239. [CrossRef]
46. Jang, H.L.; Liceaga, A.M.; Yoon, K.Y. Purification, characterisation and stability of an antioxidant peptide derived from sandfish (*Arctoscopus japonicus*) protein hydrolysates. *J. Funct. Foods* **2016**, *20*, 433–442. [CrossRef]
47. Bradford, M.M. A rapid and sensitive method for the quantification of microgram quantities of protein utilizing the principle of protein-dye binding. *Anal. Biochem.* **1976**, *72*, 248–254. [CrossRef]
48. Li, X.R.; Chi, C.F.; Li, L.; Wang, B. Purification and identification of antioxidant peptides from protein hydrolysate of scalloped hammerhead (*Sphyrna lewini*) cartilage. *Mar. Drugs* **2017**, *15*, 61. [CrossRef]
49. Zhao, Y.Q.; Zhang, L.; Tao, J.; Chi, C.F.; Wang, B. Eight antihypertensive peptides from the protein hydrolysate of Antarctic krill (*Euphausia superba*): Isolation, identification, and activity evaluation on human umbilical vein endothelial cells (HUVECs). *Food Res. Int.* **2019**, *121*, 197–204. [CrossRef]
50. Zhang, L.; Zhao, G.X.; Zhao, Y.Q.; Qiu, Y.T.; Chi, C.F.; Wang, B. Identification and active evaluation of antioxidant peptides from protein hydrolysates of skipjack tuna (*Katsuwonus pelamis*) head. *Antioxidants* **2019**, *8*, 318. [CrossRef]

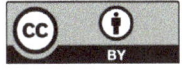

© 2019 by the authors. Licensee MDPI, Basel, Switzerland. This article is an open access article distributed under the terms and conditions of the Creative Commons Attribution (CC BY) license (http://creativecommons.org/licenses/by/4.0/).

Article

Limited Benefit of Marine Protein Hydrolysate on Physical Function and Strength in Older Adults: A Randomized Controlled Trial

Linda Kornstad Nygård [1,*], Ingunn Mundal [1,2], Lisbeth Dahl [3], Jūratė Šaltytė Benth [4,5] and Anne Marie Mork Rokstad [1,6]

1. Faculty of Health Sciences and Social Care, Molde University College, P.O. Box 2110, 6402 Molde, Norway; ingunn.p.mundal@himolde.no (I.M.); anne.m.m.rokstad@himolde.no (A.M.M.R.)
2. Department of Mental Health, Faculty of Medicine and Health Sciences, Norwegian University of Science and Technology (NTNU), P.O. Box 8905, 7491 Trondheim, Norway
3. Institute of Marine Research (IMR), P.O. Box 1870 Nordnes, 5817 Bergen, Norway; Lisbeth.Dahl@hi.no
4. Institute of Clinical Medicine, Campus Ahus, University of Oslo, P.O. Box 1171, Blindern, 0318 Oslo, Norway; jurate.saltyte-benth@medisin.uio.no
5. Health Services Research Unit, Akershus University Hospital, P.O. Box 1000, 1478 Lørenskog, Norway
6. Norwegian National Advisory Unit on Ageing and Health, Vestfold Hospital Trust, P.O. Box 2136, 3103 Tønsberg, Norway
* Correspondence: anettekornstad@gmail.com; Tel.: +47-712-14000

Abstract: Age-related muscle wasting can compromise functional abilities of the elderly. Protein intake stimulates muscle protein synthesis; however, ageing muscle is more resistant to stimuli. This double-blinded, randomized, controlled trial is one of the first registered studies to evaluate the effects of a supplement of marine protein hydrolysate (MPH) on measures of physical function and strength. Eighty-six older adults received nutritional supplements containing 3 g of MPH or a placebo for up to 12 months. Short Physical Performance Battery (SPPB), grip strength and gait speed were measured, and dietary intake was registered at baseline, 6 months, and 12 months. No difference was found between the intervention and control groups in mean change in SPPB (independent sample t-test, $p = 0.41$) or regarding time trend in SPPB, grip strength, or gait speed (linear mixed model). The participants in our study were well functioning, causing a ceiling effect in SPPB. Further, they had sufficient protein intake and were physically active. Differences in physical function between those completing the intervention and the dropouts might also have created bias in the results. We recommend that future studies of MPH be carried out on a more frail or malnourished population.

Keywords: hydrolysate; fish protein; ageing; physical function; dietary assessment; seafood intake; healthy ageing

1. Introduction

In 2019, 65-year-old Norwegian men could expect to live five years longer compared with 30 years ago [1]. With increasing lifespans, healthy ageing is crucial to maintain independence and reduce future healthcare costs for society. Maintenance of muscle strength and function plays an important role in healthy ageing [2]. Age-related muscle wasting (i.e., sarcopenia) is accompanied by loss of strength and can compromise the functional abilities and activity levels of the elderly [3,4].

One of the main mechanisms of muscle wasting is a reduction in muscle protein synthesis (MPS), and it appears that the muscles of older adults are more resistant to anabolic stimuli than the muscles of younger people. This implies that older muscles might need larger amounts of protein than younger ones to adequately stimulate MPS [2,3]. However, high protein intake might be challenging as ageing is often accompanied by decreased energy intake and loss of appetite, i.e., the anorexia of ageing [5].

Protein supplements have been shown to elicit gains in muscle strength in older people when used in combination with strength exercise [6]. However, the majority of muscle wasting happens in periods of low physical activity [7]. Thus, it is also interesting to study nutritional interventions alone, i.e., without combining them with exercise. Several signaling pathways are described where proteins, peptides, and amino acids stimulate MPS, and among the single amino acids, leucine and other branch-chained amino acids (BCAA) are especially active parts of these pathways [8]. Lean fish is a source of protein of good quality and tends to have a moderate to high content of BCAA [9]. Fish protein supplements in small doses have shown a positive effect on body composition in favor of muscle vs. fat in overweight people, both in a study using 3 g fish protein [10] and 1.4–2.8 g fish protein hydrolysate [11]. These doses are small, and the effect might be related to bioactive peptides, rather than the known effect of protein as a source of amino acids [12].

Small dose supplements could constitute a more feasible way of supplementing elderly and/or frail persons as the amount of intake is smaller and contributes less to the feeling of satiety; thus, it does not suppress micronutrient intake from other food sources. The aim of this trial was to evaluate the effects of marine protein hydrolysate (MPH) supplements on physical function and strength in the elderly. This is one of the first long-term studies of MPH and age-related changes in muscle health [12].

Our hypothesis was that a daily intake of 3 g MPH for 6 to 12 months would prevent loss of physical performance, compared with a placebo, as measured by the Short Physical Performance Battery (SPPB) and loss of muscle strength as measured by grip strength.

2. Results

The mean age of the participants in this study was 72.7 (SD 8.2) years: 72.5 (SD 8.3) and 73.1 (SD 8.2) years in women and men, respectively. Forty participants (46.5%) had higher education, and 30 participants (34.9%) lived alone. Forty-two participants (48.8%) reported that they performed strength exercises at least once a week, and 45 participants (52.3%) reported being physically active daily.

The mean protein intake was 71.8 g (SD 23.6) and 83.7 g (SD 19.0), corresponding to 1.1 g/kg BW (SD 0.4) and 1.0 g/kg BW (SD 0.2) in women and men, respectively. Energy intake was 1728 kcal (SD 542) in women and 1958 kcal (SD 498) in men.

The mean baseline values of SPPB were 10.5 points (SD 2.4): 10.3 points (SD 2.6) and 11.0 points (SD 1.8) in women and men, respectively. The top SPPB score of 12 points was reached by 44 participants (51.2%). The mean baseline value of grip strength was 33.0 kg (SD 11.6): 26.7 kg (SD 6.7) and 45.5 kg (SD 8.4) in women and men, respectively. Nine women (15.8%) had a grip strength <20 kg, and two men (6.9%) had a grip strength <30 kg. The mean baseline gait speed was 1.0 m/s (SD 0.3) in both women and men.

Characteristics of the participants in the intervention group and control group are shown in Table 1, including intake of energy, protein, and seafood, levels of 25-hydroxy vitamin D, outcome measures of physical function, and compliance with intervention/control.

At the 6-month follow-up, 26 participants reported gastrointestinal problems related to the tablets, in the form of increased gas or slight nausea, constipation or diarrhea. Further, 26 participants reported some difficulties swallowing the tablets. However, these problems were apparent in both the intervention and control groups (gastrointestinal symptoms $p = 0.64$ and swallowing difficulties $p = 0.11$), and mean compliance of tablet intake from the start to 6 months was 83.4% (SD 23.3). No compliance differences were found between intervention group and control group ($p = 0.97$).

During the study, nine participants were lost before the 6-month follow-up, and an additional 29 were lost between 6 and 12 months. The participants dropped out for the following reasons: gastrointestinal problems related to tablets (n = 9), health issues not related to the study (n = 4), lack of motivation due to the large number of tablets, no experience of effect, or just 'had enough' (n = 10). Three participants developed illnesses listed as exclusion criteria during the study. As illustrated in Table 2, dropouts were older ($p = 0.01$), had lower physical function (SPPB $p = 0.01$ and gait speed $p < 0.001$) and strength

(p = 0.01). Additionally, dropouts more often lived alone compared with participants completing the study (p = 0.03). However, there were no differences in energy, protein, or seafood intake between dropouts and participants completing the study.

According to the primary analysis based on independent samples t-test, there was no significant difference in mean change between intervention and control groups in the main outcome, SPPB, from baseline to 12 months (p = 0.41). However, this analysis does not adjust for differences in the cluster effect within each municipality, which was found to be of significance with ICC 88.7%, 37.0%, and 62.3% for SPPB, grip strength, and gait speed, respectively. Particularly, the participants recruited from homecare services were very distinct from the others.

Table 1. Demographic and clinical characteristics at the baseline, and descriptive statistics of the outcome variables of the randomized participants (N=86) at each time point, in the intervention (n = 43) * and control (n = 43) * groups.

	Intervention	Control
Demographic and clinical characteristics		
Demographic:		
Age in years, mean (SD)	73.4 (8.7)	72.0 (7.7)
Weight, kg mean (SD)	72.2 (13.1)	78.5 (14.7)
BMI, kg/m² mean (SD)	25.5 (3.8)	27.7 (4.7)
Gender, female, n (%)	29 (67.4)	28 (65.1)
Education level college/university, n (%)	21 (48.8)	19 (44.2)
Perform strength exercise weekly, n (%)	22 (51.2)	20 (46.5)
Other physical activities daily, n (%)	28 (65.1)	17 (39.5)
Live alone, n (%)	16 (37.2)	14 (32.6)
Dietary factors		
Energy intake, kcal, mean (SD)	1809 (551)	1802 (527)
Energy intake, kcal/kgBW [1], mean (SD)	26.4 (8.8)	25.2 (8.8) [a]
Protein intake, g/kgBW [1], mean (SD)	1.1 (0.3)	1.1 (0.4) [a]
Protein intake, g/1000 kcal, mean (SD)	42.3 (10.4)	43.5 (10.1)
Seafood index [2], mean (SD)	3.3 (1.4) [a]	3.4 (1.2)
Serum 25-hydroxy vitamin D, nmol/L, mean (SD)	84.2 (31.3) [c]	84.1 (31.8) [b]
Outcome variables		
SPPB [3], total points, mean (SD)		
baseline	10.7 (2.3)	10.4 (2.4)
6 months	11.0 (2.1) [d]	11.0 (1.6) [c]
12 months	11.4 (1.8) [f]	11.1 (1.8) [g]
Grip strength, kg, mean (SD)		
baseline	33.0 (11.4)	33.1 (11.9)
6 months	34.2 (12.6) [d]	34.1 (10.6) [b]
12 months	37.0 (11.5) [f]	33.9 (10.9) [g]
Gait speed, m/s, mean (SD)		
baseline	1.1 (0.3)	1.0 (0.3)
6 months	1.0 (0.3) [d]	1.0 (0.2) [c]
12 months	1.1 (0.2) [f]	1.1 (0.2) [g]
Compliance		
% of tablets taken, 0–6 months (SD)	83.5 (23.1)	83.4 (23.8)
% of tablets taken, 6–12 months (SD)	92.1 (18.4)	92.9 (5.8)
Difficulties swallowing tablets n (%)	16 (29.7) [d]	10 (25.6) [c]
Gastrointestinal effects of tablets n (%)	11 (32.4) [e]	15 (37.5) [b]

[1] BW = body weight, adjusted for over- and underweight. [2] Seafood index is computed from frequency questions regarding seafood for dinner and lunch, and it corresponds to dinner portion equivalents per week. [3] Short Physical Performance Battery. * Variables with missing values are marked with remaining n: [a] n = 42, [b] n = 40, [c] n = 39, [d] n = 37, [e] n = 34, [f] n = 28, [g] n = 20.

Table 2. Baseline characteristics of, and *p*-value for difference between, participants completing the 12-month follow-up (n = 48) and participants dropping out (n = 38).

	Completing	Drop-Out	*p*-Value
Age in years, (mean ± SD)	70.5 (6.3)	75.5 (9.5)	0.01 [2]
Female gender, n (%)	28 (58.3)	29 (76.3)	0.08 [3]
Living alone, n (%)	12 (25.0)	18 (47.4)	0.03 [3]
Education level college/university, n (%)	27 (56.3)	13 (34.2)	0.04 [3]
Intervention group, n (%)	28 (58.3)	15 (39.5)	0.08 [3]
Control group, n (%)	20 (41.7)	23 (60.5)	0.08 [3]
Nutrition			
Protein intake, g/kgBW [1]	1.1 (0.4)	1.1 (0.3)	0.98 [2]
Energy intake, kcal/kgBW [1]	25.9 (10.2)	25.8 (6.6)	0.98 [2]
Seafood intake, index	3.5 (1.3)	3.2 (1.2)	0.38 [2]
Physical function			
SPPB, points (mean ± SD)	11.2 (1.5)	9.7 (3.0)	0.01 [2]
Grip strength, kg (mean ± SD)	35.7 (11.2)	29.6 (11.3)	0.01 [2]
Gait speed, m/s (mean ± SD)	1.1 (0.3)	0.9 (0.3)	<0.001 [2]

[1] BW = body weight, adjusted for over- and underweight. [2] *p*-value for independent samples *t*-test. [3] *p*-value for χ^2-test.

According to a bivariate linear mixed model for SPPB adjusting for a cluster effect on a municipal level, there was no overall difference between the intervention group and control group regarding time trend in SPPB, grip strength, or gait speed (non-significant interactions) (Table 3). The intervention and control groups were, however, significantly different in SPPB at the baseline ($p = 0.033$) and 6-month follow-up ($p = 0.037$), but not at the 12-month follow-up ($p = 0.093$). For grip strength, groups were not significantly different at any time point. Regarding gait speed, groups were significantly different at the baseline ($p = 0.027$) and 6-month follow-up ($p = 0.027$), but not at the 12-month follow-up ($p = 0.106$). These results are illustrated with 95% confidence intervals in Figure 1.

Table 3. Results of linear mixed models assessing changes in Short Physical Performance Battery (SPPB), grip strength, and gait speed in relation to the intervention or control group. Adjusted for a cluster effect on a municipal level.

	SPPB				Grip Strength				Gait Speed			
	N = 196 (n = 85 at T0, n = 68 at T6, n = 43 at T12)				N = 197 (n = 85 at T0, n = 68 at T6, n = 43 at T12)				N = 196 (n = 85 ved T0, n = 68 ved T6, n = 43 ved T12)			
	Bivariate Models		Multiple Model		Bivariate Models		Multiple Model		Bivariate Models		Multiple Model	
	Regr.coeff (SE)	*p*-Value	Regr.coeff (SE)	*p*-Value	Regr.coeff (SE)	*p*-Value	Regr.coeff (SE)	*p*-Value	Regr.coeff	*p*-Value	Regr.coeff (SE)	*p*-Value
Intercept Time T0	10.1 (1.5) 0	0.01	11.08 (2.4) 0	<0.001	31.9 (4.0) 0	0.003	65.6 (12.2) 0	<0.001	1.0 (0.1) 0	0.01	2.4 (0.4) 0	
T6	0.2 (0.2)	0.25	0.2 (0.2)	0.23	0.4 (0.6)	0.5	0.5 (0.6)	0.45	−0.02 (0.003)	0.57	−0.01 (0.003)	0.80
T12	0.2 (0.2)	0.30	0.1 (0.2)	0.42	0.01 (0.5)	0.98	0.2 (0.6)	0.76	−0.0052 (0.04)	0.90	−0.0002 (0.04)	0.99
Group Intervention group–ref	0		0		0		0		0		0	
Control group	−0.5 (0.2)	0.030	−0.5 (0.2)	0.030	−0.7 (2.2)	0.75	−1.2 (−1.2)	0.31	−0.1 (0.04)	0.03	−0.1 (0.04)	0.02
Time x Group T0	0		0		0		0		0		0	
T6	−0.04 (0.3)	0.89	−0.1 (0.3)	0.80	−0.6 (0.8)	0.50	0.5 (0.8)	0.51	−0.01 (0.04)	0.88	−0.02 (0.04)	0.65
T12	0.03 (0.2)	0.99	0.1 (0.2)	0.83	0.2 (0.8)	0.85	0.04 (0.8)	0.96	0.01 (0.1)	0.89	−0.004 (0.1)	0.94
Age	−0.02 (0.02)	0.46	−0.02 (0.03)	0.39	−0.1 (0.3)	0.74	−0.3 (0.2)	0.07	−0.02 (0.01)	0.003	−0.02 (0.01)	0.01
Gender, female	−0.2 (0.2)	0.49	−0.2 (0.2)	0.33	−17.8 (1.2)	<0.001	−18.3 (1.3)	<0.001	0.02 (0.04)	0.61	−0.03 (0.04)	0.46
Education, higher	0.5 (0.02)	0.02	0.6 (0.2)	0.01	−1.0 (2.5)	0.70	0.4 (1.3)	0.76	0.1 (0.04)	0.07	0.1 (0.04)	0.08
Strength exercise	0.1 (0.2)	0.40	0.1 (0.2)	0.39	−4.6 (0.6)	0.51	−0.2 (0.5)	0.71	−0.1 (0.03)	0.05	0.1 (0.04)	0.02
Live Alone	−0.1 (0.2)	0.58	−0.1 (0.3)	0.85	−7.2 (2.3)	0.003	−0.2 (1.5)	0.91	−0.03 (0.04)	0.46	0.02 (0.1)	0.61
Seafood intake	−0.1 (0.1)	0.33	−0.1 (0.1)	0.40	0.3 (0.3)	0.23	0.4 (0.3)	0.09	0.01 (0.01)	0.68	0.01 (0.1)	0.57

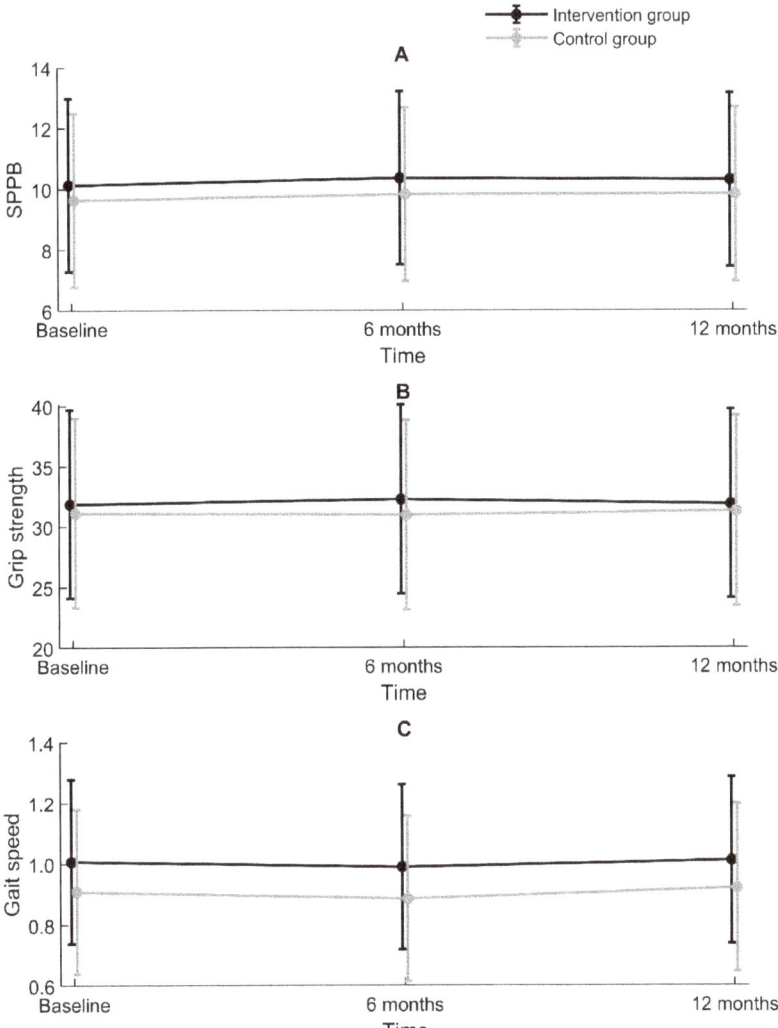

Figure 1. Differences between the intervention group and control group for (**A**) Short Physical Performance Battery (SPPB, points), (**B**) grip strength (kg), and (**C**) gait speed (m/s), with a 95% confidence interval, estimated by linear mixed models adjusting for within-participant and within-municipality correlations.

Due to dropout during the follow-up period, a number of preplanned covariates had to be reconsidered. Protein and energy intake were excluded from the model as they highly correlated with each other (r = 0.75) and were not significantly associated with the outcome variables at the baseline [13]. Vitamin D measurements were performed with 6 months between analyses to account for seasonal variation; however, 21 participants were missing one of the two measurements. Seven participants were missing both measurements of vitamin D. Thus, vitamin D was also excluded as an adjustment covariate. The results of the multiple linear mixed model reduced by Akaike's Information Criterion did not change the conclusions of the bivariate analyses.

3. Discussion

Our intervention study among elderly persons did not reveal any significant differences in measures of physical function (SPPB and gait speed) or strength (grip strength) between the intervention group receiving a supplement of MPH and the control group receiving a placebo. However, the study participants had good physical function and strength and sufficient protein intake at the starting point. We used standardized measurements and questions to collect data at several time points, ensuring comparability of results across different studies.

Mean SPPB in this study was 10.3 points in women and 11.0 points in men. In the power calculation, we anticipated the mean SPPB to be 7.5 (see methods Section 4.7). Our assumption was based on data from a more sedentary and already frail population [14] as the initial goal was to recruit participants among home care service users. The SPPB scores observed in our study were more in line with the normative scores reported by Bergland et al. [15], where the mean score in the age group of 70–74 years was 10.8 in women and 11.4 in men. Bergland's study also reports that the SPPB test has a considerable ceiling effect, where more than 20% have the highest or lowest scores. In our study, 51.2% of the participants reached the top score of 12 points. Thus, the ceiling effect of the SPPB test is a considerable shortcoming of our study as possible changes in physical function could not be identified by our primary outcome measure.

The baseline values of the secondary outcomes, grip strength and gait speed, further underline that the participants in our study sample have good physical function and strength. The mean grip strength in our study was 26.7 kg in women and 45.5 kg in men. Compared with the normative data reported by Dodds et al., this represents a level of grip strength comparable to 60-year-old women and men [16]. However, all participants in our study were >65years, with a mean age of 72.7 years. Recent studies in Norway [17] and Finland [18] show that older adults are stronger and have better grip strength now than in earlier generations, corresponding to a five-year difference, i.e., the more recently born generation of 80-year-olds have a similar mean grip strength as 75-year-olds born one generation earlier [17].

The participants in our study had a protein intake of 1.1 g/kg BW, which is higher than the recommended daily allowance (RDA) of 0.8 g/kg and in accordance with the increased dosage for elderly persons according to Nordic nutritional recommendations [19]. Protein intake is, however, lower than in other Norwegian studies such as Norkost3 [20] and the Tromsø study [21]. Energy intake in our study was in line with the results of Norkost3 in women; however, the male participants in our study reported lower energy intake compared with Norkost3. This might indicate underreporting, especially by men. Protein and energy intake were, however, assessed by a single day food recall, and this is a weakness as diet often varies from day to day. Protein and energy intake were not included in the regression model. However, their sufficient protein intake might indicate that this study population was not the appropriate target group for MPH supplementation.

Moreover, the participants in our study had a relatively high seafood intake. The mean computed seafood index corresponded to >3 meals of seafood per week, which is in accordance with the dietary guidelines in Norway [22] and in line with data from Norkost3 [20]. The seafood intake was equally high in both intervention and control groups, and thus would not influence the results in terms of difference between groups. However, the relatively high seafood intake and protein intake among the participants might indicate that they were not in need of supplementation, and thus it was difficult to notice any effects.

We anticipated that the SPPB score would decline by 0.9 points in the control group. However, we could not detect a change in physical function over time in either the control or intervention group. Bergland et al. [15] demonstrated that a decline in physical function, as measured by the SPPB, occurs in the mid-sixties, with a slightly earlier decline in women than in men. However, Hämäläinen [23] examined 6-year changes in physical performance among high-functioning older adults and found improvement in physical performance in age groups comparable to the participants in our study. Hämäläinen finds that this might be related to an increased physical activity level after recent retirement from work. In our study, more than 50% reported being physically active daily. Weekly strength exercise was also frequently reported. However, only self-reported frequency of physical activity and strength exercise was measured, not the loading or the level of activity. Strength exercise might be the most influential factor in muscle health in ageing, and nutritional supplements may support these effects [24]. We wanted to examine the effects of the MPH supplement without exercise; however, the possible high frequency of strength exercise in the group might have biased the results.

Daily physical activity was more frequent in the intervention group than in the control group, and the intervention and control groups were also significantly different in SPPB and gait speed at the baseline and the 6-month follow-up, with higher scores in the intervention group according to linear mixed model analyses adjusting for a cluster effect on a municipal level. Groups were not significantly different at the 12-month follow-up. Thus, differences between the intervention and control groups decreased with time; however, this could be related to selection bias as dropouts were significantly different from those completing the full 12-month follow-up.

Participants dropping out of the study had significantly lower scores in SPPB, grip strength, and gait speed compared with those completing the follow-up. A review of attrition in longitudinal studies among the elderly shows that dropout is associated with, e.g., higher age, fewer years of education, poor functioning, and living alone [25]. These factors are also significantly different between participants dropping out versus those completing our study. However, dietary factors did not significantly differ between dropouts and those completing the study, nor did compliance in intervention or problems related to the tablets. Compliance was high in both the intervention group and control group, despite many reported problems with swallowing and/or gastrointestinal effects related to the tablets. One out of three participants experienced gastrointestinal problems, and every fourth participant had difficulties swallowing the tablets. As there were no differences in gastrointestinal complaints or swallowing difficulties between the intervention group and control group, we believe that the problems might be related to the large number of tablets and possibly to the additives used to make the tablets look similar and be odor free.

This study did not identify differences in measures of physical performance and strength between the intervention group and control group; however, this might be related to the limitations of the study. As previously discussed, the study participants had good physical function, strength, and nutrient intake, and we could not see a decline in physical function during the study. This might indicate that they were not in need of a supplement enhancing MPS. On the other hand, one year might not be sufficient time to detect the preventive effect on muscle health. This was one of the first studies assessing MPH in relation to physical function and strength in older adults [12], and we suggest the following recommendations for future studies:

- Future studies should be performed on a frailer population or on populations with immobilized older adults. The population that is most in need of help with stimulating MPS is composed of people who are immobilized over a period of time, e.g., after injuries or illnesses affecting mobility.
- MPH might have the potential to mitigate loss of muscle function and strength in populations of older adults with lower protein and seafood intake.
- Physical activity should be measured more precisely.
- The large number of tablets was burdensome and might have caused gastrointestinal symptoms in both the intervention and control groups. The number of tablets should be reduced. The use of a soft drink, similar to the supplement used in the feasibility study by Drotningsvik et al. [26], might be a better choice. Alternatively, MPH could be used as an additive in enteral nutrition solutions or soft drink supplements.

4. Materials and Methods

This study was a randomized, controlled, double-blinded trial in which the participants received tablets containing 3 g of MPH or a placebo, with data collected at a baseline and at 6- and 12-month follow-ups. A 12-month follow-up period was planned for all participants; however, they were given the supplements for 6 months at a time, with the opportunity to withdraw at any time. Thus, statistical analyses were pre-planned to include measurements at both 6 months and 12 months of intervention. The study design is graphically illustrated in Figure 2.

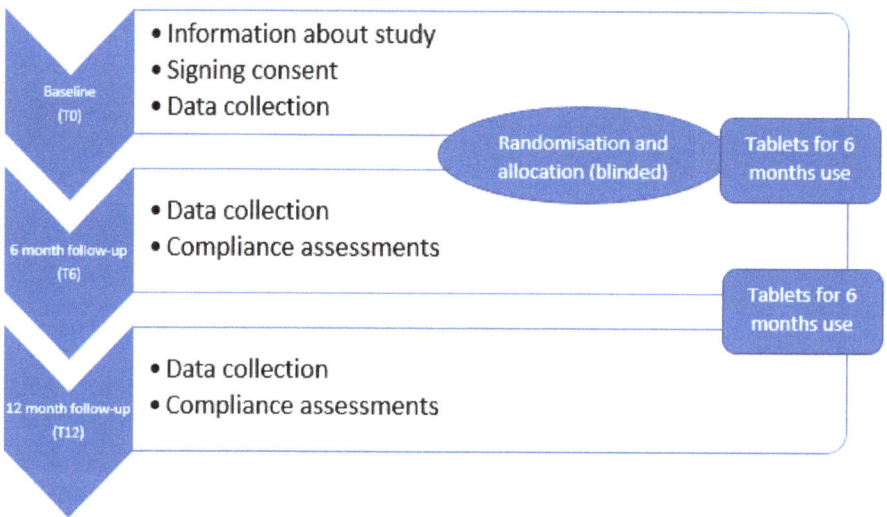

Figure 2. Study design: A randomized, controlled, double-blinded trial with data collection at the baseline, 6 months and 12 months.

4.1. Recruitment

Participants were recruited from March 2017 to May 2018, with all follow-up observations completed in January 2019. The study included adults ≥65 years old. Exclusion criteria included active cancer or progressive muscle illness (e.g., multiple sclerosis or Lou Gehrig's disease), diabetes, kidney failure, short life expectancy (<1 year), and allergies to fish protein. Mental illness or neurodegenerative illnesses were not defined as exclusion criteria, however; participants were considered competent enough to provide informed consent to participate. Initially, one of the inclusion criteria was need of home care services, and recruitment was supposed to be facilitated trough municipal healthcare services. However, this recruitment proved difficult, and after 6 months and only 16 participants recruited, we omitted the criterion of the need for municipal support and started recruitment through local media and by leaving flyers at healthcare offices and senior citizen associations. A total of 92 individuals from several municipalities on the west coast of Norway consented to participate in the study. They represented a mixed cohort of elderly receiving home care services (n = 16) and elderly who were independent in daily activities and thus were without need of municipal home care (n = 76). The predetermined sample size goal of 82 (see power calculation below) was achieved, however, we did not succeed in recruiting extra participants to account for dropouts. The flow of participant recruitment and allocation is described in Figure 3 (CONSORT flow diagram).

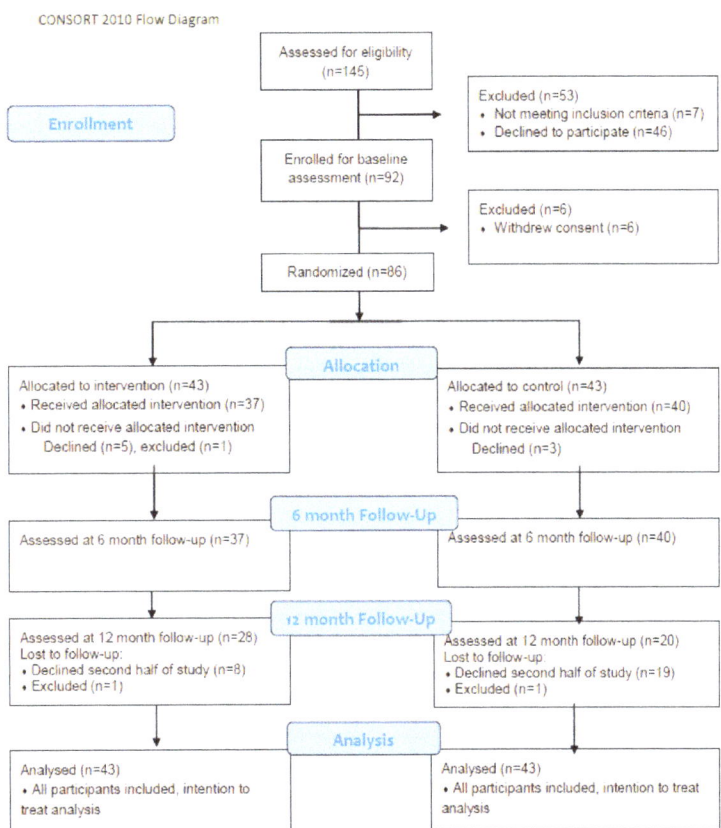

Figure 3. Consort flow diagram illustrating flow of participant recruitment and allocation.

4.2. Randomisation

Eight participants withdrew their consent, and one was excluded due to exclusion criteria occurring after inclusion, leaving 86 participants, 57 women and 29 men for randomization into the intervention group (n = 43) or control group (n = 43).

The participants were given project identification numbers and block-randomized into two groups. Blocks were based on the baseline score of the SPPB test (low score 0–6 points, medium score 7–9 points, or high score 10–12 points) and gender. The main researcher (LKN) enrolled participants and forwarded identification numbers and block information to the statistician (JSB), who performed randomization into either group A (n = 43) or group B (n = 43). Supplements and placebos were distributed in similar boxes prepared by a person not involved in the study and only marked with participants' identification numbers. Participants, care providers, outcome assessors, and data analysts were blinded for the intervention. The study investigators were blinded when analyzing the primary and secondary outcomes as the code was masked until statistical analyses were completed.

4.3. Intervention

The participants in both the intervention and control groups were instructed to take five tablets twice a day, preferably with breakfast and their evening meal. For the intervention group, each tablet contained 300 mg of MPH, which corresponds to a total dose of 3 g of protein per day (1.5 g in the morning and 1.5 g in the evening). The tablets were produced by Flexipharma AS and based on the marine peptide compound 565952 P from Firmenich Bjørge Biomarin AS (data sheet in Supplemental Material). The marine peptide compound was manufactured through the hydrolysis of fresh or fresh-frozen Atlantic cod fillet (*Gadus morhua*) using industrial food approved non-GMO proteolytic enzymes, and maltodextrin from corn was added to mask the odor and taste of fish. Hydrolysis was conducted using equipment and procedures according to regulations provided by the Norwegian Food Safety Authorities. Marine peptides are approved as a food ingredient in Norway according to EU regulations. The control group received the same number of similar-looking placebo tablets produced from gum Arabic.

4.4. Assessments

Assessments were completed in the participants' homes at the baseline and at 6- and 12-month follow-ups. The researcher filled in the questionnaires based on a structured interview with each participant. Demographic data included age, gender, living condition, and educational level, and this information was collected only at the baseline. The participants' education levels were dichotomized as having higher or lower education. Higher education was defined as education at university or college level, i.e., more than 12 years of education.

Physical activity was reported in categories based on how often participants performed strength exercises and how often they were physically active otherwise (e.g., walking, running, bicycling). Strength exercise was dichotomized into at least once a week or more seldom. Other physical activity was dichotomized into daily or more seldom.

A 24-hour food recall was conducted using a multiple pass method following the five-step protocol described by Moshfegh et al. [27], recording all food items and amounts eaten the day before the visit. To adapt the method to Norwegian participants, we used an illustrated food portion booklet with a corresponding list of weights from the Norwegian study Ungkost 2000 [28]. Energy and protein intake per day were calculated using the online diet tool from the Norwegian Directorate of Health and the Norwegian Food Safety Authority, www.kostholdsplanleggeren.no. The food database in the Diet Planner is based on the Norwegian Food Composition table, which provides an overview of the content of energy and nutrients for the most common foods eaten in Norway.

Estimated protein and energy intake were expressed in grams per kilogram (g/kg) of body weight (BW). For participants who were under- or overweight (BMI < 22.0 kg/m^2 or >27 kg/m^2), the BW was adjusted by applying the BW corresponding to a BMI of 22 or 27 kg/m^2, respectively. Higher BMI is recommended for older adults compared with adults [29,30]. The BMI cut-off values used in this study are described in the Norwegian guidelines for treatment and prevention of malnutrition [31]. This adjustment was made to let the intake represent the intake related to protein requirement rather than BW in under- and overweight individuals, as underweight persons require extra protein to build muscle tissue, while the extra weight in overweight persons is often composed of adipose tissue [32,33].

Habitual intake of seafood in the past 6 months was estimated by using a shorter version of a previously validated Food Frequency Questionnaire (FFQ) [34]. The frequency of seafood intake for dinner and frequency of seafood used as a spread in salads, as a snack, or something similar was recorded. Responses were reported as never, <1 time/month, 1–3 times/month, once/week, 2–3 times/week, and ≥4 times/week. The midpoint of categories was used to calculate frequency of meals per week, e.g., 2–3 times per week was regarded as 2.5. Frequency of seafood used as a spread in salads, as a snack, or something similar was divided by six, as six portions of seafood as spreads correspond to one dinner portion. Thus, the combined frequency of seafood consumption corresponds to a dinner portion equivalent per week. This method of making a continuous scale of seafood consumption from FFQ was developed and validated against biomarkers by Markhus et al. [35].

Body mass was recorded in light clothing to the nearest 0.1 kg using a digital scale (Seca 803), and height was measured with a tape measure (Seca 201). Furthermore, the participants were instructed to visit their general practitioner (GP) for blood sampling. Blood samples were handled at the participants' local municipality laboratories, and serum was sent to the local hospital for analysis of 25-hydroxy vitamin D as a biomarker for vitamin D status.

4.5. Main Outcome: Short Physical Performance Test (SPPB)

Muscle performance was measured with the SPPB, a test battery developed originally for the Established Populations for Epidemiologic Studies of the Elderly and translated into Norwegian in 2013 by Bergh and colleagues [36]. The test battery includes standing balance, walking speed, and repeated chair rise. Each of the three domain scores ranges from 0–4 points, yielding an integer sum score ranging from 0–12 points. A higher sum score indicates a higher level of functioning, and a change of one unit is considered a clinically meaningful change [14]. A systematic review of instruments assessing performance-based physical function in older community-dwelling persons concluded that the SPPB is highly recommended in terms of validity, reliability, and responsiveness [37]. The SPPB complements self-reported disability and may predict mortality and nursing home admission even at the high end of the functional spectrum [38]. Gait speed was calculated as meters per second (m/s) from the 4m walking test included in SPPB and used as a secondary outcome.

4.6. Secondary Outcome: Grip Strength

Grip strength was measured to the nearest 0.1 kg using the Jamar Plus+ digital hand dynamometer. The maximum value of three trials on each hand was used for analyses [16]. Grip strength is a useful and simple measure of muscle strength. It correlates with leg strength, is a clinical marker of poor mobility, and is considered a better predictor of clinical outcomes than low muscle mass [39]. Cutoff scores are set at 30 kg and 20 kg for men and women, respectively [39]. However, Dodds et al. provided normative data for grip strength across the life course [16].

4.7. Sample Size and Statistical Power Calculation

Based on an American study reporting a clinically meaningful change in the main outcome of SPPB to be 0.4–1.5 points [14], we assumed that the mean SPPB score at inclusion was 7.52 in both groups, and the standard deviation after the intervention period would be 1.42 in both groups. Freiberger et.al. [37] evaluated the responsiveness of SPPB, and the observed effect sizes in intervention studies were ranging from 0.48 to 1.25. Based on these numbers, we assumed a reduction of 0.9 (mid-point) in the control group. We also assumed that the intervention group maintained a stable SPPB score throughout the study period, so that the effect would be seen as a decrease in the control group. A sample size of 41 participants in each group was required to detect a statistically significant mean difference of 0.9 points at a significance level of 5% and with a power of 80% using a two-sided independent samples t-test. As the participants were older, we expected a 20% dropout rate and therefore aimed to include 50 participants in each group.

4.8. Statistical Analyses

The demographic and clinical characteristics of the participants in each group were described as means and standard deviations (SDs) or frequencies and percentages, as appropriate. Independent samples t-test and χ^2-test were used to assess the gender differences and differences between participants completing the study and the dropouts. As a primary analysis, independent samples t-test was used to assess the difference in change in the primary outcome, SPPB, between the intervention group and the control group.

A linear mixed model was then estimated to assess the effect of MPH on the SPPB in the intervention group and control group throughout the 12-month follow-up. The model included fixed effects for time components up to the second order to account for non-linear effects, group allocation, and interaction between the two. A significant interaction between time and group allocation would imply differences in SPPB scores between the groups throughout the follow-up. As participants were recruited from different municipalities, the data will likely exhibit a hierarchical structure. The within-municipality cluster effect was assessed using the intra-class correlation coefficient (ICC). Moreover, due to repeated measurements for each participant, the within-participant correlation will likely be present. Therefore, random effects for participants nested within the municipality were included to correctly adjust estimates for possible within-participant and within-municipality correlations. Random slopes for the time component were considered but not included as they did not improve the model fit. Pairwise comparisons were conducted by deriving individual time-point contrasts within each group with corresponding 95% confidence intervals (CIs) and p-values, and the results were illustrated graphically. The results were further adjusted for several of the pre-planned covariates: age, gender, education, living status, strength exercise, and habitual seafood intake [40]. Some of the pre-planned covariates were not included due to high correlations or many missing values. Cases with missing values on one or more covariates were excluded from regression analysis. Akaike's Information Criterion, where the smaller value means a better model, was used to reduce models for excessive adjustment variables. The secondary outcomes grip strength (kg) and gait speed (m/s) were assessed in the same way. Statistical analyses were performed using SPSS v 24 and SAS v 9.4. Results with p-values below 0.05 were considered statistically significant. The intention-to-treat principle was used in statistical analysis.

4.9. Ethical Approval and Registration

All subjects gave their informed oral and written consent for inclusion before they participated in the study, which was conducted in accordance with the Declaration of Helsinki and approved by the Regional Committee on Ethics in Medical Research (REK) in Mid-Norway in September 2016 with the registration ID 2016/1152. Changes in inclusion criteria were approved in August 2017. The study protocol has been published elsewhere [40], and the trial was pre-registered at http://www.clinicaltrials.gov with the unique identifier NCT02890290.

Supplementary Materials: The following are available online at https://www.mdpi.com/1660-3397/19/2/62/s1, Data sheet marine peptides.

Author Contributions: Conceptualisation, L.K.N.; methodology, L.K.N., L.D., I.M., and A.M.M.R.; formal analysis, J.Š.B.; investigation, L.K.N.; data curation, L.K.N.; writing—original draft preparation, L.K.N.; writing—review and editing, A.M.M.R., L.D., I.M., and J.Š.B.; visualisation, J.Š.B.; supervision, A.M.M.R. All authors have read and agreed to the published version of the manuscript.

Funding: The project is funded by a general PhD grant from Molde University College. Blood analyses are funded by The Research Council of Norway, Programme for Regional R&D and Innovation (VRI). The intervention is funded by Firmenich Bjørge Biomarin AS, who provided the marine protein hydrolysate supplement and placebo preparation. The founding sponsors had no role in the design of the study; in the collection, analyses, and interpretation of data; in the writing of the manuscript, nor in the decision to publish the results.

Institutional Review Board Statement: The study was conducted according to the guidelines of the Declaration of Helsinki, and approved by the Regional Committee on Ethics in Medical Research (REK) in Mid-Norway in Sep-tember 2016 with the registration ID 2016/1152. Changes in inclusion criteria were approved in August 2017.

Informed Consent Statement: Informed consent was obtained from all subjects involved in the study.

Data Availability Statement: The data presented in this study are available on request from the corresponding author. The data are not publicly available due to privacy restrictions.

Acknowledgments: We would like to express our very great appreciation to the participants in the study, to the healthcare staff who recruited the first 16 participants, and to public relations adviser Jan Ragnvald Eide, local media, senior citizen associations, and others who participated in further recruitment of participants. We also want to acknowledge the assistance provided by Stine Hauvik in preparing tablets and blinding the intervention and by local GPs and laboratory staff in taking the blood samples and laboratories at Molde hospital and St. Olav hospital for analysis. A special 'thank you' goes to Tore Skei at St. Olav hospital for assistance with laboratory reports.

Conflicts of Interest: The authors declare no conflict of interest.

References

1. Expectation of Lifetime, by Sex and Age 1986–2019. Available online: https://www.ssb.no/en/statbank/table/05375 (accessed on 1 October 2020).
2. Phillips, S.M. Nutrition in the elderly: A recommendation for more (evenly distributed) protein? *Am. J. Clin. Nutr.* **2017**, *106*, 12–13. [CrossRef]
3. Breen, L.; Phillips, S.M. Skeletal muscle protein metabolism in the elderly: Interventions to counteract the 'anabolic resistance' of ageing. *Nutr. Metab. (Lond.)* **2011**, *8*, 68. [CrossRef]
4. Verlaan, S.; Aspray, T.J.; Bauer, J.M.; Cederholm, T.; Hemsworth, J.; Hill, T.R.; McPhee, J.S.; Piasecki, M.; Seal, C.; Sieber, C.C.; et al. Nutritional status, body composition, and quality of life in community-dwelling sarcopenic and non-sarcopenic older adults: A case-control study. *Clin. Nutr.* **2015**, *36*, 267–274. [CrossRef]
5. Wysokiński, A.; Sobów, T.; Kłoszewska, I.; Kostka, T. Mechanisms of the anorexia of aging-a review. *Age (Dordr)* **2015**, *37*, 9821. [CrossRef]
6. Liao, C.D.; Tsauo, J.Y.; Wu, Y.T.; Cheng, C.P.; Chen, H.C.; Huang, Y.C.; Chen, H.C.; Liou, T.H. Effects of protein supplementation combined with resistance exercise on body composition and physical function in older adults: A systematic review and meta-analysis. *Am. J. Clin. Nutr.* **2017**, *106*, 1078–1091. [CrossRef]
7. Brioche, T.; Pagano, A.F.; Py, G.; Chopard, A. Muscle wasting and aging: Experimental models, fatty infiltrations, and prevention. *Mol. Asp. Med.* **2016**, *50*, 56–87. [CrossRef]
8. Galvan, E.; Arentson-Lantz, E.; Lamon, S.; Paddon-Jones, D. Protecting Skeletal Muscle with Protein and Amino Acid during Periods of Disuse. *Nutrients* **2016**, *8*, 404. [CrossRef]
9. Dale, H.F.; Madsen, L.; Lied, G.A. Fish-derived proteins and their potential to improve human health. *Nutr. Rev.* **2019**, *77*, 572–583. [CrossRef] [PubMed]
10. Vikoren, L.A.; Nygard, O.K.; Lied, E.; Rostrup, E.; Gudbrandsen, O.A. A randomised study on the effects of fish protein supplement on glucose tolerance, lipids and body composition in overweight adults. *Br. J. Nutr.* **2013**, *109*, 648–657. [CrossRef] [PubMed]
11. Nobile, V.; Duclos, E.; Michelotti, A.; Bizzaro, G.; Negro, M.; Soisson, F. Supplementation with a fish protein hydrolysate (*Micromesistius poutassou*): Effects on body weight, body composition, and CCK/GLP-1 secretion. *Food Nutr. Res.* **2016**, *60*, 29857. [CrossRef] [PubMed]
12. Lees, M.J.; Carson, B.P. The Potential Role of Fish-Derived Protein Hydrolysates on Metabolic Health, Skeletal Muscle Mass and Function in Ageing. *Nutrients* **2020**, *12*, 2434. [CrossRef] [PubMed]
13. Nygard, L.A.K.; Dahl, L.; Mundal, I.; Saltyte Benth, J.; Rokstad, A.M.M. Protein intake, protein mealtime distribution and seafood consumption in elderly Norwegians: Associations with physical function and strength. *Geriatrics* **2020**, *5*, 100. [CrossRef] [PubMed]
14. Kwon, S.; Perera, S.; Pahor, M.; Katula, J.A.; King, A.C.; Groessl, E.J.; Studenski, S.A. What is a meaningful change in physical performance? Findings from a clinical trial in older adults (the LIFE-P study). *J. Nutr. Health Aging* **2009**, *13*, 538–544. [CrossRef] [PubMed]
15. Bergland, A.; Strand, B.H. Norwegian reference values for the Short Physical Performance Battery (SPPB): The Tromsø Study. *BMC Geriatr.* **2019**, *19*, 216. [CrossRef]
16. Dodds, R.M.; Syddall, H.E.; Cooper, R.; Benzeval, M.; Deary, I.J.; Dennison, E.M.; Der, G.; Gale, C.R.; Inskip, H.M.; Jagger, C.; et al. Grip strength across the life course: Normative data from twelve British studies. *PLoS ONE* **2014**, *9*, e113637. [CrossRef]
17. Strand, B.H.; Bergland, A.; Jørgensen, L.; Schirmer, H.; Emaus, N.; Cooper, R. Do More Recent Born Generations of Older Adults Have Stronger Grip? A Comparison of Three Cohorts of 66- to 84-Year-Olds in the Tromsø Study. *J. Gerontol. Ser. A* **2018**, *74*, 528–533. [CrossRef]
18. Koivunen, K.; Sillanpää, E.; Munukka, M.; Portegijs, E.; Rantanen, T. Cohort Differences in Maximal Physical Performance: A Comparison of 75- and 80-Year-Old Men and Women Born 28 Years Apart. *J. Gerontol. Ser. A* **2020**. [CrossRef]
19. *Nordic Nutrition Recommendations 2012: Integrating Nutrition and Physical Activity*, 5th ed.; Nordic Council of Ministers: Copenhagen, Denmark, 2014; Volume 2014.
20. Totland, T.H.; Helsedirektoratet. *Norkost 3: En Landsomfattende Kostholdsundersøkelse Blant Menn og Kvinner i Norge i Alderen 18–70 år, 2010–2011*; Helsedirektoratet: Oslo, Norway, 2012.
21. Lundblad, M.W.; Andersen, L.F.; Jacobsen, B.K.; Carlsen, M.H.; Hjartaker, A.; Grimsgaard, S.; Hopstock, L.A. Energy and nutrient intakes in relation to National Nutrition Recommendations in a Norwegian population-based sample: The Tromso Study 2015-16. *Food Nutr. Res.* **2019**, *63*. [CrossRef]
22. Helsedirektoratet. *IS-1881: Kostråd for å Fremme Folkehelsen og Forebygge Kroniske Sykdommer*; Helsedirektoratet: Oslo, Norway, 2011.
23. Hämäläinen, P.; Suni, J.; Pasanen, M.; Malmberg, J.; Miilunpalo, S. Changes in physical performance among high-functioning older adults: A 6-year follow-up study. *Eur. J. Ageing* **2006**, *3*, 3–14. [CrossRef]

24. McKendry, J.; Currier, B.S.; Lim, C.; McLeod, J.C.; Thomas, A.C.Q.; Phillips, S.M. Nutritional Supplements to Support Resistance Exercise in Countering the Sarcopenia of Aging. *Nutrients* **2020**, *12*, 2057. [CrossRef]
25. Chatfield, M.D.; Brayne, C.E.; Matthews, F.E. A systematic literature review of attrition between waves in longitudinal studies in the elderly shows a consistent pattern of dropout between differing studies. *J. Clin. Epidemiol.* **2005**, *58*, 13–19. [CrossRef] [PubMed]
26. Drotningsvik, A.; Oterhals, Å.; Flesland, O.; Nygård, O.; Gudbrandsen, O.A. Fish protein supplementation in older nursing home residents: A randomised, double-blind, pilot study. *Pilot Feasibility Stud.* **2019**, *5*, 35. [CrossRef] [PubMed]
27. Moshfegh, A.J.; Rhodes, D.G.; Baer, D.J.; Murayi, T.; Clemens, J.C.; Rumpler, W.V.; Paul, D.R.; Sebastian, R.S.; Kuczynski, K.J.; Ingwersen, L.A.; et al. The US Department of Agriculture Automated Multiple-Pass Method reduces bias in the collection of energy intakes. *Am. J. Clin. Nutr.* **2008**, *88*, 324–332. [CrossRef] [PubMed]
28. Øverby, N.C.; Frost Andersen, L. *Ungkost-2000: Landsomfattende Kostholdsundersøkelse Blant Elever i 4.—og 8. Klasse i Norge*; Sosial- og Helsedirektoratet: Oslo, Norway, 2002.
29. Gulsvik, A.K.; Thelle, D.S.; Mowe, M.; Wyller, T.B. Increased mortality in the slim elderly: A 42 years follow-up study in a general population. *Eur. J. Epidemiol.* **2009**, *24*, 683–690. [CrossRef] [PubMed]
30. Winter, J.E.; MacInnis, R.J.; Wattanapenpaiboon, N.; Nowson, C.A. BMI and all-cause mortality in older adults: A meta-analysis. *Am. J. Clin. Nutr.* **2014**, *99*, 875–890. [CrossRef]
31. Helsedirektoratet. *IS-1580: Nasjonale Faglige Retningslinjer for Forebygging og Behandling av Underernæring*; Helsedirektoratet: Oslo, Norway, 2010.
32. Berner, L.A.; Becker, G.; Wise, M.; Doi, J. Characterization of dietary protein among older adults in the United States: Amount, animal sources, and meal patterns. *J. Acad. Nutr. Diet.* **2013**, *113*, 809–815. [CrossRef]
33. Wijnhoven, H.A.H.; Elstgeest, L.E.M.; de Vet, H.C.W.; Nicolaou, M.; Snijder, M.B.; Visser, M. Development and validation of a short food questionnaire to screen for low protein intake in community-dwelling older adults: The Protein Screener 55+ (Pro55+). *PLoS ONE* **2018**, *13*, e0196406. [CrossRef]
34. Dahl, L.; Maeland, C.A.; Bjorkkjaer, T. A short food frequency questionnaire to assess intake of seafood and n-3 supplements: Validation with biomarkers. *Nutr. J.* **2011**, *10*, 127. [CrossRef]
35. Markhus, M.W.; Graff, I.E.; Dahl, L.; Seldal, C.F.; Skotheim, S.; Braarud, H.C.; Stormark, K.M.; Malde, M.K. Establishment of a seafood index to assess the seafood consumption in pregnant women. *Food Nutr. Res.* **2013**, *57*, 19272. [CrossRef]
36. Bergh, S.; Lyshol, H.; Selbæk, G.; Strand, B.H.; Taraldsen, K.; Thingstad, P. Short Physical Performance Battery (SPPB). Available online: https://stolav.no/PublishingImages/Sider/Bevegelsesvansker-og-fall-hos-eldre/SPPB%20Norsk%20versjon%2006.05.13.pdf (accessed on 1 October 2020).
37. Freiberger, E.; de Vreede, P.; Schoene, D.; Rydwik, E.; Mueller, V.; Frandin, K.; Hopman-Rock, M. Performance-based physical function in older community-dwelling persons: A systematic review of instruments. *Age Ageing* **2012**, *41*, 712–721. [CrossRef]
38. Guralnik, J.M.; Simonsick, E.M.; Ferrucci, L.; Glynn, R.J.; Berkman, L.F.; Blazer, D.G.; Scherr, P.A.; Wallace, R.B. A short physical performance battery assessing lower extremity function: Association with self-reported disability and prediction of mortality and nursing home admission. *J. Gerontol.* **1994**, *49*, M85–M94. [CrossRef] [PubMed]
39. Cruz-Jentoft, A.J.; Baeyens, J.P.; Bauer, J.M.; Boirie, Y.; Cederholm, T.; Landi, F.; Martin, F.C.; Michel, J.P.; Rolland, Y.; Schneider, S.M.; et al. Sarcopenia: European consensus on definition and diagnosis: Report of the European Working Group on Sarcopenia in Older People. *Age Ageing* **2010**, *39*, 412–423. [CrossRef] [PubMed]
40. Nygard, L.A.K.; Mundal, I.; Dahl, L.; Saltyte Benth, J.; Rokstad, A.M.M. Nutrition and physical performance in older people-effects of marine protein hydrolysates to prevent decline in physical performance: A randomised controlled trial protocol. *BMJ Open* **2018**, *8*, e023845. [CrossRef] [PubMed]

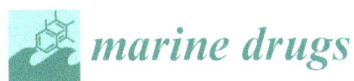

Review

Marine Bioactive Peptides—An Overview of Generation, Structure and Application with a Focus on Food Sources

Milica Pavlicevic [1], Elena Maestri [2,3,*] and Marta Marmiroli [2]

[1] Institute for Food Technology and Biochemistry, Faculty of Agriculture, University of Belgrade, 11070 Belgrade, Serbia; mpavlicevic@agrif.bg.ac.rs
[2] Department of Chemistry, Life Sciences and Environmental Sustainability, and SITEIA.PARMA, University of Parma, 42123 Parma, Italy; marta.marmiroli@unipr.it
[3] Consorzio Italbiotec, Via Fantoli 16/15, 20138 Milan, Italy
* Correspondence: elena.maestri@unipr.it

Received: 4 July 2020; Accepted: 11 August 2020; Published: 13 August 2020

Abstract: The biggest obstacles in the application of marine peptides are two-fold, as in the case of non-marine plant and animal-derived bioactive peptides: elucidating correlation between the peptide structure and its effect and demonstrating its stability in vivo. The structures of marine bioactive peptides are highly variable and complex and dependent on the sources from which they are isolated. They can be cyclical, in the form of depsipeptides, and often contain secondary structures. Because of steric factors, marine-derived peptides can be resistant to proteolysis by gastrointestinal proteases, which presents an advantage over other peptide sources. Because of heterogeneity, amino acid sequences as well as preferred mechanisms of peptides showing specific bioactivities differ compared to their animal-derived counterparts. This review offers insights on the extreme diversity of bioactivities, effects, and structural features, analyzing 253 peptides, mainly from marine food sources. Similar to peptides in food of non-marine animal origin, a significant percentage (52.7%) of the examined sequences contain one or more proline residues, implying that proline might play a significant role in the stability of bioactive peptides. Additional problems with analyzing marine-derived bioactive peptides include their accessibility, extraction, and purification; this review considers the challenges and proposes possible solutions.

Keywords: bioactive peptides; marine; secondary structure; proline; mechanism of activity; marine waste

1. Introduction

Although marine peptides have only fairly recently garnered deserved attention (especially compared to peptides from other plant/animal sources), their potential to generate classes of peptides with interesting properties such as antiaging, antituberculosis, anticoagulant, and antidiabetic makes them promising agents not only in medicine and pharmacy [1–3], but also in the cosmetic industry [4–6]. Because of the beneficial interactions of the marine peptides with phenolic compounds [7], and to the improved emulsifying and foaming properties [8], their usage in the food industry has also proven to be valuable. Attempts have also been made to employ peptides derived from seaweed in prebiotics and nutraceuticals [9]. The use of marine waste for peptide generation is not only useful from economic and ecological standpoints, but can also produce peptides with proven ACE (angiotensin-converting enzyme) inhibitory, antioxidant, and immunomodulatory activity [10–14].

However, several problems regarding wide-spread use of marine-derived peptides still need to be solved: finding optimal conditions for the isolation of peptides from their sources and creating uniform conditions for their production from particular sources; establishing correlations between structure and bioactivity; demonstrating the peptide's stability and effectiveness in vivo; and in certain cases, improving their accessibility and extraction yields. For example, in the case of marine peptides derived from seaweed, both the accessibility of source material and the inefficiency of peptide extraction present problems. Extraction of seaweed-derived peptides is additionally hindered by the presence of polysaccharides in cell walls of the seaweed [15].

Similarly to peptides of other animal and plant origin, the structures of marine bioactive peptides are highly dependent on the source from which they are isolated [16,17]. But such variations in activities and structures of marine peptides are even more pronounced because of the high taxonomic diversity among and within the five major groups of marine organisms used as food, fish, algae, bivalves, cephalopods, and crustaceans, spanning four kingdoms of living organisms.

However, unlike peptides from other sources, many marine-derived peptides are more resistant to proteolysis by gastrointestinal proteases, because of the steric factors derived from their unusual structures (branched, cyclic and possessing both D and L amino acids) [18,19].

Thus, the aim of this work is to present the current understanding of marine peptides' production, structures, and applications, and also to compare and contrast them with production, structures, and applications of peptides from other animal food sources.

In order to achieve that, we comprised a list of 253 peptides from all five groups of marine organisms used as food (Table S1), using the BIOPEP database [20] and our own survey of literature. Reason why BIOPEP was chosen for peptide selection is two-fold: first, it is currently the most inclusive database, since it encompasses all bioactive peptides, regardless of their origin, effect, or length, with 4031 entries as of August 2020. Second, it provides additional information, such as in cases of ACE inhibitors, EC50 value, and type of organism from which peptide(s) were extracted. Although other databases for marine products exist, they are either too broad, such as the marine natural product database [21] or too narrow, focusing only on a specific type of organism and class of peptides (such as PenBase [22]) or a specific length (such as PepBank [23]) or a particular bioactivity [24–29]. Thus, we decided to use BIOPEP as the database most closely appropriate and add any missing sequences found during our literature survey. Our decision to include peptides from freshwater algae [15–17] in our analysis rests on the fact that a large number of them possess interesting medicinal potential (including peptides with very efficient antithrombotic and antidiabetic properties). Decision to include peptides from freshwater algae was also driven by two additional factors: the number of marine algae-derived peptides with known sequence is relatively low and freshwater algae are often used as food.

We included peptides ranging from 2 to 40 amino acid (AA) residues in length, reporting their sequence, the source from which they were isolated, their bioactive effect, and their EC50 value (where available) (Table S1). The complete set of peptides derives from eight different phyla, and represents 14 classes, from Eubacteria, Chromista, Plantae, and Animalia. To perform statistical analysis, we followed the flow chart given in Figure 1. First, we classified peptides according to their bioactivity (ACE inhibitors, antioxidative, immunomodulatory, antimicrobial, antithrombotic, and antidiabetic). Second, we classified AA residues, as in our previous paper [30], either as aliphatic (glycine (G) alanine (A), leucine (L), isoleucine (I), proline (P), and valine (V)); as aromatic (tryptophan (W), phenylalanine (F), and tyrosine (Y)); as polar noncharged (asparagine (N), glutamine (Q), methionine (M), cysteine (C), serine (S), and threonine (T)); as positively charged (histidine (H), arginine (R), and lysine (K)); as negatively charged (aspartic acid (D) and glutamic acid (E)). Third, we calculated the percentages of each class of amino acid present in peptides of a specific activity. Then, statistical tests were performed. One-way analysis of variance (one-way ANOVA) was used to assess if there is a significant influence of amino acid composition of peptide on its activity. The effect of the type of AA residue on peptide activity was assessed using the chi-square (χ^2) test [31]. Additionally, we compared results for marine peptides with results for peptides from food of non-marine animal origin (taken from 30) to see if there are differences between sequences of peptides exhibiting the same effect in different types of food sources.

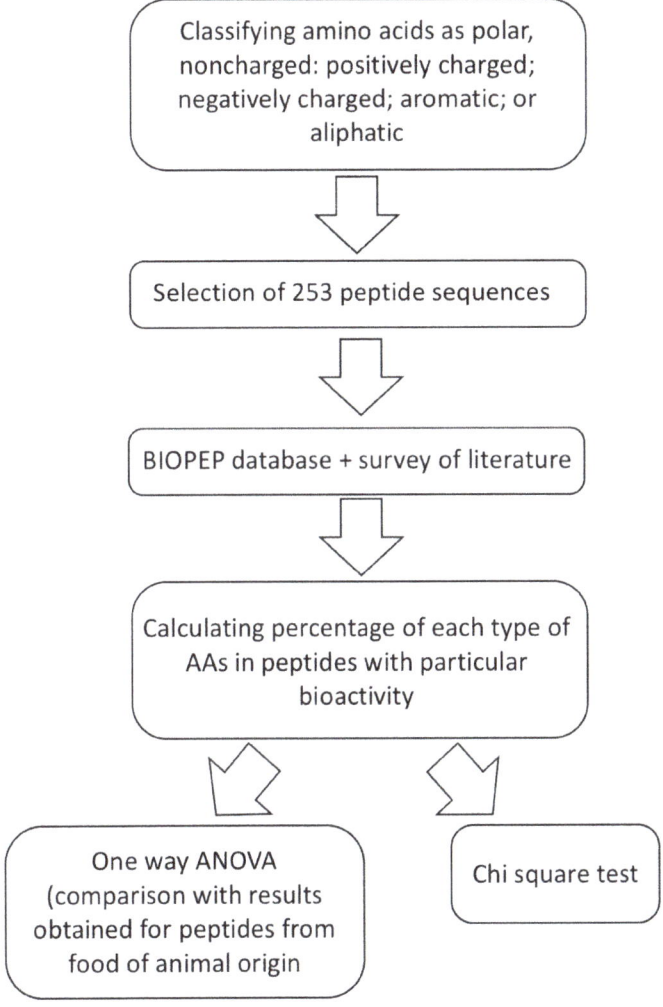

Figure 1. Flow chart for obtaining and analyzing data.

2. Isolation and Purification of Marine-Derived Peptides

The bioactive peptides may already be present in some food samples. They can also be generated either by processing (during preparation of hydrolyzates or technological operations) or released from parent protein during digestion (Figure 2). Peptides already present in products can be either ribosomal or non-ribosomal. Non-ribosomal peptides are those peptides that are synthesized by non-ribosomal peptide synthetase (NRPS) enzymes [32] rather than on ribosomes. Among the marine bioactive peptides, a significant number of the pharmacologically attractive and the most researched peptides are non-ribosomal. In marine organisms non-ribosomal peptides are present mostly in marine bacteria and sponges [33,34]. All peptides listed in Table S1 are of ribosomal origin.

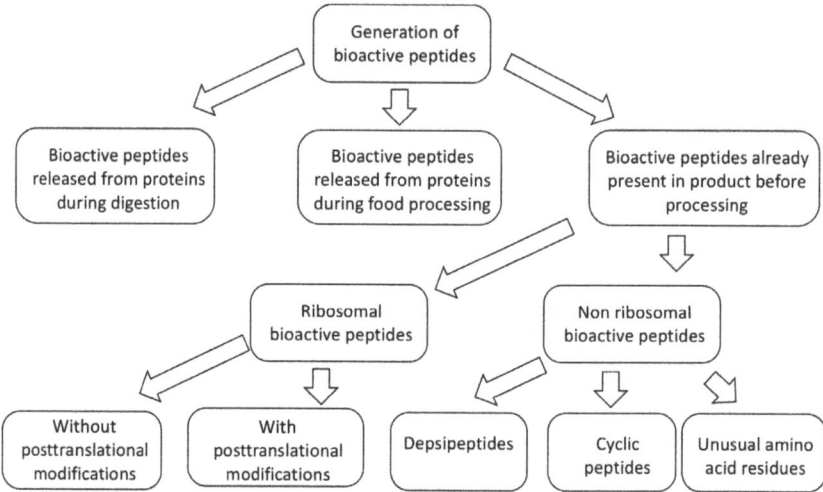

Figure 2. Generation of marine bioactive peptides.

As in the case of peptides from other animal and plant sources, isolation and production of marine-derived peptides face a few challenges. Such challenges primarily arise from (i) the lack of standardization of hydrolysis and/or extraction processes, (ii) usage of the whole hydrolyzate (instead of individual peptides) to determine activity, (iii) technological limitations in methods for purification and analysis, and (iv) as stated previously, variation in composition and primary structure of peptides between different groups of marine organisms.

Two major reasons could be identified as causes for hydrolysis standardization problems:

1. Usage of insufficiently characterized, crude enzyme preparations obtained from another organism [35–37]. Although the efficiency of this method of extraction might be high, the presence of large numbers of proteases with different specificities [38] can make reproducibility of the results questionable and hinder standardization of this extraction method.
2. Change in ratio of enzyme(s) to substrate, conditions of hydrolysis, and in ratio of proteases (if more than one protease is used) (Table 1).

Table 1. Commonly used proteases for production of marine-derived peptides.

Protease/Proteases Combination	References
Alcalase	[39–41]
Bromelain	[7,42,43]
Proteinase K + thermolysin	[44–46]
Thermolysin	[47–50]
Pepsin	[51–53]
Proteases	[54–56]
Alcalase + pepsin + chymotrypsin	[57–59]
Neutrase	[53,60,61]
Papain	[62–64]
Neutral protease + papain	[65]

Because of their different Km and specificities, such changes in enzyme/substrate ratios and/or temperature and pH will have a significant impact on the number and type of peptides produced [42,60–62].

Additionally, prior to hydrolysis, extraction is usually done by organic solvents, buffers, or water. The extract is further purified by application of often multiple types of chromatographic methods [66–74]. However, as with the often variable conditions for hydrolysis, extraction of marine peptides, even from the same class of organisms, is often done with buffers of variable compositions [72–74] or different combinations of organic solvents [75–77]. Such practice, although allowing the extraction of new peptides with different bioactivities, is adding to variability and complexity of the results.

Although hydrolyzate is usually further fractionated and individual peptides are separated, sometimes the extract as a whole is purified and analyzed further [42,67,69,70,78]. This prevents the assessment of individual peptides, and in turn the establishment of correlation between each peptide's structure and its bioactivity.

Technological limitations present another challenge when it comes to correlating structure and bioactivity of individual peptides. Those technological limitations can be broadly classified as problems with separation of bioactive peptides and problems with their analysis. Most separations are performed using either ultrafiltration or chromatographic techniques that separate peptides based on their charge, size, or hydrophobicity. Considering that peptides are often of very similar size, charge, and/or hydrophobicity, and that most of these fractionation techniques take into account only one of the mentioned characteristics, isolation of individual peptides is hindered. Proposed solutions to this problem are two-fold: employment of orthogonal or multidimensional separation systems or inclusion of additional steps, such as electrodiffusion [79]. In regard to the challenges of analyzing individual peptides, which is usually done by mass spectrometry, a solution might be found in using more sophisticated analyzers such as ion traps or triple quadrupoles [80].

As stated before, the isolation of peptides from certain classes of marine organisms requires additional steps, such as the addition of enzymes (cellulase and/or xylanase) for extractions of peptides from marine algae [15].

Because of the great variety of marine organisms, it is hard to give recommendations for one-fits-all solution that can act for extraction/hydrolysis, purification, and identification of marine peptides. Especially since, as stated before, certain organisms require additional steps in procedure or specific conditions (e.g., disruption of cell wall in algae and bacteria, multiple washing steps during organic extraction of peptides from fish via surimi process [81], etc.). However, the main question that dictates both extraction/hydrolysis step as well as purification step is whether we are performing only an exploratory search (e.g., accessing all possible activities) or whether we are looking for peptides with specific activities. This is a question of crucial importance because it determines the selection of an appropriate method. For example, both extraction with organic solvents and extraction with acids/alkaline solutions (followed by isoelectric precipitation) can lead to the production of variety of peptides, but both of these methods are time-consuming, environmentally dangerous, and require longer purification process [81,82]. Additionally, because of the harsh condition and/or changes in pH both these methods can damage proteins and could result in loss of amino acids such as tryptophan [81,82]. Fermentation can also be applied for extraction of marine peptides [41], but depending on the strain(s) used and required experimental conditions (namely, temperature and pH) this can also lead to additional reactions of amino acids and changes in hydrophobicity [83]. Application of certain techniques, such as ultrasound-assisted extraction or microwave-assisted extraction was proven to result in high number of bioactive peptides, which was especially useful for extraction of peptides from algae, since it also leads to the rupture of cell wall [82,84]. One of the problems with those methods is variable yield [82,84]. Enzymatic hydrolysis is a highly specific and reproducible technique, but as stated before, because of the complexities of marine organisms and interactions of their proteins with other components within the cell, will not produce the same peptides in all marine organisms [15,41,84]. Additionally, as discussed above, hydrolysis with multiple proteases results simultaneously in high number of peptides with different bioactivities, while application of single proteases produces fewer peptides, but with similar effects. Another important factor to consider during enzymatic hydrolysis is the level of stability of peptides. Since, as would be discussed in following sections, the presence of proline enhances the stability of peptides, the usage of trypsin for hydrolysis might be beneficial.

As discussed, purification of extract/hydrolyzate is usually done by combination of filtration and chromatographic techniques. Such procedure also carries its challenges: ultrafiltration, which is commonly used to separate peptides from larger components in the extract/hydrolyzate, is relatively a cheap and fast method (especially if used in reactors), but usually requires several repetitions (because of decrease in selectivity and accumulation of peptides on membrane surface) and does not eliminate salts and other soluble components that can interfere with chromatographic separation. Certain improvements of filtration technique, such as application of electric field, pressure gradient, and/or electrodialysis cell, have been employed (with different level of success) [85]. Chromatographic techniques use characteristics such as polarity, charge, or affinity for separation of peptides. These methods all have several major drawbacks: first, the separation efficiency is impacted by number of peptides in the hydrolyzate; second, the separation condition (especially temperature) impacts greatly on both speed and efficiency of separation (which can greatly impact reproducibility of results); third, individual types of chromatography separate peptides based on only one characteristic, so multiple different chromatographic methods must be applied for separation of complex mixtures [79,86]. A potential solution for at least one of these drawbacks is the application of multi-dimensional liquid chromatography (MD-LC) in which peptides could be simultaneously separated based on two characteristics [86].

3. Comparison of the Structures of Marine-Sourced Peptides with Other Animal-Sourced Peptides and the Impacts of Protein Structure on Their Activity

Although different classifications of effects of bioactive peptides can be found in literature, the most often mentioned ones include: ACE inhibitors, antioxidative, antimicrobial, immunomodulatory, antithrombotic, and antidiabetic peptides. Table S2 summarizes the main bioactivities and mechanisms of actions. ACE inhibitors act as inhibitors for ACE, resulting in decrease of blood pressure. Antioxidative peptides help prevent or reduce damage caused by free radicals, using different mechanisms [30] (Table S2). Antimicrobial peptides prevent growth and reproduction of microorganisms. Immunomodulatory peptides help boost adaptive immune response, and are the most heterogenous group in terms of mechanisms employed [30]. Antithrombotic peptides help prevent platelet aggregation, thus decreasing the risk of diseases like stroke, arterial sclerosis, etc. Antidiabetic peptides help decrease the concentration of glucose in the bloodstream, also by using multiple mechanisms (Table S2).

As with the peptides of non-marine animal origin [30], the percentages of bioactive marine peptides isolated from different organisms vary depending on their effect (Figure 3). Over-representation of ACE inhibitors and antioxidative peptides in the literature can be partly explained by economic incentives driving research on drugs [87,88] to fight the rise of cardiovascular and antioxidant diseases [89,90].

Often peptides can be multifunctional, exhibiting more than one effect [91–94]. There are three important reasons for such occurrence: the peptides might act like signaling molecules at a systemic level [95], or there might be connections between metabolic pathways [93,94,96–99], or peptides may utilize more than one mode of action [30,100]. For peptides of certain bioactivity, such as antioxidative or antithrombotic peptides, the mode of action is well-known and relatively simple [30,56,101,102] (Table S2). On the other hand, for some categories, such as immunomodulatory peptides, different modes of actions are exhibited simultaneously and to a different extent in different source organisms [103–107] (Table S2). Variability and complexity of marine peptides has slowed the elucidation of the mechanism behind some activities. More intriguingly, several of the proposed mechanisms for marine-derived peptide activities are quite unique and different compared to other animal-derived peptides [30]. Examples include the interaction between cytotoxic peptides from sea anemones and voltage-dependent membrane channels [108], and the antimalarial effect of C Phycocyanin (isolated from marine cyanobacteria), exhibited through binding to ferriprotoporphyrin IX [2]. These findings could show that either specificities among organism classes dictate the particular mode of action, or that the structure of the peptides themselves is different.

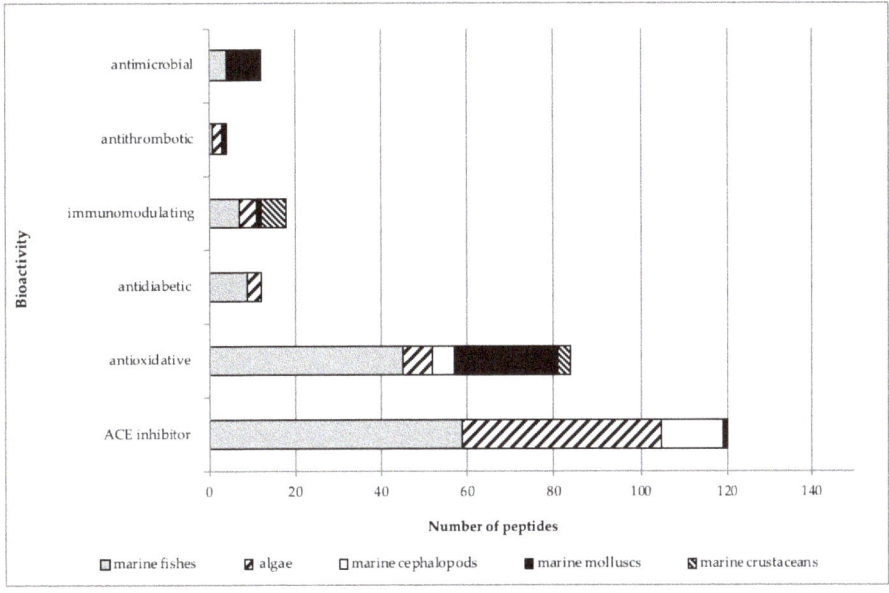

Figure 3. Distribution of bioactive peptides in the different groups of marine organisms. Peptides with multiple activities have been counted in each category.

Given these different modes of actions, different tests are used to determine specific effects of a given peptide (Table S2). This fact is especially problematic when it comes to immunomodulatory peptides, since if all aspects of immune response (cytotoxicity, activation of macrophages and neutrophils, up-regulation of caspase genes and propagation of apoptosis, etc.) were to be tested that would be both time consuming and highly costly. Additionally, even when testing for activities, such as antimicrobial, ACE inhibitory or antioxidative, for which few, well-defined assays are commonly employed, such assays often have different detection limits, specificity, reproducibility, and/or show preferential detection of compounds with given characteristic (such as polarity in the case of antioxidative tests) (Table S2). A further point of confusion is that different tests use different units to demonstrate effect (Table S2), thus making difficult any comparison of activity of different peptides. Therefore, efforts should be made to define which test should be used to monitor specific effects (and consequently in which units effects are measured) in order to obtain clear insight into peptides bioactivities.

As expected, the percentage of AA residue types in marine-derived peptides varies depending on the peptides' bioactivity (Figure 4). To confirm this, we compared observed and expected frequencies for each type of AA residues (aliphatic, aromatic, noncharged polar, and positively and negatively charged) using the χ^2 test. As in our previous paper [30], the expected frequencies were calculated using the following formula:

Expected frequency = (the number of amino acids in a given group × the total number of peptides with a particular effect)/20

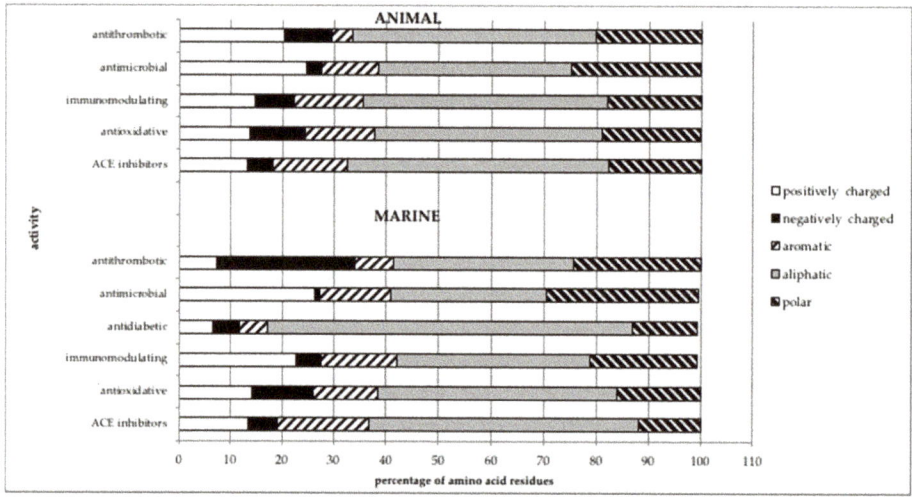

Figure 4. Comparison of amino acid distribution in bioactive peptides from different sources. Bioactive peptides from animal (non-marine) sources have been described in Maestri et al. 2019 [30]. Bioactive peptides from marine organisms are described in this paper. The five main categories of amino acids are as described in the text. Deviation from 100% can be explained by the presence of multifunctional peptides, unusual amino acid residues, etc.

The χ^2 test [31] showed significant differences for observed and expected frequencies of AA residues in specific classes of bioactive peptides (χ^2 (1,8) = 2150.07; $p = 2.52 \times 10^{-15}$).

Difference in percentages of different AA residues in peptides with particular bioactivity can be explained through correlations between structure and function. For example, a high percentage of hydrophobic (aliphatic and aromatic) AA residues in antidiabetic peptides (Figure 4) [109–111] is necessary for inhibition of dipeptidyl peptidase IV, a key enzyme involved in degradation of incretins [110,112,113], and for recognition of receptors for glucagon-like peptides [114,115]. A high percentage of negatively charged AA residues (Figure 4) has been reported in antithrombotic peptides showing both direct thrombin inhibition [116,117] and inhibition of factors in intrinsic pathways [72,118]. A high frequency of positively charged AA residues in so-called cationic antimicrobial peptides (Figure 4) [119–121] is proven to be necessary for interactions with anionic microbe membranes.

Similar to the results obtained for non-marine animal peptides [30], a significant percentage (52.7%) of examined sequences contain one or more proline residues (Table S1). This could imply that proline plays a significant role in peptide stability [18]. Therefore, the use of trypsin to generate stable peptides might be a valuable consideration [122].

When data for percentage of AA residues per category for animal-derived peptides described in our previous work [30] and marine-derived peptides (Figure 4) are compared, dependency of peptide's structure from source becomes visible and suggestive of possible peculiarities. To estimate these differences, we used the one-way ANOVA test to compare the percentages of polar noncharged, aliphatic, aromatic, and positively and negatively charged AA residues per activity (antithrombotic, antimicrobial, immunomodulating, antioxidative, and ACE inhibitors) in non-marine animal and marine sources. As previously stated, the source organisms for the marine peptides are taxonomically diversified, ranging from bacteria to plants and animals. Antidiabetic marine-derived peptides were not included because of the insufficient data for antidiabetic peptides from other animal sources. Results of one-way ANOVA showed that for each bioactivity, with the exception of the antithrombotic peptides, the percentages of AA residues of a given category were statistically different at $p = 0.05$ (ACE inhibitors: F(4,5) = 137.26; $p = 2.69 \times 10^{-5}$; antioxidative: F(4,5) = 253.87; $p = 5.86 \times 10^{-6}$;

antimicrobial: $F(4,5) = 36.32$; $p = 0.00069$; immunomodulatory: $F(4,5) = 18.40$; $p = 0.0034$; antithrombotic: $F(4,5) = 5.1$; $p = 0.052$).

There are three possible explanations for such occurrence. First, as previously stated, marine peptides come from taxonomically diverse groups of highly specific organisms, and this can have great impact on both peptide structure and function: the sample of peptides of animal origin described in [30] derives from few species in the phylum Chordata, comprised of classes Aves and Mammalia. On the contrary, the sample of marine peptides encompasses 14 different classes in 4 kingdoms. Additionally, even if not considered in this analysis, this is especially prominent in the case of peptides isolated from sponges and mollusks, which can be cyclical or composed of "unusual" amino acid residues [19,41,84,123–125]. Second, this opens the possibility that other mechanisms exist beyond those found and described in non-marine-derived peptides [30]. For example, Kouno et al. [126] found that dried bonito hydrolyzate contains peptides that regulate in vivo blood pressure by directly acting on vascular smooth muscle, instead of acting through ACE inhibition. Additionally, certain marine-derived antimicrobial peptides can also act as K^+ blockers [127] (Table S2). However, further studies showing the modes of action of different classes of marine peptides are needed. Third, as shown in Figure 3, distribution of peptides showing specific bioactivities is not uniform across all marine organisms, with a prevalence of fish, algae, and bivalves. Moreover, some categories of peptides are derived from few species (see Figure 3 and Table S1).

Because of the above mentioned factors, combined with overall differences in the literature concerning marine-derived vs. animal-derived peptides, comparisons between specific groups (for example terrestrial Chordata vs. fish) are not possible at this point. Hence, in this analysis, we chose to compare all animal-derived peptides showing particular bioactivity with all marine-derived peptides exhibiting the same effect. As stated, results of such comparison would be skewed and should be taken with caution.

Further point to be taken into account when discussing amino acid composition of peptides showing a specific effect is whether any indication exists that the mechanism of action of the marine peptide depends on the type of organism from which it is isolated [105]. Since, as we discussed, difference in preferred mechanism stems from difference in amino acid composition, this implies that inclusion of all groups of marine organisms into analysis can skew the results. For example, peptides from fish showing both antimicrobial and immunomodulatory activities, as well as immunomodulatory peptides from crustaceans, are rich in positively charged and polar amino acids (Figure 4). High percentage of polar and positively charged amino residues in marine organisms can be a consequence of certain specificities of their mechanisms of action, such as interaction with antibodies and complement system, prevention of formation of biofilms, induction of cytokine synthesis, suppression of NO production (Table S2) [105,128–130]. Since the majority of antimicrobial peptides included in this analysis are isolated from fish and bivalves (Figure 3) this could be an additional factor accounting for a large difference in content of positively charged and polar amino acids among antimicrobial peptides from marine and animal sources. Given that ACE inhibitors isolated from marine fish and algae (that made up the biggest portion of ACE inhibitory peptides in this analysis; Figure 3) also show non-competitive inhibition as a mechanism of action [131,132] this could explain a slightly higher ratio of aromatic and aliphatic amino acid residues in peptides isolated from marine sources compared to animal sources. The majority of antioxidative peptides in this analysis was isolated from marine fish and bivalves (Figure 3). Slightly higher ratio of positively and negatively charged amino acid residues in antioxidative peptides of marine origin compared to antioxidative peptides of animal origin (in which higher ratio of polar amino residues was observed, [30]) is harder to explain, since seemingly they do not show differences in mechanism of action (Table S2). One possible explanation for such discrepancy could be overrepresentation of peptides from certain marine species in the literature and in this analysis.

4. Stability of Marine-Derived Peptides In Vivo

The stability of peptides in vivo is determined by several factors, most importantly the peptides' size and structure [30,133]. Besides influencing the speed of a peptide's transport from lumen to enterocytes, the size of the peptide will also influence the mode of transport (paracellular, transcellular or via peptide transporters-PEPT1 and PEPT2) [134–136]. The type of amino acid residues, as well as the shape of the peptide, greatly influences its susceptibility to degradation by gastrointestinal proteases [137,138]. This could explain the high percentage of proline residues in examined sequences, since the presence of proline promotes increased stability toward protease degradation [18,139–141].

Marine-derived peptides have several other characteristics as well that can increase their in vivo stability compared to other animal and plant sourced peptides. These properties contribute to "unusual" structures and make peptides less likely to be recognized by digestive enzymes, thus preventing the formation of enzyme-peptide complex. These characteristics can be broadly classified as the following:

1. High percentage of proline and branched amino acid residues [18,19,142];
2. Presence of both D and L amino acids [19,84,143]
3. Cyclic structure [18,19,123–125,144–147]. Steric factors are the reason why cyclic peptides are more resistant to digestion, because of their cyclic nature neither N nor C terminus can be recognized by proteases (either during processing or in gastrointestinal tract) [148–150].
4. Peptides in form of depsipeptides. A depsipeptide is one in which one or more amide bonds are substituted with ester bonds [151–153], often leading to the formation of cyclic depsipeptides [154–158].
5. Presence of unusual AA residues, such as bromotryptophan [84,159,160]. Bromotryptophan, as brominated tryptophan, is non-coded amino acid that is usually found in non-ribosomal proteins and peptides, although some ribosomal proteins of marine origin were shown to contain 6-bromo-L-tryptophan [160,161].
6. Presence of secondary structures [41,127,162–165]. Given that formation of α helix requires only 4 amino acid residues per turn it can be formed in shorter peptides. Therefore, α helix is the most common secondary structure in marine peptides, although in longer peptides β sheets can also be present [163].

Not all groups of marine organisms produce peptides with all of these characteristics, and some of these characteristics are more common in certain groups. Cyclic peptides are often found in marine sponges and mollusks [19,84,138,145,146], while cyclic depsipeptides are often isolated from marine bacteria [153,155,157,158]. Secondary structures, especially α helix, are common in antimicrobial marine peptides [162–165], because the presence of α helix allows penetration through a microbe's membrane [163,164].

However, although all these factors contribute to the peptides' stability in vivo, bioactivities are usually tested during in vitro experiments. Correlating results obtained in in vitro experiments with the conditions existing in the human gastrointestinal tract presents a major challenge in determining the in vivo stability. Certain factors that can influence both the stability and the digestibility of peptides in vivo are often not considered during in vitro generation. These factors include: Using enzymes that are very different from digestive enzymes in their structures/activities or using them in ratios different than physiological ones; not accounting for the effects of technological processing (effects of temperature, pressure or fermentation); not considering changes in pH between different parts of the gastrointestinal tract; not analyzing the "matrix effect"(the interaction with other components in food or the body); and not counting the effect of peristaltics. Some attempts to use gastrointestinal proteases for peptide generation in the same ratio present in the human duodenum have been made [166,167]. But changes in pH, the "matrix effect" and the effect of peristaltics still cannot be properly assessed, especially with the static digestion models that are commonly being employed.

Fortunately, because of the significant number of antitumor, antidiabetic, and antihypertensive peptides isolated from marine sources [41,84,168–174], epidemiological studies and clinical trials are now under way. Therefore, at least for these types of peptides, the relative influence of different factors affecting peptides' activity and correlation between in vitro and in vivo effects will be determined in the near future.

An additional point should be considered here: increased stability of a peptide diminishes its digestibility. Decreased digestibility, although important in preserving peptide's activity, can lead to allergic reactions [175,176].

5. Usage of Whole Hydrolyzate vs. Purified Peptides vs. Synthetic Peptides in Production of Food and Marine Drugs

Marine peptides and hydrolyzates can be utilized in two principal ways: as food/feed supplements and as drugs [2,41,82,84,177–187]. Whole hydrolyzates of marine-derived proteins are usually applied in food/feed preparations, where they serve different functions, as antioxidants [178], hypolipidemic agents [181,182], enhancing physical performance in elderly people [177], and preventing hair loss [180]. Although all these activities have been verified by clinical trials, there are several problems with using whole protein hydrolyzates. First, the composition of the hydrolyzates (the type and content of individual amino acids) is greatly dependent on the type and ratio of enzymes used for hydrolysis as well as on the pH during hydrolysis [188,189]. Second, in whole hydrolyzates it is hard to determine which peptides are biologically active. Third, because of complex compositions, it becomes hard to predict their behaviors in vivo. However, there are two significant advantages in using whole hydrolyzates: cost and time. The methods and chemicals necessary to isolate and characterize individual peptides (such as the use of chromatographic techniques and mass spectrometry) both prolong and add expenses to the creation of products able to be tested for in vivo activity. Research to improve the extraction step can enhance the number of peptides with more pronounced and/or different bioactivities in hydrolyzate. For example, microwave assisted extraction [82] has proven to be a good method for enhancing peptide's bioactivity.

Individual peptides require identification, purification, and analysis before being used in food preparation or drugs. Therefore, their cost is higher compared to hydrolyzates. This is a particular problem with antimicrobial peptides that are more expensive to produce than "commercial" antibiotics [84], and thus a less attractive option. Another problem is when the mode of action of an individual peptide is unknown [183,185], as it leads to unexpected results due to metabolic pathway interconnections [95]. Such is the case with antidiabetic peptides from salmon skin which, although they caused decrease in blood level glucose, also increased levels of HDL (high-density lipoproteins) [171]. Furthermore, certain peptides exhibit their effect preferentially in specific tissues [190]. Because of the "matrix effect" and problematic correlations with animal models, peptides that showed particular bioactivity in vitro or in animal models can show variable results in clinical trials [41]. Since such variations in activity can be partially ascribed to decreased stability, encapsulation and the use of different carriers are methods being considered and employed [191–194]. Conversely, these methods can lead to difficulty in a peptide's release and therefore hinder its activity [193,194].

Because of the prevalence of cancer and diabetes mellitus type 2, antidiabetic and anticancer peptides are the most interesting targets for synthesis [41,84,183–185]. Since most of the peptides exhibiting anticancer effects have cyclical structures [29,84,145,154,167,170,173,174], this makes production of synthetic anticancer peptides difficult. Also, as said previously, although the stability of such cyclic peptides is high, their digestibility is lower than linear peptides. This can prevent their transport into enterocytes and from enterocytes into capillaries, thus hindering their activity.

In all of these cases, one important point has not received the attention it deserves. A large number of in vivo studies are still performed on rats and mice [36,62,84,126,169,171,181]. Given the clear differences in anatomy and physiology, correlation between animal models and humans is questionable [195,196]. Additionally, since age, health, nutrition, and hormonal status [197–199] of the subject can all influence the peptides'/hydrolyzates' effects, precaution should be taken during selection of subjects for clinical trials.

6. Conclusions

Although there are still many challenges to be solved, mainly harmonization of extraction methods and hydrolysis, as well as correlation between in vitro and in vivo results, marine organisms have proven to be invaluable sources of peptides with unique structures and diverse bioactivities. Because marine peptide research has only recently gotten its fair share of attention, many of their mechanisms of action are still unknown. In future, as more marine-derived peptides are isolated and characterized, comparisons of structures and activities with counterparts from other organisms will become more informative. However, the construction of databases, such as StraPep [200] (http://isyslab.info/StraPep/, accessed August 2020), that correlate the structures of bioactive peptides with their functions will help solve this problem. Additionally, correlating structures with mechanism of action will help not only with constructing proper peptide carriers and predicting their release and possible undesired effects in clinical trials, but can also provide useful guidance in searching for peptides with the same potential.

Supplementary Materials: The following are available online at http://www.mdpi.com/1660-3397/18/8/424/s1: Table S1: Sequences, activity, source material, EC50 (where applicable), and length of the 253 marine-derived peptides used for analysis in this paper. Table S2: Description of main bioactivities of peptides, mechanisms of action and bioassays for testing.

Author Contributions: Authors M.P. and E.M. researched literature, wrote the manuscripts, and performed the statistical analysis. Author M.M. researched literature and critically revised the manuscript. All authors have read and agreed to the published version of the manuscript.

Funding: This research was funded by EU FP7 project, Grant Agreement No.316004 (REGPOT-AREA) and by POR FESR 2014-2020 Region Emilia-Romagna, project BIOWAFER.

Acknowledgments: The authors wish to acknowledge Nelson Marmiroli (Univ. Parma) and Renee Stoops (Plant Allies) for critical reading of the manuscript.

Conflicts of Interest: The authors declare no conflict of interest.

References

1. Rangel, M.; de Santana, C.J.C.; Pinheiro, A.; dos Anjos, L.; Barth, T.; Rodrigues Pires Júnior, O.; Fontes, W.; Castro, M.S. Marine depsipeptides as promising pharmacotherapeutic agents. *Curr. Protein Pept. Sci.* **2017**, *18*, 72–91. [CrossRef] [PubMed]
2. Anjum, K.; Abbas, S.Q.; Akhter, N.; Shagufta, B.I.; Shah, S.A.A.; Hassan, S.S.U. Emerging biopharmaceuticals from bioactive peptides derived from marine organisms. *Chem. Biol. Drug Des.* **2017**, *90*, 12–30. [CrossRef] [PubMed]
3. Mayer, A.M.S.; Rodríguez, A.D.; Taglialatela-Scafati, O.; Fusetani, N. Marine pharmacology in 2009–2011: Marine compounds with antibacterial, antidiabetic, antifungal, anti-inflammatory, antiprotozoal, antituberculosis, and antiviral activities; affecting the immune and nervous systems, and other miscellaneous mechanisms of action. *Mar. Drugs* **2013**, *11*, 2510–2573. [CrossRef]
4. Kim, S.W.; Wijesekara, I. Development and biological activities of marine-derived bioactive peptides: A review. *J. Funct. Food* **2010**, *2*, 1–9. [CrossRef]
5. Venketasan, J.; Anil, S.; Kim, S.W.; Shim, M.S. Marine fish proteins and peptides for cosmeceuticals: A review. *Mar. Drugs* **2017**, *15*, 143. [CrossRef]
6. Corinaldesi, C.; Barone, G.; Marcellini, F.; Dell'Anno, A.; Danovaro, R. Marine microbial-derived molecules and their potential use in cosmeceutical and cosmetic products. *Mar. Drugs* **2017**, *15*, 118. [CrossRef]
7. Wang, H.M.D.; Li, X.C.; Lee, D.J.; Chang, J.S. Potential biomedical applications of marine algae. *Bioresour. Technol.* **2017**, *244*, 1407–1415. [CrossRef]
8. Halim, N.R.A.; Yusof, H.M.; Sarbon, N.M. Functional and bioactive properties of fish protein hydolysates and peptides: A comprehensive review. *Trends Food Sci. Techol.* **2016**, *51*, 24–33. [CrossRef]
9. Charoensiddhi, S.; Conlon, M.A.; Franco, C.M.M.; Zhang, W. The development of seaweed-derived bioactive compounds for use as prebiotics and nutraceuticals using enzyme technologies. *Trends Food Sci. Techol.* **2017**, *70*, 20–33. [CrossRef]

10. Lemes, A.C.; Sala, L.; da Costa Ores, J.; Cavalcante Braga, A.R.; Buranelo Egea, M.; Fernandes, K.F. A review of the latest advances in encrypted bioactive peptides from protein-rich waste. *Int. J. Mol. Sci.* **2016**, *17*, 950. [CrossRef]
11. Sheih, I.C.; Wu, T.K.; Fang, T.J. Antioxidant properties of a new antioxidative peptide from algae protein waste hydrolysate in different oxidation systems. *Bioresour. Technol.* **2009**, *100*, 3419–3425. [CrossRef] [PubMed]
12. Cian, R.E.; Alaiz, M.; Vioque, J.; Drago, S.R. Enzyme proteolysis enhanced extraction of ACE inhibitory and antioxidant compounds (peptides and polyphenols) from *Porphyra columbina* residual cake. *J. Appl. Phycol.* **2013**, *25*, 1197–1206. [CrossRef]
13. Gajanan, P.G.; Elavarasan, K.; Shamasundar, B.A. Bioactive and functional properties of protein hydrolysates from fish frame processing waste using plant proteases. *Environ. Sci. Pollut. Res. Int.* **2016**, *23*, 24901–24911. [CrossRef] [PubMed]
14. Gildberg, A. Enzymes and bioactive peptides from fish waste related to fish silage, fish feed and fish sauce production. *J. Aquat. Food Prod. Technol.* **2008**, *13*, 3–11. [CrossRef]
15. Admassu, H.; Gasmalla, M.A.A.; Yang, R.; Zhao, W. Bioactive peptides derived from seaweed protein and their health benefits: Antihypertensive, antioxidant, and antidiabetic properties. *J. Food Sci.* **2018**, *83*, 6–16. [CrossRef]
16. Mayer, A.M.S.; Rodríguez, A.D.; Taglialatela-Scafati, O.; Fusetani, N. Marine pharmacology in 2012–2013: Marine compounds with antibacterial, antidiabetic, antifungal, anti-inflammatory, antiprotozoal, antituberculosis, and antiviral activities; affecting the immune and nervous systems, and other miscellaneous mechanisms of action. *Mar. Drugs* **2017**, *15*, 273. [CrossRef]
17. Blunt, J.W.; Carroll, A.R.; Copp, B.R.; Davis, R.A.; Keyzers, R.A.; Prinsep, M.R. Marine natural products. *Nat. Prod. Rep.* **2018**, *35*, 8–53. [CrossRef]
18. Shinnar, A.E.; Butler, K.L.; Park, H.J. Cathelicidin family of antimicrobial peptides: Proteolytic processing and protease resistance. *Bioorg. Chem.* **2003**, *31*, 425–436. [CrossRef]
19. Phyo, Y.Z.; Ribeiro, J.; Fernandes, C.; Kijjoa, A.; Pinto, M.M.M. Marine natural peptides: Determination of absolute configuration using liquid chromatography methods and evaluation of bioactivities. *Molecules* **2018**, *23*, 306. [CrossRef]
20. Minkiewicz, P.; Dziuba, J.; Iwaniak, A.; Dzuiba, M.; Darewicz, M. BIOPEP database and other programs for processing bioactive peptide sequences. *J. Aoac Int.* **2008**, *91*, 965–980. [CrossRef]
21. Lei, J.; Zhou, J. A marine natural product database. *J. Chem. Inf. Comput. Sci.* **2002**, *42*, 742–748. [CrossRef] [PubMed]
22. Gueguen, Y.; Garnier, J.; Robert, L.; Lefranc, M.P.; Mougenot, I.; de Lorgeril, J.; Janech, M.; Gross, P.S.; Warr, G.W.; Cuthbertson, B.; et al. PenBase, the shrimp antimicrobial peptide penaeidin database: Sequence-based classification and recommended nomenclature. *Dev. Comp. Immunol.* **2006**, *30*, 283–288. [CrossRef] [PubMed]
23. Shtatland, T.; Guettler, D.; Kossodo, M.; Pivovarov, M.; Weissleder, R. PepBank—A database of peptides based on sequence text mining and public peptide data sources. *Bmc Bioinform.* **2007**, *8*, 280. [CrossRef] [PubMed]
24. Kapoor, P.; Singh, H.; Gautam, A.; Chaudhary, K.; Kumar, R.; Raghava, G.P.S. TumorHoPe: A database of tumor homing peptides. *PLoS ONE* **2012**, *7*, e35187. [CrossRef]
25. Kumar, R.; Chaudhary, K.; Sharma, M.; Nagpal, G.; Chauhan, S.; Singh, S.; Gautam, A.; Raghava, G.P.S. AHTPDB: A comprehensive platform for analysis and presentation of antihypertensive peptides. *Nucleic Acids Res.* **2014**, *43*, 956–962. [CrossRef] [PubMed]
26. Gautam, A.; Chaudhary, K.; Singh, S.; Joshi, A.; Anand, P.; Tuknait, A.; Mathur, D.; Varshney, G.; Raghava, G.P.S. Hemolytik: A database of experimentally determined hemolytic and non-hemolytic peptides. *Nucleic Acid Res.* **2013**, *42*, 444–449. [CrossRef]
27. Piotto, S.; Sessa, L.; Concilio, S.; Iannelli, P. YADAMP: Yet another database of antimicrobial peptides. *Int. J. Antimicrob. Agents* **2012**, *39*, 346–351. [CrossRef]
28. Quareshi, A.; Thakur, N.; Kumar, M. HIPdb: A database of experimentally validated HIV inhibiting peptides. *PLoS ONE* **2013**, *8*, e54908. [CrossRef]

29. Tyagi, A.; Tuknait, A.; Anand, P.; Gupta, S.; Sharma, M.; Mathur, D.; Joshi, A.; Singh, S.; Gautam, A.; Raghava, G.P.S. CancerPPD: A database of anticancer peptides and proteins. *Nucleic Acids Res.* **2015**, *43*, D837–D843. [CrossRef]
30. Maestri, E.; Pavlicevic, M.; Montorsi, M.; Marmiroli, N. Meta-analysis for correlating structure of bioactive peptides in foods of animal origin with regard to effect and stability. *Compr. Rev. Food Sci. Food Saf.* **2019**, *18*, 3–30. [CrossRef]
31. McHugh, M.L. The Chi-square test of independence. *Biochem. Med.* **2013**, *23*, 143–149. [CrossRef]
32. Martínez-Núñez, M.A.; López, V.E.L. Nonribosomal peptides synthetases and their applications in industry. *Sustain. Chem. Process.* **2016**, *4*, 13. [CrossRef]
33. Matsunaga, S.; Fusetani, N. Nonribosomal peptides from marine sponges. *Curr. Org. Chem.* **2003**, *7*, 945–966. [CrossRef]
34. Agrawal, S.; Acharya, D.; Adholeya, A.; Barrow, C.J.; Deshmukh, S.K. Nonribosomal peptides from marine microbes and their antimicrobial and anticancer potential. *Front. Pharmacol.* **2017**, *8*, 828. [CrossRef]
35. Aissaoui, N.; Abidi, F.; Hardouin, J. ACE inhibitory and antioxidant activities of novel peptides from *Scorpaena notata* by-product protein hydrolysate. *Int. J. Pept. Res. Ther.* **2017**, *23*, 13–23. [CrossRef]
36. Balti, R.; Bougatef, A.; Sila, A.; Guillochon, D.; Dhulster, P.; Nedjar-Arroume, N. Nine novel angiotensin I-converting enzyme (ACE) inhibitory peptides from cuttlefish (*Sepia officinalis*) muscle protein hydrolysates and antihypertensive effect of the potent active peptide in spontaneously hypertensive rats. *Food Chem.* **2015**, *170*, 519–525. [CrossRef] [PubMed]
37. Wu, R.; Chen, L.; Liu, D.; Huang, J.; Zhang, J.; Xiao, X.; Lei, M.; Chen, Y.; He, H. Preparation of antioxidant peptides from salmon byproducts with bacterial extracellular proteases. *Mar. Drugs* **2017**, *15*, 4. [CrossRef]
38. Shahidi, F.; Zhong, Y. Bioactive peptides. *J. Aoac Int.* **2008**, *91*, 914–931. [CrossRef]
39. Aleman, A.; Gimenez, B.; Perez-Santin, E.; Gomez-Guillen, M.C.; Montero, P. Contribution of Leu and Hyp residues to antioxidant and ACE-inhibitory activities of peptide sequences isolated from squid gelatin hydrolysate. *Food Chem.* **2011**, *125*, 334–341. [CrossRef]
40. Kong, Y.Y.; Chen, S.S.; Wei, J.Q.; Chen, Y.P.; Lan, W.T.; Yang, Q.W.; Huang, G.R. Preparation of antioxidative peptides from Spanish mackerel (*Scomberomorus niphonius*) processing byproducts by enzymatic hydrolysis. *Biotechnology* **2015**, *14*, 188–193. [CrossRef]
41. Cheung, R.C.; Ng, T.B.; Wong, J.H. Marine peptides: Bioactivities and applications. *Mar. Drugs* **2015**, *13*, 4006–4043. [CrossRef] [PubMed]
42. Auwal, M.S.; Zarei, M.; Abdul-Hamid, A.; Saari, N. Optimization of bromelain-aided production of angiotensin I-converting enzyme inhibitory hydrolysates from stone fish using response surface methodology. *Mar. Drugs* **2017**, *15*, 104. [CrossRef] [PubMed]
43. Salampessy, J.; Phillips, M.; Seneweera, S.; Kailasapathy, K. Release of antimicrobial peptides through bromelain hydrolysis of leatherjacket (*Meuchenia* sp.) insoluble proteins. *Food Chem.* **2010**, *120*, 556–560. [CrossRef]
44. Ghassem, M.; Arihara, K.; Salam, A.; Said, M.; Ibrahim, S. Purification and identification of ACE inhibitory peptides from Haruan (*Channa striatus*) myofibrillar protein hydrolysate using HPLC–ESI-TOF MS/MS. *Food Chem.* **2011**, *129*, 1770–1777. [CrossRef]
45. Sánchez, A.; Vázquez, A. Bioactive peptides: A review. *Food Qual. Saf.* **2017**, *1*, 29–46. [CrossRef]
46. Ryan, J.T.; Ross, R.P.; Bolton, D.; Fitzgerald, G.F.; Stanton, C. Bioactive peptides from muscle sources: Meat and fish. *Nutrients* **2011**, *3*, 765–791. [CrossRef]
47. Fujita, H.; Yoshikawa, M. LKPNM: A prodrug-type ACE-inhibitory peptide derived from fish protein. *Int. J. Immunopharmacol.* **1999**, *44*, 123–127. [CrossRef]
48. Ono, S.; Hosokawa, M.; Miyashita, K.; Takahashi, K. Isolation of angiotensin-I converting enzyme inhibitory effect derived from hydrolysate of upstream chum salmon muscle. *J. Food Sci.* **2003**, *68*, 1611–1614. [CrossRef]
49. Lee, S.Y.; Hur, S.J. Antihypertensive peptides from animal products, marine organisms, and plants. *Food Chem.* **2017**, *228*, 506–517. [CrossRef]
50. Panjaitan, F.C.A.; Gomez, H.L.R.; Chang, Y.W. In silico analysis of bioactive peptides released from Giant grouper (*Epinephelus lanceolatus*) roe proteins identified by proteomics approach. *Molecules* **2018**, *23*, 2910. [CrossRef]

51. Je, J.Y.; Park, P.J.; Kwon, J.Y.; Kim, S.K. A novel angiotensin-I converting enzyme inhibitory peptide from Allaska pollack (*Theragra chalcogramma*) frame protein hydrolysate. *J. Agric. Food Chem.* **2004**, *52*, 7842–7845. [CrossRef] [PubMed]
52. Lee, S.H.; Qian, Z.J.; Kim, S.K. A novel angiotensin-I converting enzyme inhibitory peptide from tuna frame protein hydrolysate and its antihypertensive effect in spontaneously hypertensive rats. *Food Chem.* **2010**, *118*, 96–102. [CrossRef]
53. Qian, Z.J.; Je, J.Y.; Kim, S.K. Antihypertensive effect of angiotensin-I converting enzyme-inhibitory peptide from hydrolysates of bigeye tuna dark muscle, *Thunnus obesus*. *J. Agric. Food Chem.* **2007**, *55*, 8398–8403. [CrossRef] [PubMed]
54. Bougatef, A.; Nedjar-Arroume, N.; Ravallec-Ple, R.; Leroy, Y.; Guillochon, D.; Barkia, A.; Nasri, M. Angiotensin I-converting enzyme (ACE) inhibitory activities of sardinelle (*Sardinella aurita*) by-products protein hydrolysates obtained by treatment with microbial and visceral fish serine proteases. *Food Chem.* **2008**, *111*, 350–356. [CrossRef]
55. Wu, H.; He, H.L.; Chen, X.L.; Sun, C.Y.; Zhang, Y.Z.; Zhou, B.C. Purification and identification of novel angiotensin-I-converting enzyme inhibitory peptides from shark meat hydrolysate. *Process. Biochem.* **2008**, *43*, 457–461. [CrossRef]
56. He, S.; Zhang, Y.; Sun, H.; Du, M.; Qiu, J.; Tang, M.; Sun, X.; Zhu, B. Antioxidative peptides from proteolytic hydrolysates of false abalone (*Volutharpa ampullacea perryi*): Characterization, identification, and molecular docking. *Mar. Drugs* **2019**, *17*, 116. [CrossRef]
57. Kim, S.K.; Ravichandran, Y.D.; Khan, S.B.; Kim, Y.T. Prospective of the cosmeceuticals derived from marine organisms. *Biotechnol. Bioprocess. Eng.* **2008**, *13*, 511–523. [CrossRef]
58. Thomas, N.V.; Kim, S.K. Beneficial effects of marine algal compounds in cosmeceuticals. *Mar. Drugs* **2013**, *11*, 146–164. [CrossRef]
59. Kim, S.K. Marine cosmeceuticals. *J. Cosmet. Dermatol.* **2014**, *13*, 56–67. [CrossRef]
60. Jun, S.Y.; Park, P.J.; Jung, W.K.; Kim, S.K. Purification and characterization of an antioxidative peptide from enzymatic hydrolysate of yellowfin sole (*Limanda aspera*) frame protein. *Eur. Food Res. Technol.* **2004**, *219*, 20–26. [CrossRef]
61. Qian, Z.-J.; Heo, S.-J.; Oh, C.H.; Kang, D.-H.; Jeong, S.H.; Park, W.S.; Choi, I.-W.; Jeon, Y.-J.; Jung, W.K. Angiotensin I-converting enzyme (ACE) inhibitory peptide isolated from biodiesel byproducts of marine microalgae, *Nannochloropsis Oculata*. *J. Biobased Mater. Bioenergy* **2013**, *7*, 135–142. [CrossRef]
62. Ko, S.-C.; Kang, N.; Kim, E.-A.; Kang, M.C.; Lee, S.-H.; Kang, S.-M.; Lee, J.-B.; Jeon, B.-T.; Kim, S.-K.; Park, S.-J.; et al. A novel angiotensin I-converting enzyme (ACE) inhibitory peptide from a marine *Chlorella ellipsoidea* and its antihypertensive effect in spontaneously hypertensive rats. *Process. Biochem.* **2012**, *47*, 2005–2011. [CrossRef]
63. Barkia, I.; Al-Haj, L.; Hamid, A.A.; Zakaria, M.; Saari, N.; Zadjali, F. Indigenous marine diatoms as novel sources of bioactive peptides with antihypertensive and antioxidant properties. *Int. J. Food Sci. Technol.* **2019**, *54*, 1514–1522. [CrossRef]
64. Ngo, D.H.; Kim, S.H. Marine bioactive peptides as potential antioxidants. *Curr. Protein Pept. Sci.* **2013**, *14*, 189–198. [CrossRef] [PubMed]
65. Hu, Z.; Yang, P.; Zhou, C.; Li, S.; Hong, P. Marine collagen peptides from the skin of Nile Tilapia (*Oreochromis niloticus*): Characterization and wound healing evaluation. *Mar. Drugs* **2017**, *15*, 102. [CrossRef]
66. Michael, P.; Hansen, K.Ø.; Isaksson, J.; Andersen, J.H.; Hansen, E. A novel brominated alkaloid Securidine A, isolated from the marine Bryozoan *Securiflustra securifrons*. *Molecules* **2017**, *22*, 1236. [CrossRef]
67. Samarakoon, K.W.; Ko, J.Y.; Shah, M.R.; Lee, J.H.; O-Nam, K.; Lee, J.B.; Jeon, Y.J. In vitro studies of anti-inflammatory and anticancer activities of organic solvent extracts from cultured marine microalgae. *Algae* **2013**, *28*, 1–9. [CrossRef]
68. Liaset, B.; Madsen, L.; Hao, Q.; Criales, G.; Mellgren, G.; Marschall, H.U.; Hallenborg, P.; Espe, M.; Frøyland, L.; Kristiansen, K. Fish protein hydrolysate elevates plasma bile acids and reduces visceral adipose tissue mass in rats. *Biochim. Biophys. Acta* **2009**, *1791*, 254–262. [CrossRef]
69. Mendonça, S.; Saldiva, P.H.; Cruz, R.J.; Arêas, J.A.G. Amaranth protein presents cholesterol-lowering effect. *Food Chem.* **2009**, *116*, 738–742. [CrossRef]

70. Wergedahl, H.; Liaset, B.; Gudbrandsen, O.A.; Lied, E.; Espe, M.; Muna, Z.; Mørk, S.; Berge, R.K. Fish protein hydrolysate reduces plasma total cholesterol, increases the proportion of HDL cholesterol, and lowers acyl-CoA:cholesterol acyltransferase activity in liver of Zucker rats. *J. Nutr.* **2004**, *134*, 1320–1327. [CrossRef]
71. Mitta, G.; Hubert, F.; Noël, T.; Roch, P. Myticin, a novel cysteine-rich antimicrobial peptide isolated from haemocytes and plasma of the mussel *Mytilus galloprovincialis*. *Eur. J. Biochem.* **1999**, *265*, 71–78. [CrossRef] [PubMed]
72. Jung, W.K.; Kim, S.K. Isolation and characterisation of an anticoagulant oligopeptide from blue mussel, *Mytilus Edulis*. *Food Chem.* **2009**, *117*, 687–692. [CrossRef]
73. Jung, W.K.; Je, J.Y.; Kim, H.J.; Kim, S.K. A novel anticoagulant protein from *Scapharca broughtonii*. *J. Biochem. Mol. Biol.* **2002**, *35*, 199–205. [CrossRef] [PubMed]
74. Tao, J.; Zhao, Y.Q.; Chi, C.F.; Wang, B. Bioactive peptides from cartilage protein hydrolysate of spotless smoothhound and their antioxidant activity in vitro. *Mar. Drugs* **2018**, *16*, 100. [CrossRef] [PubMed]
75. Park, C.B.; Lee, J.H.; Park, I.Y.; Kim, M.S.; Kim, S.C. A novel antimicrobial peptide from the loach, *Misgurnus anguillicaudatus*. *FEBS Lett.* **1997**, *411*, 173–178. [CrossRef]
76. Sepčić, K.; Kauferstein, S.; Mebs, D.; Turk, T. Biological activities of aqueous and organic extracts from tropical marine sponges. *Mar. Drugs* **2010**, *8*, 1550–1566. [CrossRef]
77. Purushottama, G.B.; Venkateshvaran, K.; Pani Prasad, K.; Nalini, P. Bioactivities of extracts from marine sponge Halichondria panicea. *J. Venom. Anim. Toxins Incl. Trop. Dis.* **2009**, *15*, 444–459. [CrossRef]
78. Samarakoon, K.W.; O-Nam, K.; Ko, J.Y.; Lee, J.H.; Kang, M.C.; Kim, D.; Lee, J.B.; Lee, J.S.; Jeon, Y.J. Purification and identification of novel angiotensin-I converting enzyme (ACE) inhibitory peptides from cultured marine microalgae (*Nannochloropsis oculata*) protein hydrolysate. *J. Appl. Phycol.* **2013**, *25*, 1595–1606. [CrossRef]
79. Acquah, C.; Chan, Y.W.; Pan, S.; Agyei, D.; Udenigwe, C.C. Structure-informed separation of bioactive peptides. *J. Food Biochem.* **2019**, *43*, e12765. [CrossRef]
80. Mora, L.; Gallego, M.; Reig, M.; Toldrà, F. Challenges in the quantitation of naturally generated bioactive peptides in processed meats. *Trends Food Sci. Technol.* **2017**, *69*, 306–314. [CrossRef]
81. Le Gouic, A.V.; Harnedy, P.A.; FitzGerald, R.J. Bioactive peptides from fish protein by-products. In *Bioactive Molecules in Food*; Mérillon, J.-M., Ramawat, K., Eds.; Springer International Publishing AG: Cham, Switzerland, 2019; pp. 355–388. [CrossRef]
82. Wang, X.; Yu, H.; Xing, R.; Li, P. Characterization, preparation, and purification of marine bioactive peptides. *Biomed. Res. Int.* **2017**, *2017*, 9746720. [CrossRef] [PubMed]
83. Wolfenden, R.; Lewis, C.A.; Yuan, Y.; Carter, C.W. Temperature dependence of amino acid hydrophobicities. *Proc. Natl. Acad. Sci. USA* **2015**, *112*, 7484–7488. [CrossRef] [PubMed]
84. Sable, R.; Parajuli, P.; Joi, S. Peptides, peptidomimetics, and polypeptides from marine sources: A wealth of natural sources for pharmaceutical applications. *Mar. Drugs* **2017**, *15*, 124. [CrossRef] [PubMed]
85. Bazinet, L.; Firdaous, L. Membrane processes and devices for separation of bioactive peptides. *Recent Pat. Biotechnol.* **2009**, *3*, 61–72. [CrossRef] [PubMed]
86. Cavaliere, C.; Capriotti, A.L.; La Barbera, G.; Montone, C.M.; Piovesana, S.; Laganà, A. Liquid chromatographic strategies for separation of bioactive compounds in food matrices. *Molecules* **2018**, *23*, 3091. [CrossRef] [PubMed]
87. Haggag, Y.A.; Donia, A.A.; Osman, M.A.; El-Gizawy, S.A. Peptides as drug candidates: Limitations and recent development perspectives. *Biomed. J. Sci. Technol. Res.* **2018**, 6659–6662. [CrossRef]
88. Lau, J.L.; Dunn, M.K. Therapeutic peptides: Historical perspectives, current development trends, and future directions. *Bioorg. Med. Chem.* **2018**, *26*, 2700–2707. [CrossRef]
89. Luepker, R.V. Cardiovascular disease: Rise, fall, and future prospects. *Annu. Rev. Public Health* **2011**, *32*, 1–3. [CrossRef]
90. Liu, Z.; Ren, Z.; Zhang, J.; Chuang, C.C.; Kandaswamy, E.; Zhou, T.; Zuo, L. Role of ROS and nutritional antioxidants in human diseases. *Front. Physiol.* **2018**, *9*, 477. [CrossRef]
91. Meisel, H. Multifunctional peptides encrypted in milk proteins. *Biofactors* **2004**, *21*, 55–61. [CrossRef]
92. Aguilar-Toalá, J.E.; Santiago-López, L.; Peres, C.M.; Peres, C.; Garcia, H.S.; Vallejo-Cordoba, B.; González-Córdova, A.F.; Hernández-Mendoza, A. Assessment of multifunctional activity of bioactive peptides derived from fermented milk by specific *Lactobacillus plantarum* strains. *J. Dairy Sci.* **2017**, *100*, 65–75. [CrossRef] [PubMed]

93. Bali, A.; Randhawa, P.K.; Jagg, A.S. Interplay between RAS and opioids: Opening the Pandora of complexities. *Neuropeptides* **2014**, *48*, 249–256. [CrossRef] [PubMed]
94. Udenigwe, C.C.; Aluko, R.E. Food protein-derived bioactive peptides: Production, processing, and potential health benefits. *J. Food Sci.* **2012**, *77*, R11–R24. [CrossRef] [PubMed]
95. Boonen, K.; Creemers, J.W.; Schoofs, L. Bioactive peptides, networks and systems biology. *Bioessays* **2009**, *31*, 300–314. [CrossRef]
96. Shou, I.; Wang, L.N.; Suzuki, S.; Fukui, M.; Tomino, Y. Effects of antihypertensive drugs on antioxidant enzyme activities and renal function in stroke-prone spontaneously hypertensive rats. *Am. J. Med. Sci.* **1997**, *314*, 377–384. [CrossRef]
97. Godsel, L.M.; Leon, J.S.; Engman, D.M. Angiotensin converting enzyme inhibitors and angiotensin II receptor antagonists in experimental myocarditis. *Curr. Pharm. Des.* **2003**, *9*, 723–735. [CrossRef]
98. Kucharewicz, I.; Pawlak, R.; Matys, T.; Pawlak, D.; Buczko, W. Antithrombotic effect of captopril and losartan is mediated by angiotensin-(1-7). *Hypertension* **2002**, *40*, 774–779. [CrossRef]
99. Ruiz-Ortega, M.; Lorenzo, O.; Egido, J. Angiotensin III increases MCP-1 and activates NF-κB and AP-1 in cultured mesangial and mononuclear cells. *Kidney Int.* **2000**, *57*, 2285–2298. [CrossRef]
100. Izadpanah, A.; Gallo, R.L. Antimicrobial peptides. *J. Am. Acad. Derm.* **2005**, *52*, 381–390. [CrossRef]
101. Zou, T.B.; He, T.P.; Li, H.B.; Tang, H.W.; Xia, E.Q. The structure-activity relationship of the antioxidant peptides from natural proteins. *Molecules* **2016**, *21*, 72. [CrossRef]
102. Xiong, J.; Fang, W.; Fang, W.; Bai, L.; Huo, J.; Kong, Y.; Yunman, L. Anticoagulant and antithrombotic activity of a new peptide pENW (pGlu-Asn-Trp). *J. Pharm. Pharmacol.* **2009**, *61*, 89–94. [CrossRef] [PubMed]
103. Haney, E.F.; Hancock, R.E. Peptide design for antimicrobial and immunomodulatory applications. *Biopolymers* **2013**, *100*, 572–583. [CrossRef] [PubMed]
104. Bowdish, D.M.; Davidson, D.J.; Scott, M.G.; Hancock, R.E. Immunomodulatory activities of small host defense peptides. *Antimicrob. Agents Chemother.* **2005**, *49*, 1727–1732. [CrossRef] [PubMed]
105. Kang, H.K.; Lee, H.H.; Seo, C.H.; Park, Y. Antimicrobial and immunomodulatory properties and applications of marine-derived proteins and peptides. *Mar. Drugs* **2019**, *17*, 350. [CrossRef] [PubMed]
106. Lombardi, V.R.M.; Corzo, L.; Carrera, I.; Cacabelos, R. The search for biomarine-derived compounds with immunomodulatory activity. *J. Explor. Res. Pharmacol.* **2018**, *3*, 30–41. [CrossRef]
107. Zheng, L.H.; Wang, Y.J.; Sheng, J.; Wang, F.; Zheng, Y.; Lin, X.H.; Sun, M. Antitumor peptides from marine organisms. *Mar. Drugs* **2011**, *9*, 1840–1859. [CrossRef]
108. Aneiros, A.; Garateix, A. Bioactive peptides from marine sources: Pharmacological properties and isolation procedures. *J. Chromatogr. B Anal. Technol. Biomed. Life Sci.* **2004**, *803*, 41–53. [CrossRef]
109. Ramadhan, A.H.; Nawas, T.; Zhang, X.; Pembe, W.M.; Wenshui, X.; Xu, Y. Purification and identification of a novel antidiabetic peptide from Chinese giant salamander (*Andrias davidianus*) protein hydrolysate against α-amylase and α-glucosidase. *Int. J. Food Prop.* **2017**, *20*, S3360–S3372. [CrossRef]
110. Xia, E.Q.; Zhu, S.S.; He, M.J.; Luo, F.; Fu, C.Z.; Zou, T.B. Marine peptides as potential agents for the management of type 2 diabetes mellitus-a prospect. *Mar. Drugs* **2017**, *15*, 88. [CrossRef]
111. Marthandam Asokan, S.; Wang, T.; Su, W.T.; Lin, W.T. Antidiabetic effects of a short peptide of potato protein hydrolysate in STZ-induced diabetic mice. *Nutrients* **2019**, *11*, 779. [CrossRef]
112. McIntosh, C.H.; Demuth, H.U.; Pospisilik, J.A.; Pederson, R. Dipeptidyl peptidase IV inhibitors: How do they work as new antidiabetic agents? *Regul. Pept.* **2005**, *128*, 159–165. [CrossRef] [PubMed]
113. Kehinde, B.A.; Sharma, P. Recently isolated antidiabetic hydrolysates and peptides from multiple food sources: A review. *Crit. Rev. Food Sci. Nutr.* **2020**, *60*, 322–340. [CrossRef] [PubMed]
114. Nauck, M. Incretin therapies: Highlighting common features and differences in the modes of action of glucagon-like peptide-1 receptor agonists and dipeptidyl peptidase-4 inhibitors. *Diabet. Obes. Metab.* **2016**, *18*, 203–216. [CrossRef] [PubMed]
115. Bhat, V.K.; Kerr, B.D.; Flatt, P.R.; Gault, V.A. A novel GIP-oxyntomodulin hybrid peptide acting through GIP, glucagon and GLP-1 receptors exhibits weight reducing and anti-diabetic properties. *Biochem. Pharmacol.* **2013**, *85*, 1655–1662. [CrossRef] [PubMed]
116. Azoulay, Z.; Rapaport, H. The assembly state and charge of amphiphilic β-sheet peptides affect blood clotting. *J. Mater. Chem. B* **2016**, *4*, 3859–3867. [CrossRef] [PubMed]
117. Qiao, M.; Tu, M.; Wang, Z.; Mao, F.; Chen, H.; Qin, L.; Du, M. Identification and antithrombotic activity of peptides from Blue Mussel (*Mytilus edulis*) protein. *Int. J. Mol. Sci.* **2018**, *19*, 138. [CrossRef]

118. Rajapakse, N.; Jung, W.K.; Mendis, E.; Moon, S.H.; Kim, S.K. A novel anticoagulant purified from fish protein hydrolysate inhibits factor XIIa and platelet aggregation. *Life Sci.* **2005**, *76*, 2607–2619. [CrossRef]
119. Leoni, G.; De Poli, A.; Mardirossian, M.; Gambato, S.; Florian, F.; Venier, P.; Wilson, D.N.; Tossi, A.; Pallavicini, A.; Gerdol, M. Myticalins: A novel multigenic family of linear, cationic antimicrobial peptides from marine mussels (*Mytilus* spp.). *Mar. Drugs* **2017**, *15*, 261. [CrossRef]
120. Omardien, S.; Brul, S.; Zaat, S.A. Antimicrobial activity of cationic antimicrobial peptides against gram-positives: Current progress made in understanding the mode of action and the response of bacteria. *Front. Cell Dev. Biol.* **2016**, *4*, 111. [CrossRef]
121. Jiang, Z.; Vasil, A.I.; Hale, J.D.; Hancock, R.E.W.; Vasil, M.L.; Hodges, R.S. Effects of net charge and the number of positively charged residues on the biological activity of amphipathic α-helical cationic antimicrobial peptides. *Biopolymers* **2008**, *90*, 369–383. [CrossRef]
122. Rodriguez, J.; Gupta, N.; Smith, R.D.; Pevzner, P.A. Does trypsin cut before proline? *J. Proteome Res.* **2008**, *7*, 300–305. [CrossRef] [PubMed]
123. Di Cosmo, A.; Polese, G. Molluscan Bioactive Peptides. In *Handbook of Biologically Active Peptides*, 2nd ed.; Kastin, A.J., Ed.; Academic Press Inc.: Cambridge, MA, USA, 2013; pp. 276–286. [CrossRef]
124. Pangestuti, R.; Kim, S.K. Bioactive peptide of marine origin for the prevention and treatment of non-communicable diseases. *Mar. Drugs* **2017**, *15*, 67. [CrossRef]
125. Lee, Y.; Phat, C.; Hong, S.C. Structural diversity of marine cyclic peptides and their molecular mechanisms for anticancer, antibacterial, antifungal, and other clinical applications. *Peptides* **2017**, *95*, 94–105. [CrossRef] [PubMed]
126. Kouno, K.; Hirano, S.; Kuboki, H.; Kasai, M.; Hatae, K. Effects of dried bonito (katsuobushi) and captopril, an angiotensin I-converting enzyme inhibitor, on rat isolated aorta: A possible mechanism of antihypertensive action. *Biosci. Biotechnol. Biochem.* **2005**, *69*, 911–915. [CrossRef]
127. Semreen, M.H.; El-Gamal, M.I.; Abdin, S.; Alkhazraji, H.; Kamal, L.; Hammad, S.; El-Awady, F.; Waleed, D.; Kourbaj, L. Recent updates of marine antimicrobial peptides. *Saudi Pharm. J.* **2018**, *26*, 396–409. [CrossRef]
128. Masso-Silva, J.A.; Diamond, G. Antimicrobial peptides from fish. *Pharmaceuticals* **2014**, *7*, 265–310. [CrossRef]
129. Valero, Y.; Saraiva-Fraga, M.; Costas, B.; Guardiola, F.A. Antimicrobial peptides from fish: Beyond the fight against pathogens. *Rev. Aquacult.* **2020**, *12*, 224–253. [CrossRef]
130. Raheem, N.; Straus, S.K. Mechanisms of action for antimicrobial peptides with antibacterial and antibiofilm functions. *Front. Microbiol.* **2019**, *10*, 2866. [CrossRef]
131. Pujiastuti, D.Y.; Ghoyatul Amin, M.N.; Alamsjah, M.A.; Hsu, J.-L. Marine organisms as potential sources of bioactive peptides that inhibit the activity of angiotensin I-converting enzyme: A review. *Molecules* **2019**, *24*, 2541. [CrossRef]
132. Deng, Z.; Liu, Y.; Wang, J.; Wu, S.; Geng, L.; Sui, Z.; Zhang, Q. Antihypertensive effects of two novel angiotensin I-converting enzyme (ACE) inhibitory peptides from *Gracilariopsis lemaneiformis* (Rhodophyta) in spontaneously hypertensive rats (SHRs). *Mar. Drugs* **2018**, *16*, 299. [CrossRef]
133. Wang, B.; Xie, N.; Li, B. Influence of peptide characteristics on their stability, intestinal transport, and in vitro bioavailability: A review. *J. Food Biochem.* **2019**, *43*, 12571. [CrossRef]
134. Assimakopoulos, S.F.; Papageorgiou, I.; Charonis, A. Enterocytes' tight junctions: From molecules to diseases. *World J. Gastrointest. Pathophysiol.* **2011**, *2*, 123–137. [CrossRef] [PubMed]
135. Brodin, B.; Nielsen, C.U.; Steffansen, B.; Frokjaer, S. Transport of peptidomimetic drugs by the intestinal di/tri-peptide transporter, PepT1. *Pharmacol. Toxicol.* **2002**, *90*, 285–296. [CrossRef] [PubMed]
136. Segura-Campos, M.; Chel-Guerrero, L.; Betancur-Ancona, D.; Hernandez-Escalante, V.M. Bioavailability of bioactive peptides. *Food Rev. Int.* **2011**, *27*, 213–226. [CrossRef]
137. FitzGerald, R.J.; Meisel, H. Milk protein-derived peptide inhibitors of angiotensin-I-converting enzyme. *Br. J. Nutr.* **2000**, *84*, S33–S37. [CrossRef] [PubMed]
138. Van der Pijl, P.C.; Kies, A.K.; Ten Have, G.A.M.; Duchateau, G.S.M.J.E.; Deutz, N.E.P. Pharmacokinetics of proline-rich tripeptides in the pig. *Peptides* **2008**, *29*, 2196–2202. [CrossRef]
139. Foltz, M.; Meynen, E.E.; Bianco, V.; van Platerink, C.; Koning, T.M.M.G.; Kloek, J. Angiotensin converting enzyme inhibitory peptides from a lactotripeptide-enriched milk beverage are absorbed intact into the circulation. *J. Nutr.* **2007**, *137*, 953–958. [CrossRef]
140. Jambunathan, K.; Galande, A.K. Design of a serum stability tag for bioactive peptides. *Protein Pept. Lett.* **2014**, *21*, 32–38. [CrossRef]

141. Apostolovic, D.; Stanic-Vucinic, D.; de Jongh, H.H.J.; de Jong, G.A.H.; Mihailovic, J.; Radosavljevic, J.; Radibratovic, M.; Nordlee, J.A.; Baumert, J.L.; Milcic, M.; et al. Conformational stability of digestion-resistant peptides of peanut conglutins reveals the molecular basis of their allergenicity. *Sci. Rep.* **2016**, *6*, 29249. [CrossRef]
142. Arai, M.; Yamano, Y.; Fujita, M.; Setiawan, A.; Kobayashi, M. Stylissamide X, a new proline-rich cyclic octapeptide as an inhibitor of cell migration, from an Indonesian marine sponge of *Stylissa* sp. *Bioorg. Med. Chem. Lett.* **2012**, *22*, 1818–1821. [CrossRef]
143. Zagon, J.; Dehne, L.I.; Bögl, K.W. D-amino acids in organisms and food. *Nutr. Res.* **1994**, *14*, 445–463. [CrossRef]
144. Schultz, A.W.; Oh, D.C.; Carney, J.R.; Williamson, R.T.; Udwary, D.W.; Jensen, P.R.; Gould, S.J.; Fenical, W.; Moore, B.S. Biosynthesis and structures of cyclomarins and cyclomarazines, prenylated cyclic peptides of marine actinobacterial origin. *J. Am. Chem. Soc.* **2008**, *130*, 4507–4516. [CrossRef] [PubMed]
145. Sparidan, R.W.; Stokvis, E.; Jimeno, J.M.; López-Lázaro, L.; Schellens, J.H.; Beijnen, J.H. Chemical and enzymatic stability of a cyclic depsipeptide, the novel, marine-derived, anti-cancer agent kahalalideF. *Anticancer Drugs* **2001**, *12*, 575–582. [CrossRef]
146. Guan, L.L.; Sera, Y.; Adachi, K.; Nishida, F.; Shizuri, Y. Isolation and evaluation of nonsiderophore cyclic peptides from marine sponges. *Biochem. Biophys. Res. Commun.* **2001**, *283*, 976–981. [CrossRef] [PubMed]
147. Ibrahim, A.H.; Attia, Z.E.; Hajjar, D.; Anany, M.A.; Desoukey, S.Y.; Fouad, M.A.; Kamel, S.M.; Wajant, H.; Gulder, T.A.M.; Abdelmohsen, U.R. New cytotoxic cyclic peptide from the marine sponge-associated *Nocardiopsis* sp. UR67. *Mar. Drugs* **2018**, *16*, 290. [CrossRef]
148. Gang, D.; Kim, D.W.; Park, H.-S. Cyclic peptides: Promising scaffolds for biopharmaceuticals. *Genes* **2018**, *9*, 557. [CrossRef]
149. Joo, S.-H. Cyclic peptides as therapeutic agents and biochemical tools. *Biomol. Ther.* **2012**, *20*, 19–26. [CrossRef]
150. Sharma, M.; Singhvi, I.; Ali, Z.M.; Kumar, M.; Dev, S.K. Synthesis and biological evaluation of natural cyclic peptide. *Future J. Pharm. Sci.* **2018**, *4*, 220–228. [CrossRef]
151. Stawikowski, M.; Cudic, P. Depsipeptide Synthesis. In *Peptide Characterization and Application Protocols*; Fields, G.B., Ed.; Humana Press: New York, NY, USA, 2007; Volume 386, pp. 321–339. [CrossRef]
152. Nguyen, M.M.; Ong, N.; Suggs, L. A general solid phase method for the synthesis of depsipeptides. *Org. Biomol. Chem.* **2013**, *11*, 1167–1170. [CrossRef]
153. Vining, O.B.; Medina, R.A.; Mitchell, E.A.; Videau, P.; Li, D.; Serrill, J.D.; Kelly, J.X.; Gerwick, W.H.; Proteau, P.J.; Ishmael, J.E.; et al. Depsipeptide companeramides from a Panamanian marine cyanobacterium associated with the coibamide producer. *J. Nat. Prod.* **2015**, *78*, 413–420. [CrossRef]
154. Kitagaki, J.; Shi, G.; Miyauchi, S.; Murakami, S.; Yang, Y. Cyclic depsipeptides as potential cancer therapeutics. *Anti-Cancer Drug* **2015**, *26*, 259–271. [CrossRef] [PubMed]
155. Ding, C.Y.G.; Ong, J.F.M.; Goh, H.C.; Coffill, C.R.; Tan, L.T. Benderamide A, a cyclic depsipeptide from a Singapore collection of marine cyanobacterium cf. *Lyngbya* sp. *Mar. Drugs* **2018**, *16*, 409. [CrossRef]
156. Pelay-Gimeno, M.; Tulla-Puche, J.; Albericio, F. "Head-to-side-chain" cyclodepsipeptides of marine origin. *Mar. Drug* **2013**, *11*, 1693–1717. [CrossRef]
157. Oku, N.; Kawabata, K.; Adachi, K.; Katsuta, A.; Shizuri, Y. Unnarmicins A and C, new antibacterial depsipeptides produced by marine bacterium *Photobacterium* sp. MBIC06485. *J. Antibiot.* **2008**, *61*, 11–17. [CrossRef] [PubMed]
158. Ratnayake, A.S.; Bugni, T.S.; Feng, X.; Harper, M.K.; Skalicky, J.J.; Mohammed, K.A.; Andjelic, C.D.; Barrows, L.R.; Ireland, C.M. Theopapuamide, a cyclic depsipeptide from a Papua New Guinea lithistid sponge *Theonella swinhoei*. *J. Nat. Prod.* **2006**, *69*, 1582–1586. [CrossRef]
159. Nguyen, B.; Caer, J.P.; Mourier, G.; Thai, R.; Lamthanh, H.; Servent, D.; Benoit, E.; Molgó, J. Characterization of a novel *Conus bandanus* conopeptide belonging to the M-superfamily containing bromotryptophan. *Mar. Drugs* **2014**, *12*, 3449–3465. [CrossRef]
160. Jimenez, E.C. Bromotryptophan and its analogs in peptides from marine animals. *Protein Pept. Lett.* **2019**, *26*, 251–260. [CrossRef]
161. Bittner, S.; Scherzer, R.; Harlev, E. The five bromotryptophans. *Amino Acids* **2007**, *33*, 19. [CrossRef]

162. Zhang, S.K.; Song, J.W.; Gong, F.; Li, S.B.; Chang, H.Y.; Xie, H.M.; Gao, H.W.; Tan, Y.X.; Ji, S.P. Design of an α-helical antimicrobial peptide with improved cell-selective and potent anti-biofilm activity. *Sci. Rep.* **2016**, *6*, 27394. [CrossRef]
163. Ravichandran, S.; Kumaravel, K.; Rameshkumar, G.; AjithKumar, T.T. Antimicrobial peptides from the marine fishes. *Res. J. Immunol.* **2010**, *3*, 146–156. [CrossRef]
164. Partridge, A.W.; Kaan, H.Y.K.; Juang, Y.C.; Sadruddin, A.; Lim, S.; Brown, C.J.; Ng, S.; Thean, D.; Ferrer, F.; Johannes, C.; et al. Incorporation of putative helix-breaking amino acids in the design of novel stapled peptides: Exploring biophysical and cellular permeability properties. *Molecules* **2019**, *24*, 2292. [CrossRef]
165. Falanga, A.; Lombardi, L.; Franci, G.; Vitiello, M.; Iovene, M.R.; Morelli, G.; Galdiero, M.; Galdiero, S. Marine antimicrobial peptides: Nature provides templates for the design of novel compounds against pathogenic bacteria. *Int. J. Mol. Sci.* **2016**, *17*, 785. [CrossRef] [PubMed]
166. Bougatef, A.; Hajji, M.; Balti, R.; Lassoued, I.; Triki-Ellouz, Y.; Nasri, M. Antioxidant and free radical-scavenging activities of smooth hound (*Mustelus mustelus*) muscle protein hydrolysates obtained by gastrointestinal proteases. *Food Chem.* **2018**, *114*, 1198–1205. [CrossRef]
167. Suarez-Jimenez, G.M.; Burgos-Hernandez, A.; Ezquerra-Brauer, J.M. Bioactive peptides and depsipeptides with anticancer potential: Sources from marine animals. *Mar. Drugs* **2012**, *10*, 963–986. [CrossRef] [PubMed]
168. Zhu, C.F.; Li, G.Z.; Peng, H.B.; Zhang, F.; Chen, Y.; Li, Y. Treatment with marine collagen peptides modulates glucose and lipid metabolism in Chinese patients with type 2 diabetes mellitus. *Appl. Physiol. Nutr. Metab.* **2010**, *35*, 797–804. [CrossRef] [PubMed]
169. Tu, A.T. Sea snake venoms and neurotoxins. *J. Agric. Food Chem.* **1974**, *22*, 36–43. [CrossRef] [PubMed]
170. Negi, B.; Kumar, D.; Rawat, D.S. Marine peptides as anticancer agents: A remedy to mankind by nature. *Curr. Protein Pept. Sci.* **2017**, *18*, 885–904. [CrossRef]
171. Zhu, C.F.; Peng, H.B.; Liu, G.Q.; Zhang, F.; Li, Y. Beneficial effects of oligopeptides from marine salmon skin in a rat model of type 2 diabetes. *Nutrition* **2010**, *26*, 1014–1020. [CrossRef]
172. Marr, A.K.; Gooderham, W.J.; Hancock, R.E. Antibacterial peptides for therapeutic use: Obstacles and realistic outlook. *Curr. Opin. Pharmacol.* **2006**, *6*, 468–472. [CrossRef] [PubMed]
173. Dyshlovoy, S.A.; Honecker, F. Marine compounds and cancer: 2017 updates. *Mar. Drugs* **2018**, *16*, 41. [CrossRef]
174. Simmons, T.L.; Andrianasolo, E.; McPhail, K.; Flatt, P.; Gerwick, W.H. Marine natural products as anticancer drugs. *Mol. Cancer Ther.* **2005**, *4*, 333–342. [CrossRef] [PubMed]
175. Bøgh, K.L.; Madsen, C.B. Food allergens: Is there a correlation between stability to digestion and allergenicity? *Crit. Rev. Food Sci. Nutr.* **2016**, *56*, 1545–1567. [CrossRef] [PubMed]
176. Foster, E.S.; Kimber, I.; Dearman, R.J. Relationship between protein digestibility and allergenicity: Comparisons of pepsin and cathepsin. *Toxicology* **2013**, *309*, 30–38. [CrossRef] [PubMed]
177. Nygård, L.A.K.; Mundal, I.; Dahl, L.; Šaltytė Benth, J.; Rokstad, A.M.M. Nutrition and physical performance in older people-effects of marine protein hydrolysates to prevent decline in physical performance: A randomised controlled trial protocol. *Bmj Open* **2018**, *8*, 023845. [CrossRef] [PubMed]
178. Guerard, F.; Sumaya-Martinez, M.T.; Linard, B.; Dufosse, L. Marine protein hydrolysates with antioxidant properties. *Agro Food Ind. Hi Tech.* **2005**, *16*, 16–18.
179. Delcroix, J.; Gatesoupe, F.-J.; Desbruyères, E.; Huelvan, C.; Le Delliou, H.; Le Gall, M.-M.; Quazuguel, P.; Mazurais, D.; Zambonino-Infante, J.L. The effects of dietary marine protein hydrolysates on the development of sea bass larvae, *Dicentrarchus labrax*, and associated microbiota. *Aquac. Nutr.* **2015**, *21*, 98–104. [CrossRef]
180. Rizer, R.L.; Stephens, T.J.; Herndon, J.H.; Sperber, B.R.; Murphy, J.; Ablon, G.R. A marine protein-based dietary supplement for subclinical hair thinning/loss: Results of a multisite, double-blind, placebo-controlled clinical trial. *Int. J. Trichol.* **2015**, *7*, 156–166. [CrossRef]
181. Drotningsvik, A.; Vikøren, L.A.; Mjøs, S.A.; Oterhals, Å.; Pampanin, D.; Flesland, O.; Gudbrandsen, O.A. Water-soluble fish protein intake led to lower serum and liver cholesterol concentrations in obese Zucker fa/fa rats. *Mar. Drugs* **2018**, *16*, 149. [CrossRef]
182. Vildmyren, I.; Cao, H.J.V.; Haug, L.B.; Valand, I.U.; Eng, Ø.; Oterhals, Å.; Austgulen, M.H.; Halstensen, A.; Mellgren, G.; Gudbrandsen, O.A. Daily intake of protein from cod residual material lowers serum concentrations of nonesterified fatty acids in overweight healthy adults: A randomized double-blind pilot study. *Mar. Drugs* **2018**, *16*, 197. [CrossRef]

183. Ruiz-Ruiz, F.; Mancera-Andrade, E.I.; Iqbal, H.M. Marine-derived bioactive peptides for biomedical sectors: A review. *Protein Pept. Lett.* **2017**, *24*, 109–117. [CrossRef]
184. Barbie, P.; Kazmaier, U. Total synthesis of cyclomarins A, C and D, marine cyclic peptides with interesting anti-tuberculosis and anti-malaria activities. *Org. Biomol. Chem.* **2016**, *14*, 6036–6054. [CrossRef] [PubMed]
185. Reen, F.J.; Gutiérrez-Barranquero, J.A.; Dobson, A.D.; Adams, C.; O'Gara, F. Emerging concepts promising new horizons for marine biodiscovery and synthetic biology. *Mar. Drugs* **2015**, *13*, 2924–2954. [CrossRef]
186. Kang, H.K.; Choi, M.C.; Seo, C.H.; Park, Y. Therapeutic properties and biological benefits of marine-derived anticancer peptides. *Int. J. Mol. Sci.* **2018**, *19*, 919. [CrossRef]
187. Andrade, L.M.; Andrade, C.J.; Dias, M.; Nascimento, C.A.O.; Mendes, M.A. *Chlorella* and *Spirulina* microalgae as sources of functional foods, nutraceuticals, and food supplements; an overview. *Moj Food Process. Technol.* **2018**, *6*, 00144. [CrossRef]
188. Je, J.-Y.; Qian, Z.-J.; Byun, H.-G.; Kim, S.-K. Purification and characterization of an antioxidant peptide obtained from tuna backbone protein by enzymatic hydrolysis. *Process. Biochem.* **2007**, *42*, 840–846. [CrossRef]
189. Kim, G.; Jang, H.; Kim, C. Antioxidant capacity of caseinophosphopeptides prepared from sodium caseinate using Alcalase. *Food Chem.* **2007**, *104*, 1359–1365. [CrossRef]
190. Matsui, T.; Imamura, M.; Oka, H.; Osajima, K.; Kimoto, K.-I.; Kawasaki, T.; Matsumoto, K. Tissue distribution of antihypertensive dipeptide, Val-Tyr, after its single oral administration to spontaneously hypertensive rats. *J. Pept. Sci.* **2004**, *10*, 535–545. [CrossRef]
191. Mohan, A.; Rajendran, S.R.C.K.; He, Q.S.; Bazinet, L.; Udenigwe, C.C. Encapsulation of food protein hydrolysates and peptides: A review. *RSC Adv.* **2015**, *5*, 79270–79278. [CrossRef]
192. Chakrabarti, S.; Guha, S.; Majumder, K. Food-derived bioactive peptides in human health: Challenges and opportunities. *Nutrients* **2018**, *10*, 1738. [CrossRef]
193. Ochnio, M.E.; Martínez, J.H.; Allievi, M.C.; Palavecino, M.; Martínez, K.D.; Pérez, O.E. Proteins as nano-carriers for bioactive compounds. The case of 7S and 11S soy globulins and folic acid complexation. *Polymers* **2018**, *10*, 149. [CrossRef]
194. Keservani, R.K.; Sharma, A.K.; Jarouliya, U. Protein and peptide in drug targeting and its therapeutic approach. *Ars. Pharm.* **2015**, *56*, 165–177. [CrossRef]
195. Musther, H.; Olivares-Morales, A.; Hatley, O.J.; Liu, B.; Rostami Hodjegan, A. Animal versus human oral drug bioavailability: Do they correlate? *Eur. J. Pharm. Sci.* **2014**, *57*, 280–291. [CrossRef] [PubMed]
196. Shanks, N.; Greek, R.; Greek, J. Are animal models predictive for humans? *Philos. Ethics Hum. Med.* **2009**, *4*, 2. [CrossRef] [PubMed]
197. Bauer, J.; Biolo, G.; Cederholm, T.; Cesari, M.; Cruz-Jentoft, A.J.; Morley, J.E.; Phillips, S.; Sieber, C.; Stehle, P.; Teta, D.; et al. Evidence-based recommendations for optimal dietary protein intake in older people: A position paper from the PROT-AGE study group. *J. Am. Med. Dir. Assoc.* **2013**, *14*, 542–559. [CrossRef] [PubMed]
198. Chen, H.; Pan, Y.; Wong, E.A.; Webb, K.E. Dietary protein level and stage of development affect expression of an intestinal peptide transporter (cPepT1) in chickens. *J. Nutr.* **2005**, *135*, 193–198. [CrossRef]
199. Sharkey, K.A.; Mawe, G.M. Neurohormonal signalling in the gastrointestinal tract: New frontiers. *J. Physiol.* **2014**, *592*, 2923–2925. [CrossRef]
200. Wang, J.; Yin, T.; Xiao, X.; He, D.; Xue, Z.; Jiang, X.; Wang, Y. StraPep: A structure database of bioactive peptides. *Database* **2018**, *2018*, 038. [CrossRef]

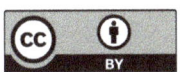

© 2020 by the authors. Licensee MDPI, Basel, Switzerland. This article is an open access article distributed under the terms and conditions of the Creative Commons Attribution (CC BY) license (http://creativecommons.org/licenses/by/4.0/).

MDPI
St. Alban-Anlage 66
4052 Basel
Switzerland
Tel. +41 61 683 77 34
Fax +41 61 302 89 18
www.mdpi.com

Marine Drugs Editorial Office
E-mail: marinedrugs@mdpi.com
www.mdpi.com/journal/marinedrugs

www.ingramcontent.com/pod-product-compliance
Lightning Source LLC
LaVergne TN
LVHW070412100526
838202LV00014B/1444